IMPROVING MEDICAL OUTCOMES

IMPROVING MEDICAL OUTCOMES

The Psychology of Doctor-Patient Visits

**Jessica Leavitt
and
Fred Leavitt**

ROWMAN & LITTLEFIELD PUBLISHERS, INC.
Lanham • Boulder • New York • Toronto • Plymouth, UK

Published by Rowman & Littlefield Publishers, Inc.
A wholly owned subsidiary of The Rowman & Littlefield Publishing Group, Inc.
4501 Forbes Boulevard, Suite 200, Lanham, Maryland 20706
http://www.rowmanlittlefield.com

Estover Road, Plymouth PL6 7PY, United Kingdom

British Library Cataloguing in Publication Information Available

Library of Congress Cataloging-in-Publication Data

Leavitt, Jessica, 1970–
   Improving medical outcomes : the psychology of doctor-patient visits / Jessica Leavitt and Fred Leavitt.
      p. ; cm.
   Includes bibliographical references and index.
   Summary: "The ability of doctors to properly diagnose and treat patients is often colored by nonspecific factors that can affect outcomes in profound ways. Communication between doctors and patients is key, but often what is left unsaid is just as important, and messages from outside sources such as medical journals, drug companies, and other patients can affect how a doctor treats any one patient at any one time. This book outlines the nonspecific factors that come into play when doctors and patients interact, how both doctors and patients can overcome these messages to focus in on the health of the person sitting on the table, and how psychological factors in both the doctor and the patient can affect medical outcomes. Anyone hoping to improve the medical care they give or the medical care they get will find in these pages strategies for improving those results" — Provided by publisher.
   ISBN 978-1-4422-0303-7 (cloth : alk. paper) — ISBN 978-1-4422-0305-1 (electronic)
   1. Physician and patient. 2. Patient participation. 3. Medical offices. 4. Patients—Psychology. 5. Physicians—Psychology. I. Leavitt, Fred. II. Title.
   [DNLM: 1. Physician-Patient Relations. 2. Office Visits. 3. Patient Participation. 4. Patients—psychology. 5. Physicians—psychology. 6. Treatment Outcome. W 62]
   R727.3.L34 2011
   610.696—dc23

                                                                            2011013594

Printed in the United States of America

We couldn't have written this book without the love and support of Diane (wife of Fred, mom of Jessica), the willingness to listen, and kid-watch, of Melanie and Jodi (daughter/sister and friend, respectively), the inspirational model of curiosity and exploration of Ma'Tia and Elijah (grandkids/kids), and the endless patience and generosity of Ian (son-in-law/husband).

This book is dedicated to all of you, with love.

CONTENTS

Introduction   ix

1   Doctor-Patient Communication   1

2   Interpreting Medical Information   23

3   Decisions: Overview   43

4   Decisions: Biases   57

5   Medical Diagnosis: The Problems   79

6   Reducing Diagnostic Errors   99

7   Prescriptions for Prescribing   121

8   Expectation Effects: Power to the Placebo   139

9   Complementary and Alternative Medicine   175

10 Patient Outlook and Social Connectedness   189

11 Healing Environments   201

Appendix 1: Psychiatric Diagnosis   215

Appendix 2: Darwinian Medicine   219

Appendix 3: Wellness Strategies   229

Notes   253

Index   303

INTRODUCTION

The problems faced by medical doctors and automobile mechanics are in some ways quite similar—something isn't working correctly and must be fixed. They must both figure out the cause of malfunctions and determine the appropriate treatments. For the mechanic, the difference between what a car engine should be doing and is doing is a factor that, if appropriately addressed, can turn a nonfunctioning car into a functional one. The specific mechanical factors are the only ones that come into play. Mechanics have no need to worry about an automobile's psyche, but in health care, the factors influencing outcomes are broader. Many nonspecific factors have profound effects, and they constitute the major topics of this book.

What do we mean by nonspecific factors? Well, instead of a damaged car, imagine a damaged appendix. The specific factor is whatever is physically wrong with the appendix. But whereas mechanics don't expect cars to describe their symptoms, doctors in most cases must communicate effectively with patients to properly diagnose the problem. The information they receive is oftentimes incomplete or inaccurate. Doctor-patient communication, which includes the doctor's demeanor, is a nonspecific factor that may greatly affect outcomes.

Another nonspecific factor is the doctor's ability to interpret the ever-expanding medical literature. Doctors should be able to distinguish between correlational and experimental studies and to appreciate the difference between statistical and clinical significance. The research articles and advertisements they read typically present data in ways that make a treatment's effectiveness seem greater than it really is. Doctors who understand various quantitative measures, such as number needed to treat, odds ratios, absolute versus relative risks, and survival versus mortality rates (all discussed on pp. 36–40), are better equipped to evaluate the data and recommend appropriate treatments.

Drug companies are in business to make money, and they use powerful and often well-disguised marketing techniques to promote their products. Promotions are directed at laypersons, students in medical school, and practicing doctors. Doctors should accept that the findings presented in published articles, even articles in prestigious medical journals, are often distorted by the researcher's financial concerns. Being aware of potential conflicts of interest may help doctors prescribe more appropriately.

People often make decisions that are far from optimal. The consequences of a poor decision are often trivial, but in a medical context they may mean the difference between life and death. We discuss several unconscious biases that lead to poor decision making; these can be overcome, but only if doctors are aware of them.

When a mechanic works on a car, the car receives the attention passively. A car will never have its radiator fixed simply by being told that the work has been done. But nonspecific factors, such as the placebo effect and other expectation effects, are real and powerful for human patients and even nonhuman animals. Furthermore, personality characteristics of patients, such as degree of optimism/pessimism and sense of control, impact outcomes. So do environmental factors—the light, sound, images, and sense of privacy in the spaces in which patients are treated. All have measurable effects on how quickly and well the patients heal.

This book includes three appendices. Appendix 1 deals with psychiatric diagnosis, which we believe is sufficiently different from other medical diagnosis to warrant a separate discussion. Appendix 2 introduces Darwinian medicine, a relatively new and innovative approach that focuses on diagnosing and treating medical problems from an evolutionary perspective. Appendix 3 offers general suggestions for maintaining a healthful lifestyle.

①

DOCTOR-PATIENT COMMUNICATION

The single biggest problem in communication is the illusion that it has taken place.

—George Bernard Shaw

Accurate and effective diagnoses and treatment decisions depend on good communication between doctors and patients. But interpersonal communication is difficult, and the doctor-patient context can raise every difficult aspect. In visits that often feel, at least for the patient, rushed, emotional, and frightening, doctors and patients may also have to contend with negotiating power and decision-making control and with accommodating demographic and cultural differences. The outcomes of these conversations have huge impacts on people's lives, so the stakes are high, and significant stress can result.

It's a wonder that communication in this context is as good as it is. But it is not very good. Studies have found that[1]

- In more than 25 percent of all visits, patients and doctors don't agree on the main presenting problem.
- Almost 50 percent of patient medical problems and more than 50 percent of patient worries about those problems are not communicated.

- In 50 percent of patients with severe depression, their depression is unrecognized by their doctor.
- Doctors give full medication dosing instructions for less than 60 percent of all medications and tell patients the duration of intake and adverse effects only one-third of the time.
- Patients immediately forget between 40 and 80 percent of information provided by health-care practitioners.
- Around 40 percent of patients don't adhere to treatment recommendations.
- Although more than 60 percent of patients cannot explain the meaning of one or more words used in their medical visit, only 15 percent tell their doctor they don't understand a term.
- In about 20 percent of primary care visits, a new problem is introduced during the visit's closing minutes.

In this chapter we'll first discuss why communication matters, offer a general approach for how it can be improved, and suggest several specific tools doctors can employ. We will end by discussing two areas of particular challenge for doctors: discussing pain and delivering bad news.

COMMUNICATION MATTERS

Bad communication in all contexts is frustrating. In the context of medical care it can also have enormous negative consequences for both patients and doctors. As we'll discuss in this section, bad communication for patients is associated with lower satisfaction with medical care, lower adherence to treatment recommendations, and worse health outcomes. Assessment of these associations is complicated, however, and we conclude this section with a cautionary note regarding their interpretation. For doctors, bad communication can lead to lower job satisfaction, more stress, and a higher risk of malpractice complaints.

Patient Satisfaction

Patient satisfaction is important as a predictor of compliance with treatment and improved outcomes. It is also a valuable outcome itself. Patients are increasingly seen as consumers of medical care who are paying for a service they expect to be high quality. In addition, dissatisfied patients are less likely to return for visits and more likely to switch doctors, and dissatisfaction with a doctor can undermine the placebo effects discussed in chapter 8 that a successful medical encounter can deliver.

It has been claimed that good communication is the most important factor in determining a patient's overall satisfaction with his or her medical care.[2] Several communication elements affect patients' satisfaction, including their doctor's communication style, the way in which visits are run, and whether their doctor likes them.

Doctor Communication Style Both nonverbal[3] and verbal doctor communication styles are linked with patient satisfaction. In a study that assessed doctors' ability at tasks requiring nonverbal skills, such as recognizing emotion in videotaped faces or communicating emotion through expression and voice tone, researchers found that patients of doctors who did well on the tasks were more satisfied than patients of less-adept doctors.[4] Patient satisfaction is also higher when doctors set a friendly, engaged tone for the patient interaction. This happens when doctors, for example, lean forward, make frequent eye contact, and often nod.[5] When doctors sit during medical visits, patients believe the visit lasted longer than it did and are more satisfied with their care.[6] Patients also perceive doctors who sit when breaking bad news as more compassionate. When doctors engage in behavior with patients that patients identify as indicating friendliness, warmth, concern, and a nonjudgmental approach to the patient, patient satisfaction is also increased.[7] Greater patient satisfaction is associated with better communication independent of the nature of the patient's medical problem.[8]

Way Visit Is Run The way a doctor runs the doctor-patient interaction predicts patient satisfaction. Doctor dominance of the interaction leads to lower patient satisfaction; this is true whether dominance is measured by assessing whether the doctor talks more than the patient, by patient ratings of dominance, or by vocal tone assessments.[9] Visits in which doctors engage patients in some nonmedical conversation are associated with greater patient satisfaction.[10] Patients like information about their medical care, and patients whose doctors provide more information in the course of the doctor-patient interaction are more satisfied than patients whose doctors provide less.[11]

Another issue related to doctor management of doctor-patient inter-actions is the degree to which patients are encouraged to participate in medical decision making. As discussed below, patients have different preferences for such participation. Most patients want to be involved and are less satisfied with their doctors and their medical care if they are not.[12] Some patients say they prefer to have little or no involvement in decision making about their care, but if encouraged to participate, they report greater satisfaction.[13]

Doctor Liking of Patient   A final communication element related to patients' satisfaction is whether or not their doctors respect and like them. Patients are generally accurate about their doctors' opinions of them and more satisfied with doctors who like them.[14] Doctors use a more positive communication style with, and give more information to, patients they respect.[15] Doctor liking of patients and patient liking of doctors are both associated with better patient health and patient ratings of a doctor's behavior, higher patient and doctor satisfaction with the visit, and decreased likelihood of the patient changing doctors within the following year.[16]

Patient Adherence

Drugs don't work in patients who don't take them.

—C. Everett Koop

If the goal is to heal, then doctors must do more than merely diagnose their patients' conditions and devise appropriate treatment plans. They must convince their patients to follow the plans. A huge number of patients, around 40 percent, don't.[17] This number almost doubles when plans are complicated and/or require lifestyle changes.[18] Nonadherence can happen because a doctor's advice is forgotten, misunderstood, or ignored.

Consequences of nonadherence are significant. Medications that are not used properly can lead to increased health-care costs, disease pro-gression, or even death. Although doctors have little control over fac-tors such as patients' forgetfulness, other priorities, deliberate omission of doses, and emotional issues,[19] doctors' communication style impacts adherence in a number of ways. Adherence is better when doctors and patients agree on a treatment plan, doctors give adequate information about prescribed treatment plans, and the patient believes that the doctor is credible.

Agreement on Treatment Plan Doctor-patient agreement on treatment plans increases adherence. Patients differ considerably in ways that impact which treatment will fit comfortably in the context of their lives. Their beliefs, abilities, needs, fears, and resources may all affect a plan's success. Patients allowed to collaborate in decisions about treatment can make choices that best fit their lives.[20] For example, a patient without easy access to transportation will have a harder time following through with frequent physical therapy appointments than a patient with highly accessible transportation. If doctors don't understand the factors in patients' lives that may impact adherence to treatment plans, patients are less likely to adhere.[21]

Not all treatment challenges can be dealt with by considering the context in which the patient operates. (The patient without transportation might still need to go to *some* physical therapy sessions, and a chosen medication may still have *some* difficult side effects.) Still, if doctors and patients work together to decide how to deal with the challenges arising from a treatment plan, adherence is much better than if patients are only told what to do and expected to confront the challenges on their own.[22]

True collaboration matters here. A supportive, patient-centered style on the doctor's part is not enough to generate greater treatment agreement and adherence. The best predictor of agreement and adherence is whether the patient was truly given the opportunity to discuss relevant information and share in the decision making.[23] Collaboration enables patients to ensure that their preferences and concerns are taken into account; it also helps them buy into a treatment plan through increased understanding of their medical condition and the rationale and importance of the plan.

Adequate and Appropriate Information Patients who do not understand a treatment protocol cannot comply with it. Two sources of misunderstanding exist: the extent to which patients can understand and retain medical information and the extent to which doctors successfully and fully convey the information.

First, approximately half of U.S. adults have only limited ability to obtain, process, and understand the health information they need to make informed decisions about health care.[24] Patients must understand what they need to do before they can do it, and without adequate health literacy, they cannot easily comply.[25] For example, one study found that 26 percent of patients couldn't understand information about when their next appointment was scheduled, 42 percent couldn't understand directions for taking medication on an empty stomach, and 60 percent did not understand a standard informed consent form.[26] Compounding the problem, those with limited health literacy are less likely to ask questions during the visit, seek written information, or understand medical terminology.[27] Doctors should always assess patient comprehension of new information and concepts.[28]

Second, doctors may give inadequate information to patients at all literacy levels.[29] Often, they don't give enough information. Tarn and colleagues found that when prescribing new medications, doctors addressed adverse effects and duration of medication use for only about one-third of the medications.[30] Doctors told only 55 percent of patients the number of tablets to take and only 58 percent the frequency and timing of the dosage. Patients who receive inadequate information about their treatment protocol may not adhere because they don't understand it.

Even when doctors communicate all the necessary information and patients are not challenged by health literacy issues, patients still may have difficulty understanding and retaining all relevant information; patients immediately forget 40–80 percent of the medical information given them, and almost half of what they retain is incorrect.[31]

It can be difficult to determine whether a patient has adhered to a treatment plan. Some nonjudgmental ways to ask about compliance are:

- Do you find it difficult to take your medications?
- What percentage of your medications would you say you take?
- Do you ever forget to take your medications?
- Do you ever stop taking your medications when you feel better? When you feel worse?

Patient Trust in Doctor   Effective doctor-patient communication increases patient confidence about the doctor's credibility, and increased doctor credibility positively influences patient adherence to recommended treatments.[32] If patients trust that their doctors have both the technical skills and the willingness to find an appropriate treatment plan, adherence is generally improved.[33]

Patient Health Outcomes

Achieving satisfaction and treatment adherence are important for both doctors and patients. But it is important to ask whether communication makes a difference *medically*. Do communication differences create differences in health outcomes? The answer is yes.

Effective communication on a doctor's part means being informative, facilitating patient participation, ensuring that patients are satisfied with the completeness of discussions, and responding to a patient's emotional state.[34] Those forms of better communication correlate with improved patient health outcomes[35] such as

- emotional health and anxiety;
- symptom resolution;
- pain;
- physiologic measures;
- length of hospital stay;
- functional status.

The mechanisms by which doctor-patient communication impacts patient health are not well understood.[36] Roter and Hall suggest a number of possibilities to explain how patients receive these benefits.[37] First, improved communication may increase the nonspecific healing mechanisms of the doctor-patient visit (as discussed in chapter 8). Second, as discussed above, improved communication increases adherence to treatment plans, and better adherence predicts better outcomes. Finally, some communications (e.g., shared decision making) may increase a patient's feelings of self-confidence and motivation, leading the patient to act more healthfully and become healthier.

Street and colleagues address this issue by positing seven ways in which communication can lead to better health: increased access to care, greater patient knowledge and shared understanding, higher-quality medical decisions, enhanced therapeutic alliances, increased social support, patient agency and empowerment, and better management of emotions.[38] They argue that "clinicians and patients should maximize the therapeutic effects of communication by explicitly orienting communication to achieve intermediate outcomes (e.g., trust, mutual understanding, adherence, social support, self-efficacy) associated with improved health."

A Cautionary Note Although the literature linking communication with positive patient outcomes is strong and abundant, the linkages don't necessarily reveal causation; other factors may be confounds. Hall gives an example.[39] Since doctors like sick patients less than healthy patients, the doctors' dislike may play out in ways that lessen sick patients' satisfaction. Alternatively, sicker patients may be more dissatisfied with life in general, and their pervasive dissatisfaction may explain their dissatisfaction with their doctors.

Franks and colleagues found the expected positive association between patients' perceptions of their doctors and reported health status, but little evidence linking doctors' behaviors to health status.[40] The authors note that patient factors may account for *both* the patients' ratings of their doctors and their reported health status. For example, patients who express negative affect tend to report worse health and worse health care. Self-efficacy may influence both health status and doctor ratings, and patients with more negative stereotypes of doctors report lower satisfaction and adherence.

Doctor Outcomes

Poor doctor-patient communication also affects doctors. This is important in its own right and also because doctors who are satisfied with work are more likely to have patients satisfied with their care. Conversely, a doctor's poor mental health may negatively impact the quality of care given to patients.[41] Furthermore, dissatisfied doctors may employ riskier prescribing practices. They also may leave their practice, creating challenges for continuity of care.[42]

Job Satisfaction and Stress Doctor job satisfaction and job stress are inversely related; in fact, job satisfaction appears to prevent job stress.[43] The most important determinant of doctor satisfaction is the doctor-patient relationship.[44] Doctors tend to get satisfaction from the same types of communication as patients: they are less satisfied with visits in which they are dominant and more satisfied with patient-centered visits.[45]

Malpractice   One event that can certainly lead to increased stress and lessened job satisfaction for doctors is being sued for malpractice. Although adverse outcomes resulting from medical errors are necessarily present in such suits, many patients who suffer adverse outcomes do not litigate. Patient (dis)satisfaction with doctor communication is an important factor, and a doctor's chance of receiving patient complaints and being sued for malpractice is tightly linked with his or her communication skills.[46] A study of patient depositions from settled malpractice suits found that relationship and communication problems (i.e., deserting the patient, poor delivery of information, failing to understand and/or value the patient/family perspective) were factors in 71 percent of them.[47]

Doctors with a history of malpractice lawsuits, compared with doctors without such a history, have shorter average visits with patients, less patient participation, and less effectiveness at educating patients on what to expect from the interaction.[48] Another study evaluated audio-taped 10-second speech segments of surgeons talking to their patients during office visits; doctors whose emotional tone was assessed as more dominant and less concerned and anxious were more likely to have been sued.[49] Yet another study found that patients whose doctors had prior malpractice claims, compared with patients of doctors who had none, had twice as many complaints about things like being rushed, ignored, or given inadequate information.[50]

In a study of 642 sued doctors, nonsued doctors, and suing patients, all respondents viewed improved doctor-patient communication as the most effective method of preventing malpractice actions.[51]

IMPROVING COMMUNICATION

One overarching way to improve communication is to recognize that each patient is unique and that each patient's uniqueness should be respected and accommodated. Specific approaches to improving communication include agenda setting, presenting a demeanor that patients find reassuring and accessible, giving information successfully, and encouraging patient participation in decision making.

A General Approach: There Is No
One-Size-Fits-All Best Way to Communicate

An underlying theme in doctor-patient communication research is that optimal communication depends on who the patient is and who the doctor is. Patients differ from one another in significant ways. The differences may be demographic (age, gender, ethnicity, socioeconomic status), personality based, or health based (severity of illness, presence or absence of depression). Patients have varying degrees of health literacy. They have varying resources and lifestyles and varying fears, expectations, and needs. All of these differences may impact how doctors and patients communicate as well as the type of communication patients *want*. The same communication style that works perfectly with a patient who is a wealthy, elderly, African American woman with no serious health concerns might not work as well with a young Caucasian man coping with depression and a chronic and serious illness.

A fundamental strategy for doctors to employ, therefore, is to try to understand and accommodate the uniqueness of their individual patients. This strategy is often discussed in relation to the concept and goal of *patient-centered* care, which has been described as the "standard for high-quality interpersonal care."[52] As formulated by Stewart, the first two elements of patient-centered care are: (1) exploring the patient's illness experience, and (2) understanding the whole person.[53] Exploring a patient's illness experience means understanding his or her feelings and ideas about the illness, the ways in which the illness affects the patient's life, and the expectations the patient has of the doctor.[54] Understanding the whole person means understanding the context in which a patient and his/her illness exist, including a patient's personality, background, family, community, and physical environment.[55]

Another influential approach to improving medical care has been called *cultural competence*, a term used to describe an approach to improving health care based on awareness of and concern about racial and ethnic disparities.[56] Cultural differences may impact health-care preferences and choices; ignoring these differences can create problems, including inappropriate decision making, negative emotions surrounding doctor-patient interactions, and patient dissatisfaction.[57] A primary goal of cultural competence is to ensure that health-care providers are sensitive to and respect the legitimacy of a patient's cultural context, including health-care beliefs, treatment preferences, and language. Cultural competence shares many values and goals with patient-centered care: seeing the patient as a unique person, building effective rapport, exploring patients' beliefs, values, and understanding of illness, and finding common ground regarding treatment plans.

Patients prefer to be treated as unique individuals, and doctors who understand how experiences and communication preferences differ can tailor their approach to best suit a particular patient. Some doctors are insufficiently sensitive to these issues. For example, they give less information to lower-income patients, interrupt unattractive patients more than attractive ones, and spend more time with Caucasian than minority patients. These biases and assumptions can impact medical care.

Patients Prefer This Approach   Patient-centered care is appealing to patients. Little and colleagues found that patients want a patient-centered approach and are "less satisfied, less enabled, and may have greater symptom burden and higher rates of referral" if they don't get it.[58] In a study that surveyed patients on their preferences as they waited to be seen by a doctor, the very large majority wanted a patient-centered approach.[59]

This Approach Is Effective   Patient-centered care is effective. It is associated with improved health status and increased efficiency of care (diagnostic tests and referrals are half as frequent when doctors employ a patient-centered care approach).[60] The whole-person dimension of patient-centered care is associated with greater medication adherence. Beach and colleagues found that a patient's perception of being "known as a person" improved adherence to antiretroviral therapy. The authors suggest that actions such as "remembering a patient's name, establishing good rapport, listening carefully, asking questions to learn about their lives, and later remembering and following up on this information with patients" might generate a patient's feelings of being known as a person.[61]

Recognizing Inappropriate Responses to Patient Characteristics May Help Reduce Them   A host of patient and doctor characteristics play into doctor-patient communication. For example:

- Doctors give female patients more information than male patients.[62]
- Female doctors spend more time with patients, ask more questions, actively facilitate more patient participation, and engage in more emotional talk than male doctors.[63]
- Patients speak more and disclose more information to female doctors.[64]
- Female doctors report liking their patients more than male doctors do, and patients report liking their female doctors more than they like their male doctors.[65]
- Female/female dyads are associated with the longest and most patient-centered consultations.[66]
- Doctors are more empathetic with Caucasian patients than with patients of color.[67]
- African American patients rate their medical visits as significantly less participatory than do Caucasian patients.[68]
- Doctors are more contentious with African American patients than with Caucasian or Hispanic patients, and they perceive African American patients to be less effective communicators and less satisfied.[69]
- Asian Americans are least likely (of Asian Americans, Caucasians, African Americans, and Latinos) to receive preventive health services, feel that their doctor understands their background, have confidence in their doctor, and be as involved in decision making as they would like.[70]
- Doctors are more verbally dominant and engage in less patient-centered communication with African American than white patients.[71]
- Race-concordant visits last longer and have higher ratings of patient positive affect.[72] Patients in race-concordant visits are more satisfied and view their doctors as more participatory, independent of the doctor's patient-centered communication behaviors.[73]

- Due to language barriers with doctors, almost 20 percent of Spanish-speaking U.S. residents did not seek care when they needed it.[74]
- Doctors like healthier patients more than they do sick ones.[75] Sicker patients behave more negatively[76] and are less satisfied with their care.[77]
- Patients of lower socioeconomic status receive less information, directions, and socioeconomic and partnership-building utterances from their doctors than patients with higher socioeconomic status.[78]
- Better-educated patients receive more reassurance and information than less-educated patients.[79]
- Doctors are rated more highly on interviewing, nonverbal attention, and courtesy when with well-groomed patients.[80] Doctors interrupt well-groomed patients less than patients who are not.

Not all the behaviors and attitudes cited above indicate inappropriate doctor bias. Doctor-patient communication reflects the personalities and communication styles of both doctors and their patients. For example, patients who ask fewer questions are likely to get less information. Still, although doctors may not be at fault for any biased treatments of patients, the biases may have substantial medical consequences. Doctors who are aware of the ways that patient characteristics impact doctor-patient communication can take steps to correct potential problems. Hooper and colleagues wrote that "the recognition that patient characteristics influence physician behavior should stimulate physicians to examine their reactions in order to insure that all types of patients receive thorough, courteous and empathic care."[81]

Specific Tools: There *Are* One-Size-Fits-Many Ways to Communicate

The section above made the point that patients are unique, and discovering and working with that uniqueness is an important prerequisite to successful communication. Still, some aspects of doctor-patient communication improve communication in most, if not all, relationships. We'll address agenda setting, doctor demeanor, providing information, and shared decision making.

Agenda Setting: "What Concerns Do You Have?" Primary care doctors are generally presented with three to six concerns per visit.[82] It's not always possible to address all concerns in detail, so collaborative prioritizing is an important step in maximizing the effectiveness and efficiency of interactions. Prioritizing can be done through eliciting patients' complete lists of concerns. This is an underused strategy; doctors solicit patients' full agendas in only about one-quarter of clinical interviews.[83]

One reason that doctors interrupt patients before their agenda is fully stated is visit time constraints. But Marvel and colleagues found that patients allowed to complete their full statement of agendas took an average of only six seconds more than the average time taken by patients not allowed to finish.[84] Failing to elicit complete agendas prevents doctors from prioritizing. In addition, they learn of fewer concerns and must deal with more end-of-visit issues.[85]

Agenda Setting Continued: "Is There Something Else?" The way in which patient agendas are solicited matters. A 2007 study gave doctors one of two scripted questions to ask after patients presented their primary concern.[86] One group of doctors asked, "Is there anything else you want to address in the visit today?" while the other group asked, "Is there something else you want to address in the visit today?" The "anything else" group could not be significantly distinguished from the nonintervention group. In contrast, the "something else" group eliminated 78 percent of patients' unmet concerns. Neither intervention affected visit length.

Demeanor and Attitude toward Patient As noted above, patients are more satisfied with doctors whose nonverbal and verbal approach suggests they are friendly, engaged, and nonjudgmental. When doctors sit down for the visit, patients believe the visit lasts longer than when the doctor stands. Patients prefer that a doctor include some brief nonmedical conversation. Patients who feel "known as a whole person" have increased satisfaction and better outcomes. Most patients prefer doctors who are not dominant in doctor-patient interactions.

Beach and colleagues found that respondents who reported being treated with dignity were more likely to report higher levels of satisfaction, adherence to therapy, and receipt of optimal preventive services. The authors suggest that treating someone with dignity "primarily involves recognizing inherent value in that person." They encourage clinicians to consider how to foster attitudes of respectfulness toward patients.[87]

Providing Information Doctors cannot reliably identify those patients with inadequate health literacy, and even patients with adequate health literacy may face difficulties in understanding and recalling medical information. So communication should be as clear and accessible as possible for all patients. Several steps can aid communication.

- *Use clear language.* Use clear, familiar, nonmedical language. For example, say *harmless* instead of *benign, test* instead of *screening, tired* instead of *fatigued.*
- *Limit and repeat key content.* Prioritize what needs to be discussed, and try to limit it to three to five key points. Repeat those points. As discussed above, a huge factor in patient compliance with prescriptions is their understanding of the medical condition, the reasons for the medication, and the instructions for medication use, so this information should be carefully covered.
- *Support spoken information with written or visual material.* Medical advice is generally communicated orally, and much is forgotten. Written information is better remembered and leads to better satisfaction and adherence.[88] Written information, however, presents challenges to patients who have low literacy or who are not given materials in their native language. Video and graphics (cartoons, drawings, and illustrations) may be useful adjuncts.[89] Doctors should not assume that patients will review educational materials on their own; doctors should always review the materials with patients and encourage spoken discussions about them.
- *Encourage patients to ask questions.* Martin and colleagues found that the most powerful things doctors can do to reassure patients that their involvement is welcome are to ask open-ended questions and be responsive to patients' questions.[90] Friendly body language can make it easier for patients to ask questions: doctors should sit, make eye contact, and present themselves as having time to listen. They should actively solicit questions. "What questions do you still have?" is a good approach because it conveys to the patient that the doctor assumes there are questions. "Do you have any questions?"

doesn't convey that assumption and is not a good way to draw a
patient out.

- *Confirm patients' understanding.* Confirm patients' understanding
  in a way that does not put the onus on them if understanding isn't
  there. Say, for example, "I want to make sure I was clear. Can you
  tell me your understanding of what I just told you?" The idea is
  not to test the patient's knowledge but to test how well the doctor
  conveyed the information. Do not ask yes/no questions like, "Do
  you understand?" It is worth noting that visits in which the doctor
  confirms recall are not longer.[91]

- *Consider using patient decision aids.* For some medical conditions,
  there is no single best treatment but rather a set of options, all with
  good and bad aspects to them (e.g., for women experiencing menopause, hormone replacement therapy alleviates some symptoms but
  increases the risk of developing certain serious medical conditions).
  Individual patients may differ on how they weigh those good and
  bad aspects. For those cases, patient decision aids (ptDAs) can be
  helpful adjuncts in helping patients choose the best treatment option for their values and preferences. PtDAs are tools that provide
  patients information about all viable treatment options and the risks
  and benefits of each. They help patients clarify their values. They
  can be paper based or electronic. Most developers are moving toward Internet-based tools.[92] The Cochrane Collaboration Team's
  inventory is available at http://decisionaid.ohri.ca/AZinvent.php.

A 2007 meta-analysis of ptDAs found that they improved decision
quality (defined as decisions being informed and based on personal values) and increased patients' feelings of being informed and clear about
their personal values.[93] In addition, the use of ptDAs reduces elective
surgical procedures in favor of more conservative treatment options—
without negative effects on health outcomes, patient satisfaction, or
patient anxiety.[94] On the other hand, there is little evidence that ptDAs
improve health outcomes, quality of life, or survival.[95]

Some potential barriers to the use of ptDAs have been identified and
include concern about their comprehensiveness and currentness, lack
of awareness about or access to them, too much complexity for patients
with low literacy levels, and practitioner expense in supplying ptDAs to

their patients. Those concerns have been addressed: Cochrane Review developed an assessment tool (CREDIBLE criteria) that includes evaluation of currentness; ptDAs are widely accessible online; most ptDAs are developed for general audiences (eighth-grade reading level); and ptDAs reduce demand for invasive procedures—this reduction likely saves health-care organizations money overall even if they spend some up front on using ptDAs.[96]

Shared Decision Making   Collaboration with doctors in decision making helps patients consider the seriousness of the condition to be prevented or treated, understand the risks, benefits, and alternative options for diagnosis and treatment, and include their beliefs and values as factors in the decision-making process. Shared decision making does not preclude clear recommendations based on a doctor's understanding of the evidence. Patients typically want to know what their doctor recommends and would do in their place.

As discussed above, shared decision making leads to better adherence with treatment plans. It is also associated with symptom resolution, patient satisfaction, better quality of life, increased trust in the doctor, increases in patients' sense of self-efficacy, and fewer doctor-ordered unnecessary tests or treatments.[97]

Most patients *want* to be involved in decision making about their health care. A 2006 survey of patients in Israel asked which features of medical care were important to them; more than one-quarter said that getting more information and taking part in decisions were their first priorities.[98] When possible, then, doctors and patients should work together to define health problems and establish the goals of treatment.

Not all patients want to participate significantly in decisions about their care. Swenson and colleagues compared patient preferences for a patient-centered approach with an approach in which the doctor is more directive. Sixty-nine percent preferred the patient-centered communication style and 31 percent, a traditional, directive style.[99] Furthermore, although most patients want to be able to share information with their doctors and be informed about treatment options, they vary considerably in the extent to which they want to be involved in final decision making.[100]

Factors that predict a preference for increased participation include younger age, female gender, higher education, less-serious illness, and personality traits of conscientiousness and openness to experience.[101]

As discussed above, patients may benefit from participating even if they express a preference for nonparticipation. Diabetic patients who participated most in decision making were the most satisfied—even those who had not wanted to be heavily involved.[102] The authors suggest that some patients may not recognize how much they want to participate. It might be useful for doctors to tell patients about the benefits of participating and that some patients find it more satisfying than they expect to.

Jahng and colleagues found that physician-patient preference similarity for patient involvement positively impacts satisfaction and perceptions of general health.[103] Physician-patient congruence was more important in predicting adherence to treatment plans than demographic factors like ethnicity, age, or gender. These findings support the argument that each doctor/patient relationship needs to be developed in light of the unique personhood of the patient. Jahng and colleagues suggest that patients be prescreened for their preferences and paired with doctors who have similar styles and preferences.

DISCUSSING PAIN AND DELIVERING BAD NEWS

Two challenging areas of communication for many doctors are preparing patients for pain and delivering bad news. We discuss these types of communication in this section.

Preparing Patients for Pain

Patients benefit from being prepared for what to expect related to their medical care. A much-replicated 1964 study analyzed the impact of doctors having brief conversations with patients the night before surgery to discuss the postoperative pain they should expect.[104] Patients who had this preparation needed about half the usual pain medication.

When preparing patients for what to expect, it is important to

- Emphasize the steps that will be taken to keep the patient comfortable and pain-free.

- Use precise language. Words such as "stinging," "dull ache," "pressure," and "jabbing pain" convey a much better sense of what patients can expect and will ease anxiety when these sensations are experienced. If the terms "pain" and "hurt" are used, the patient may imagine a more uncomfortable experience than is actually the case.
- Break procedures and associated pain into components; many procedures are painful for only a portion of the time.

Delivering Bad News

Breaking bad news is a difficult, often emotional part of the job of health-care professionals and one for which they are often undertrained.[105] Studies have identified various ways in which health professionals can best meet the needs of patients in these situations.

Be Informative and Honest   In a study that looked at the preferences of 351 patients, the most important of forty-six aspects of an initial diagnosis of cancer or a diagnosis of a recurrence were

1. Their doctor being up to date on research about their condition
2. Being told their best treatment options
3. Having their doctor take time to answer their questions
4. Believing their doctor is honest about the severity of their condition[106]

For patients to make appropriate treatment decisions, their communication with their doctor has to be honest. This is not always how bad news communications play out. In one study, doctors said they would provide a frank survival estimate only 37 percent of the time and would provide no estimate, a conscious overestimate, or a conscious underestimate most of the time (63 percent).[107]

Allow Adequate Time for Patient Questions   Patients want to be able to ask all their questions and have them answered fully.[108]

Be Clear and Unambiguous   Patients want their doctors to use unambiguous language. Although doctors sometimes are ambiguous in an attempt to make their message less painful, ambiguity can have the unintended consequence of causing patients to misunderstand their diagnosis and outlook.[109] A survey asked surviving family members of trauma patients who died to rank fourteen aspects of bad news delivery on their importance. Seventy percent ranked clarity of the message as most important.[110]

Another big source of patient misunderstandings is unclear technical language. For example, if patients do not understand what "median survival" means (and one study found that 70 percent of women diagnosed with breast cancer did not), they cannot successfully interpret the information they've been given.[111]

Give News Privately   In the study of surviving family members of deceased trauma patients, 65 percent ranked privacy as most important.[112]

Consider Using Recall Aids   Recall aids can help doctors give bad news. Both audiotapes of the doctor-patient interaction and written summaries of the information that was conveyed can improve recall of important information and reduce anxiety.[113]

Be Caring   Patients want their doctors to be caring, concerned, and sensitive to their experience. In one study of parents of children in developmental day cares, the parents' strongest preference for doctor behavior was for doctors to show caring.[114]

TIPS ESPECIALLY FOR PATIENTS

In this chapter, we have discussed how the quality of doctor-patient interactions impacts patient outcomes. A doctor may be a brilliant diagnostician, an excellent surgeon, or the most knowledgeable person in the world about a given disease but still not offer the best medical care if she or he cannot communicate effectively with patients. Patients, therefore, should try to find doctors with whom they feel comfortable and confident. When possible, patients should choose doctors whom they perceive as friendly and engaged. Patients are more satisfied with their medical care when their doctors have this demeanor.

Treatment plan adherence is a challenge for many patients. Patients typically adhere to plans more closely if they feel they've had the opportunity to give information relevant to the choice of treatment plan and participated in the decision. Patients should select a doctor with whom they feel comfortable sharing information and participating in decision making.

Patients should make sure they understand what the treatment plan *is*. Adherence is understandably reduced if patients don't know what they need to do. It might be helpful during an appointment for patients to write down what the doctor advises. This would give them the opportunity to review their understanding with the doctor before leaving. Patients should ask questions until they're confident they fully understand what the doctor expects them to do. Patients may also want to consider bringing someone with them (a family member, friend, or professional "health advocate") who can also ask questions and help patients understand and remember treatment plans.

We discussed the concept of agenda setting and encouraged doctors to ensure that agendas are clearly discussed and agreed upon at the outset of a medical visit. Patients can help this process by determining in advance the concerns they wish to discuss and communicating that list to their doctors.

At times patients must choose between treatment options that offer different advantages and disadvantages. If faced with this type of decision, a patient might want to ask whether the doctor knows of any patient decision aids.

LOOKING AHEAD

In this chapter we have addressed the importance of doctors correctly interpreting and responding to patient concerns and communication. The following chapter discusses challenges surrounding interpretation of a dramatically different type of information also of great significance for health-care practices: medical research results. This vast body of information of varying quality and reliability can be difficult for people to make sense of, especially when, as is true for many doctors, they don't have a strong background in research methodology.

②

INTERPRETING
MEDICAL INFORMATION

Although medical technology and research methodology have advanced considerably in recent years, they have not eliminated controversy. Many once widely accepted medical beliefs and health practices have been overturned by new evidence. Following is a very incomplete list:

- For decades, surgeons treated breast cancer with radical mastectomy. They now prefer the much less invasive lumpectomy.
- Stress was once believed to be a major cause of peptic ulcers, and stress reduction was a key component of treatment. We know now that bacteria cause more than 80 percent of ulcers; antibiotics are used to kill the bacteria.
- For years, nutritionists advised people to avoid eggs, coconuts, butter, chocolate, nuts, and coffee. Now, many list those foods on the positive side of the health ledger.
- Babies should sleep on their sides or on their backs until about one year of age, not on their stomachs, as previously advised.
- For decades it was believed that following childbirth, surgery, heart attack, back pain, and several other conditions, patients should get total bed rest. Doctors today urge patients to get out of bed and move about.

- Antifever drugs such as aspirin and acetaminophen may prolong, not reduce, symptoms of the flu.
- Many drugs once hailed as miracles have been taken off the market. A partial list since 1997 includes Bextra, Duract, Hismanal, Lotronex, Pondimin, Posicor, Propulsid, Raxar, Reductil, Redux, Rezulin, Seldane, Serzone, and Vioxx.
- Playing sports during menstruation does not damage reproductive organs.
- Neither iodine nor alcohol should be applied to cuts and scratches.
- Autism is not caused by lack of parental affection.
- Arthritic pain does not vary with humidity, storms, or atmospheric pressure.
- The proper first aid for minor burns is to run cold water over the burned area. Greasy ointments should not be used.
- The benefits of tonsillectomy in preventing throat infections in children are not worth the risks and costs of surgery.
- Hormone replacement therapy probably does not help protect women against heart disease.

Several reasons account for past and, almost certainly, future reversals of medical practices. First, the scientific literature is vast and constantly increasing so that true mastery of all available information on any given medical topic is likely impossible. Second, much of the published material is of questionable value because of conflicts of interest that impact the information presented. Third, most medical schools do not require rigorous courses in research methodology. As a result, doctors may overlook critical factors such as the difference between experimental and correlational designs and between statistical and clinical significance. They may not know how to compute or evaluate number needed to treat, odds ratio, relative versus absolute risk, and survival rate versus mortality rate.

THE SCIENTIFIC LITERATURE

Even the most dedicated physicians cannot possibly read more than a small fraction of the burgeoning medical literature. Each year more than six million articles are published in more than one hundred thousand scientific journals, and biomedical knowledge doubles approximately every twenty years.[1] The Medline database contains more than twelve million articles and adds more than two thousand daily.[2] As of July 4, 2010, Medline lists 17,584 articles about attention deficit hyperactivity disorder. Assuming twenty minutes on average to read each article, reading all would take about 5,860 hours—more than 730 eight-hour days for just that one condition.

CONFLICTS OF INTEREST

Even if physicians had the time to read everything, they might still end up misinformed. A popular conception of scientists is that they are dispassionate seekers after the truth. Unfortunately, not all scientists fit the stereotype. Many, including heads of major university departments and editors of influential journals, are hired, own stock in, or are subsidized by drug or medical device companies. Their incomes are affected by sales of the company's products. As a result, their published research and public speeches cannot always be trusted.

Most drug studies are designed by drug company researchers, and they typically do not allow independent researchers to see the data. Their goal is to give the company's products an edge over those of their competitors. A favorable article published in a peer-reviewed medical journal confers many benefits. The drug company can cite it in advertisements, promotional materials, and opinion pieces published in other journals.[3] So the companies use many tricks to get published. For example, they may pay professional ghostwriters to generate outlines for possible articles. If an outline is approved by company executives, the ghostwriter is asked to write a manuscript. Then the sponsor pays a well-known medical researcher to put his or her name on the manuscript. The researcher can amend it, but unless the final product is favorable to the company's goals, it will not be published—and the researcher won't get paid. The researcher submits the manuscript to a medical journal in which the company runs full-page ads—and readers believe they are reading scientifically validated articles that reached favorable conclusions about the drugs. In testimony before a British Parliament health committee, eminent psychiatrist David Healy said he believes that at least half the articles on drug efficacy that appear in the *British Medical Journal*, the *Lancet*, and the *New England Journal of Medicine* are ghostwritten by drug companies. He said that distinguished authors from prestigious universities put their names to the articles without ever seeing the raw data.[4] Following are several of a much greater number of possible examples:

Ghostwriting:

- Pfizer used a ghostwriting agency to produce nearly ninety articles for its antidepressant Zoloft.
- Wyeth paid ghostwriters to author journal articles praising its hormone replacement therapy drug Prempro. One article was published as an "Editors' Choice" feature in May 2003 in the *American Journal of Obstetrics and Gynecology*, more than a year after a large federal study linked Prempro, a combination of estrogen and progestin, to breast cancer.[5]

Bias against publishing unfavorable results:

- A substantial proportion of completed studies are never published. One reason for nonpublication is that the drug or other product being tested was ineffective.[6] Cardiologist Peter Wilmshurst testified that he was offered large bribes not to publish results unfavorable to the drug under investigation. He knew three cardiology professors who did not publish their findings after the sponsoring drug manufacturer saw the unfavorable results.[7] This bias against publishing unfavorable results causes meta-analysts to overestimate treatment effects.
- The medical community learns about drugs in part from studies published in medical journals. They do not see the FDA conclusions from materials submitted to the FDA based on those studies. But, as Turner and colleagues found, the FDA's conclusions often differ substantially from those in the published studies.[8] From seventy-four FDA-registered studies on twelve antidepressant drugs, Turner and colleagues identified fifty-one published articles that had the same drug name, dose, groups, sample size, active comparator (if used), duration, and name of principal investigator.

The authors of forty-eight of the fifty-one reported positive results. It is likely that many and probably most of the missing twenty-three had negative results. According to the FDA, only thirty-eight of their seventy-four studies had positive results, and all but one of the thirty-eight were published.

The FDA deemed thirty-six of the studies to be either negative (twenty-four) or questionable (twelve). Only three of those were published as negative; thirty-three were either not published (twenty-two) or published as positive (eleven) in conflict with the FDA's conclusion. Overall, it appeared from the published literature that 94 percent of the studies were positive. By contrast, the FDA analysis showed only 51 percent as positive.

- Rising and colleagues looked at all the new-drug applications approved by the FDA in 2001 and 2002 and then checked whether, five years later, details on all the studies on the drug had made it into print.[9] Only three-quarters of the original studies had been published. Those with positive outcomes were nearly five times as likely as those with negative outcomes to be published. Forty-one outcomes appeared in filings to the FDA but not in a journal. And on several occasions, the published conclusions differed from those reported to the FDA in ways that favored the new drugs.

Focus only on supporting data:

Many researchers focus only on data that support their claims. For example, Spiro described a study on a drug for peptic ulcers: "At the end of two weeks, the ulcer crater had healed in more than half the patients given the active drug and in only a third of patients taking placebos; that one observation point provided the desired statistical significance to permit the claim that the active drug, in this case cimetidine, 'speeded the healing' of peptic ulcer. . . . But at every other period of assessment, cimetidine and the placebo proved equally effective."[10]

Unfair comparisons:

- Drug company researchers don't make fair comparisons. Bodenheimer gave several examples of designs biased in favor of the sponsoring company's drug.[11] For example, Pfizer funded a study comparing its antifungal drug fluconazole with a competitor's amphotericin B. Both drugs were administered orally, which is the appropriate route of administration for fluconazole but not for amphotericin B.

Impact of source of funding on results:

- Bero and colleagues examined 192 published results of trials comparing one cholesterol-lowering statin drug to another or to a nonstatin drug.[12] The reported results favored the funding company's drug about twenty times more often than the comparison company's drug. The interpretation of results favored the funding company's drug about thirty-five times more often than the comparison company's drug.
- Huss and colleagues examined whether the source of funding of studies of the effects of low-level radio frequency radiation from mobile phones is associated with the results.[13] They found that studies funded exclusively by industry were least likely to report a harmful effect.
- Influential articles about nutritional research are often funded by industry and are four to eight times more likely to reach conclusions that find in favor of its products.[14]
- Cochrane reviews[15] were compared with industry-supported analyses of the same drugs for the same disease. Seven of the eight industry-supported reviews had conclusions, and they recommended the experimental drug without reservations. None of the Cochrane reviews or the sixteen reviews that were not industry supported did so.
- New drugs are protected by patent, so drug companies prefer having them turn out superior to older ones. In studies comparing new with old drugs, 43 percent funded by a drug company and only 13 percent funded from other sources favored the new. Furthermore, "In no case was a therapeutic agent manufactured by the sponsoring company found to be inferior to an alternative product manufactured by another company."[16] Ninety-eight percent of published studies favored the drug produced by the company funding the research.[17]

- Walton located 164 published papers on the artificial sweetener aspartame (NutraSweet). All of the seventy-four studies funded by the manufacturers of NutraSweet reported that aspartame is safe; eighty-three of the other ninety studies identified potentially serious health problems caused by aspartame.[18]

Impact of advertising:

- Editors of scientific journals are pressured by advertisers to reject material harmful to the advertiser's products. For example, a leading nephrology journal (*Transplantation and Dialysis*) rejected an editorial questioning the efficacy of epoetin in end-stage renal disease because it feared losing advertising. The journal editor wrote the author, saying he had been "overruled by our marketing department."[19]

Financial ties with industry:

- Yank analyzed seventy-one reviews of antihypertensive drugs. Authors who disclosed (as required) financial ties with the drug industry were five times more likely than authors funded by other sources to report conclusions favoring the study drug when such conclusions were not supported by the results.[20]
- Members of FDA advisory committees often have contracts or grants of more than $100,000 with the companies that produce the drugs under evaluation. At least one committee member disclosed a conflict of interest in 73 percent of the 221 advisory committee meetings held from January 1, 2001, to December 31, 2004. Only 1 percent of committee members were recused over that period. For every member with a financial connection to the manufacturer of the drug being evaluated or to a competitor company, there was a 10 percent greater likelihood that the final vote would be in favor of the product being discussed.[21]
- The National Cholesterol Education Program called for sharply lowering the desired levels of "bad" cholesterol. Only later was it revealed that eight of nine members of the panel writing the recommendations had financial ties to the makers of cholesterol-lowering drugs.[22]

Union of Concerned Scientists and Public Employees for Environmental Responsibility:

- In 2006, the Union of Concerned Scientists and Public Employees for Environmental Responsibility distributed a 38-question survey to 5,918 FDA scientists in order to examine the state of science at the FDA. The results are chilling.[23]
  - Eighteen percent answered "yes" to the statement "I have been asked, for non-scientific reasons, to inappropriately exclude or alter technical information or my conclusions in an FDA scientific document."
  - Sixty-one percent knew of cases in which "Department of Health and Human Services or FDA political appointees have inappropriately injected themselves into FDA determinations or actions."
  - Sixty percent knew of cases "where commercial interests have inappropriately induced or attempted to induce the reversal, withdrawal or modification of FDA determinations or actions."
  - Twenty percent said they "have been asked explicitly by FDA decision makers to provide incomplete, inaccurate or misleading information to the public, regulated industry, media, or elected/senior government officials."
  - Twenty-six percent feel that FDA decision makers implicitly expect them to "provide incomplete, inaccurate, or misleading information."
  - Forty percent said they could not publicly express "concerns about public health without fear of retaliation."
  - Thirty-six percent did not feel they could do so even inside the confines of the agency.
  - Only forty-seven percent think that the "FDA routinely provides complete and accurate information to the public."

Most major research journals have tried to minimize biased reporting by requiring that both authors of original research and meta-analysts identify all their sources of funding. But the journals don't require that the meta-analysts distinguish between studies that were and were not funded by drug companies. Roseman and her colleagues analyzed 29 meta-analyses from high-impact biomedical journals that together included information from 509 studies.[24] Only two reported the funding sources of the studies they were evaluating. Yet 219 of the 318 studies that reported funding sources were industry funded. Thus, the meta-analysts' conclusions leave out clues to influence by parties with a financial interest in an outcome.

METHODOLOGICAL ISSUES

When a manuscript is submitted to a respectable medical journal, the editor sends it to one or more experts in the relevant area to evaluate for importance and methodological quality. Despite that safeguard, many poor-quality articles make it into print. People who don't read critically are likely to end up misinformed.

Consider the astonishing and frightening work of John Ioannidis. Ioannidis examined forty-nine of the most widely cited studies published between 1990 and 2003 in three of the world's most prestigious generalist medical journals—*Journal of the American Medical Association*, the *Lancet*, and the *New England Journal of Medicine*—and in leading specialty journals.[25] He then tracked whether or not the studies' main findings held true over time. One out of every three was either refuted or seriously weakened by subsequent research.

Ioannidis published a second article with the provocative title "Why Most Published Research Findings Are False."[26] Using simulations, he convincingly showed that for most study designs and settings, a research claim is more likely false than true. He charged that as much as 90 percent of the published medical information that doctors rely on is flawed, in large part because of conflicts of interest.[27]

Experimental versus Correlational Studies

Imagine a hypothetical research project in which one hundred volunteers are randomly assigned to receive either a caffeine pill or an identical-looking placebo. That is, each volunteer has an equal chance of getting caffeine or placebo, to be determined by a random process such as flipping a coin. While waiting for the caffeine to take effect, the researcher asks the volunteers whether they smoke. Half of the people in each group are nonsmokers, and half smoke exactly one pack per day. (Hypothetical data are great to work with.) The four groups of twenty-five are asked to lift weights, with the following results:

1. caffeine/smoker   100 pounds lifted
2. caffeine/nonsmoker   80 pounds lifted
3. placebo/smoker   60 pounds lifted
4. placebo/nonsmoker   40 pounds lifted

Combining groups 1 and 2 and comparing them with combined groups 3 and 4 gives the difference between caffeine and placebo, independent of smoking habits. Comparing 1 and 3 with 2 and 4 gives the difference between smokers and nonsmokers, independent of caffeine.

> QUESTION: Assuming that the study was well done (another virtue of hypothetical research) and the data are statistically significant, what conclusions can be drawn about the effects of caffeine and smoking on weight-lifting ability?
>
> ANSWER: It's possible that all the heavy lifters received caffeine and the weaklings placebo, but random assignment makes such an outcome unlikely. The researcher could safely assume that the subjects were approximately equal in weight-lifting ability prior to swallowing their pills. So any subsequent differences between them would best be explained as a caffeine effect. If a study had actually been done with the results indicated, the researcher could be confident that caffeine increases weight-lifting ability.

But subjects were not randomly assigned to the smoking/nonsmoking groups. They had selected themselves prior to participating in the study, because of factors such as gender, genetics, stress, exposure to cigarette advertising, and desire to project a certain image. Those same or other unknown factors may have made them unequal in weight-lifting ability before treatment began. If a study had been done with the results indicated, the researcher could safely conclude that smokers lift more weight than do nonsmokers; but it would not be appropriate to conclude that smoking is the reason.

Consider the results of a real study: Puccio and colleagues asked people about their caffeine consumption.[28] Drinkers of caffeinated coffee were less healthy than others, which suggests that coffee drinking impairs health. But drinkers of caffeinated coffee were more likely than nondrinkers to smoke tobacco. They also drank more alcohol, had more saturated fats and cholesterol in their diets, and exercised less. No matter what the effects of coffee on health, coffee drinkers might be less healthy.

The examples illustrate a major distinction between two legitimate types of research. Experiments require that subjects be randomly assigned to groups. In correlational studies, there is no random assignment. As a consequence, only results from experiments justify statements such as "Treatment X benefits condition Y." More generally, whereas correlational research can show relationships between two variables, only experiments can prove that one variable causes a change in the other.

Epidemiologists study factors associated with disease and health. Epidemiological research serves as the foundation for interventions made in the interest of public health and preventive medicine. However, as noted at the beginning of the chapter, many of their recommendations have been challenged and reversed. The reason is that epidemiologists rarely have the luxury of doing experiments. Instead, they must rely on correlational data such as "People who follow the Mediterranean diet tend to live longer than people who don't." Smith and Ebrahim cited a few instances in which researchers have been able to do experiments to test epidemiological hypotheses.[29] The experiments have generally refuted the hypotheses.

Double-Blind Studies

Good scientists maximize the probability that their interpretation is correct by eliminating as many plausible alternatives as possible, so they typically use many subjects and randomly assign some to a control group. They treat experimental and control subjects exactly the same except for the treatment itself. Then, subsequent differences between the groups can reasonably be attributed to the treatment. To prevent bias, researchers do not let subjects know which group they are in, nor do they themselves know until after the data have been collected. The procedure, called the double-blind randomized controlled trial (RCT), is the most rigorous design available to medical researchers. It is the evidentiary gold standard.

But many studies are double-blind in name only. Both researchers and subjects can observe clinical improvement and side effects and thus correctly guess which group the subjects are in.[30] Furthermore, when Schulz quizzed four hundred researchers after promising them anonymity, more than half admitted opening unsealed envelopes containing the group assignments, cracking codes meant to hide the identity of the groups, searching for a master list of codes, or holding sealed envelopes up to the light.[31] That, of course, subverts the purpose of double blinding.

Fergusson and colleagues randomly sampled two hundred placebo-controlled trials from general medical and psychiatric journals. (Nine trials were discarded as they were not placebo controlled, despite being identified as such in the literature.) Only seven of the ninety-seven general medicine trials provided evidence on the success of blinding, with five reporting imperfect success. In psychiatric journals, evidence on success was reported in only eight of the ninety-four trials, with four reporting imperfect blinding.[32]

To ensure blindness in drug trials, investigators give placebos to control subjects. But the FDA has no rules regarding the composition of placebos. Golomb and colleagues reviewed 167 placebo-controlled trials published in peer-reviewed medical journals. In only 26.7 percent of the studies with pills and 8.2 percent of the studies with injections or other treatments did the investigators disclose the composition of the study placebo.[33] Yet placebos are not completely inert, and some have significant negative effects on certain individuals. So if a drug has no effects or even adverse effects, subjects in the drug group may nevertheless fare better than placebo subjects. Consequently, a useless drug will appear efficacious. Golomb and colleagues cited a study in which megestrol acetate seemed to benefit cancer patients with gastrointestinal symptoms. However, a lactose placebo was used, and lactose intolerance is prevalent in cancer patients. AIDS patients are often lactose intolerant and, despite (or maybe because of) that, they have frequently been tested with placebos made of lactose.

Statistical and Clinical Significance

Suppose a coin is flipped ten times. If it's a fair coin, the most likely outcome is five heads and five tails. A six/four split would not be surprising, or even a seven/three. But with a fair coin and no cheating, a nine/one split would be very unlikely—such an outcome should occur only about 1 percent of the time. Still, even a fair coin might occasionally turn up heads ten times in a row, and a badly nicked coin that strongly favors one side may nevertheless turn up identical numbers of heads and tails. If the coin were flipped one thousand times, the likelihood of making an incorrect decision about fairness or bias would be greatly reduced but not eliminated. Medical researchers face a similar problem when they analyze data on the effectiveness of a treatment. The more subjects they test, the more confident they can be about results. But no matter how many are tested, the researchers may, through no fault of their own, incorrectly conclude that an ineffective treatment has worked or that an effective one has not.

So most scientific journals have adopted a convention that can be illustrated by returning to the coins. Start by assuming that a coin is perfectly fair. Then, if a series of flips results in a pattern so unusual that it would occur by chance only 5 percent of the time or less, reject the assumption and call the results statistically significant. A split of nine/one or ten/zero would be called statistically significant, but eight/two would not quite make it—with a fair coin, an eight/two split should occur slightly more than 5 percent of the time.

Statistically significant results convey the important information that a real difference exists between sides of a coin or, more importantly, treatment and control groups. But statistical significance tells nothing about the size of the difference, which is at least as important. The likelihood that a fair coin, just by chance, would turn up heads at least 5,100 times out of 10,000 flips is only 2 percent. But for a casual gambler betting on a few tosses of a coin, such a statistically significant result would be irrelevant. Similarly, if large numbers of subjects are used in a medical experiment, even a small difference between groups will reach statistical significance although the clinical relevance might be minimal.

To avoid conflating statistical with clinical significance, readers of scientific articles should always consider effect size—the size of the difference between treated and control groups. Kirsch and colleagues brought the point home when they analyzed studies testing the effects of new antidepressant drugs. Although many results were statistically significant, few reached the recommended criteria for clinical significance.[34]

An additional problem is that researchers, reviewers of manuscripts, and editors of journals are all biased toward publishing studies that reach statistical significance. So such research is published more often and more quickly than studies with results that exceed the .05 level.[35] If meta-analysts are unaware of unpublished though methodologically sound studies, their conclusions will be compromised. Sutton and colleagues suggested that this type of publication bias may be present to some degree in about 50 percent of meta-analyses in medical journals and strongly indicated in about 20 percent.[36] As a result, the published literature often overestimates the effects of a treatment, with potentially serious consequences. For example, sixteen published studies indicated a significant survival advantage of a two-drug combination to treat a certain type of cancer. The combination became a popular treatment option. But the apparent advantage disappeared when the results of several unpublished studies were located and combined with those of the first group. The unpublished studies were much more likely to have yielded negative results.[37]

There is another reason for tempering enthusiasm about new medical treatments. A favorable report of a new treatment typically stimulates further research. The new research often shows that the true treatment effects are much smaller than the effects initially reported.[38]

Number Needed to Treat (NNT)

Most clinical studies compare how much better people would fare with a particular treatment than without it. The NNT statistic answers a slightly different and often overlooked question: "How many patients need to take this treatment, compared with patients in a control group, in order to achieve one additional good outcome?" The NNT statistic is simple to compute, reflects effect size, and can be a good complement to statistical significance analysis. Unfortunately, it is not typically presented in research articles or drug advertisements, so many doctors don't know about it.

To compute the NNT, subtract the percent improvement rate in the control group from the percent improvement rate in the treatment group, and divide the difference into 1. For example, suppose that a treatment cures 70 percent of recipients and a placebo cures 50 percent. The NNT would be $1 / (.7 - .5) = 5$. (Five patients would have to get the new rather than the old treatment for one patient to benefit.) A treatment that benefited every patient would have an NNT of 1.

Statin drugs such as Lipitor are prescribed to people with risk factors for heart disease. Lipitor is expensive and causes side effects in many users. But the ads of its manufacturer, Pfizer, make the costs seem worthwhile. One such ad reads, "Lipitor reduces the risk of heart attack by 36 percent . . . in patients with multiple risk factors for heart disease." Hoffman pointed out that the data seem very impressive—except when considered in terms of NNT.[39] For every one hundred people in the Lipitor trial, which lasted three years and four months, three people on placebos and two people on Lipitor had heart attacks. So, to spare one person a heart attack, one hundred people had to take Lipitor for more than three years. The other ninety-nine got no measurable benefit. Recent studies suggest an NNT for statins at 250 and up for lower-risk patients, even if they take it for five years or more.

Drugs are often tested on people with multiple risk factors for the condition under consideration. An NNT may mislead if the drug is then marketed for people with low risk factors. Aside from NNT, doctors must consider the negative consequences of a treatment—financial expense plus adverse side effects. Hoffman said, "What if you put 250 people in a room and told them they would each pay $1,000 a year for a drug they would have to take every day, that many would get diarrhea and muscle pain, and that 249 would have no benefit? And that they could do just as well by exercising? How many would take that?"

Bridge and colleagues analyzed twelve studies that included 2,862 children who received either an antidepressant or a placebo. Taken together, 49 percent of children responded to placebo and 57 percent to an antidepressant. A doctor would have to give antidepressants to ten children to see an advantage over placebo in one of them.[40]

Question   To test your understanding of the computation of NNT, try the following problem.

QUESTION: Suppose that two hundred people are randomly assigned to receive either a new treatment or an old one. Suppose that eighty of the first group and fifty of the second are cured. What is the NNT for the new treatment compared with the old one?

ANSWER: 80 percent of the first group and 50 percent of the second are cured. 1 / (.8 − .5) = 1/.3 = 3.33. 3.33 people must be treated for one to benefit.

Odds Ratio

Medical researchers often present results as an odds ratio, which is an alternative measure of effect size that compares the probability of an event in two groups. If the event is equally likely in both groups, the odds ratio is 1. An odds ratio greater than 1 implies that the event is more likely to occur in one group. Suppose that fifteen of twenty people who receive a treatment, and ten of thirty who don't, are cured. The likelihood that a treated person will be cured is 15 / 20 = .75. The likelihood that a person in the control group will be cured is 10 / 30 = .33. The odds ratio is .75 / .33 = 2.27. There is a 2.27 greater chance of someone in the treated group being cured than someone in the control group.

Relative versus Absolute Risk

Gigerenzer and colleagues discussed a different problem, that of relative versus absolute risk, and presented data showing that many doctors fail to understand the concept.[41] Suppose that mammography screening reduces the risk of dying from breast cancer by 25 percent. They wrote, "Many people believe this to mean that the lives of 250 out of 1,000 women are saved, whereas a group of Swiss gynecologists' interpretations varied between one in 1,000 and 750 in 1,000." But out of a thousand women screened and a thousand not screened, three in the first group and four in the second died of breast cancer within about ten years. Thus, whereas the relative risk reduction is 25 percent, the absolute risk reduction is one out of one thousand women, or only 0.1 percent. Presenting information as absolute risk gives a much clearer picture of the value of screening. "Of every one thousand women who undergo screening, one will be saved from dying of breast cancer." The NNT is also useful here: "To prevent one death from breast cancer, one thousand women need to undergo screening for ten years."

When physicians evaluated the Helsinki Heart Trial, those who saw the outcomes presented as NNT gave much lower ratings of treatment effectiveness than those who saw the same outcomes framed in terms of either relative or absolute risk.[42] In 1995, British medical personnel received a warning from a government committee that newer oral contraceptive pills doubled the risk of potentially life-threatening blood clots.[43] The subsequent media attention persuaded many women to stop taking the newer pills. The studies on which the warning was based had shown that of every seven thousand women who took the earlier oral contraceptive pills, about one had a thrombosis; this number increased to two among women who took the newer ones. That is, although the newer contraceptives increased relative risk by 100 percent, they increased absolute risk by only one in seven thousand. Had the report presented absolute risks, it probably would have had little impact. Instead, women's confidence in oral contraceptives was undermined, and pill sales fell sharply. This led to an estimated thirteen thousand additional abortions in the following year in England and Wales. For every additional abortion, there was also one extra birth, with some eight hundred additional conceptions among girls under sixteen years of age. Abortions and pregnancies are associated with an increased risk of thrombosis that exceeds that of the newer pill.

Forrow and colleagues asked practicing physicians to read two sets of results of published medical research. One set was presented as a relative change in outcome rate, one set as an absolute change. The results were identical but presented in different ways. Almost half (46 percent) responded differently to the two summaries; of those, 89.8 percent indicated a stronger inclination to treat patients after reading of the relative change in outcome rate.[44]

Gigerenzer and colleagues encouraged the use of absolute risks, either alone or together with relative risks. They noted that drug companies and public health agencies prefer presenting benefits as relative risk reductions, as they are bigger, more impressive figures. But patients make better choices if data are presented as absolute risks. Carling and colleagues randomized patients to receive information in various formats on costs and benefits of statins for preventing coronary heart disease. Among patients given the information in terms of relative risk reduction, 74 percent chose to take statins. Among those quoted various absolute summary statistics, no more than 56 percent chose statins. Furthermore, far more of the latter believed that their understanding of the information was greater; and they were more satisfied with and confident in their decisions. The authors concluded that absolute summary statistics are the preferable way of communicating risks and risk reductions.[45]

Survival Rates and Mortality Rates

Gigerenzer and colleagues described another frequently misunderstood statistic—survival rate. Former New York City mayor Rudy Giuliani claimed that the chance of surviving prostate cancer is 82 percent in the United States and only 44 percent in England. But survival rate (the proportion of people in a study or treatment group who are still alive after a given period following diagnosis) is misleading. The mortality rate (number of deaths within a population) from prostate cancer is approximately the same in the United States and the United Kingdom. Mortality rate is the more important statistic. The difference between the survival rates in the United States and the United Kingdom is largely due to the widespread use of prostate-specific antigen (PSA) screening in the United States but not in the United Kingdom.

- Imagine two groups of men who all die at age seventy of prostate cancer. The men in the first group do not participate in PSA screening, and their cancer is detected from symptoms at age sixty-seven; thus, their five-year survival rate is 0 percent. The second group undergoes screening, and their cancers are detected at age sixty, resulting in a five-year survival rate of 100 percent. The survival rates are different but the mortality rates identical.

- PSA screening may detect an abnormality that meets the definition of cancer but never progresses to cause symptoms. Nonprogressive cancers inflate survival rates.

TIPS ESPECIALLY FOR PATIENTS

At least four problems make it impossible for anyone to be completely knowledgeable in even the narrowest of medical fields. First, the scientific literature is vast and constantly increasing. Second, researchers often have strong conflicts of interest so that the information they present is biased. Third, practical and ethical concerns prevent them from doing experiments—they are restricted for the most part to correlational studies, which are subject to multiple interpretations. Fourth, a substantial proportion of completed studies are never published. Therefore, although doctors are the experts, patients need not be passive about their medical care. They should ask questions. Ambitious patients might even turn to the medical literature. See page 116 on the Cochrane collaboration.

Questions to Ask

- Are there any effective older drugs for my condition?

    New drugs are protected by patent, so drug companies have often slanted research to make it seem that their new drugs are superior to older ones. But the older drugs are generally less expensive. More importantly, any adverse effects they produce can be anticipated. The adverse effects of new drugs are often not recognized until large numbers of people have taken them.
- How many patients need to take this treatment, compared with patients in a control group, in order to achieve one additional good outcome?

    The number needed to treat statistic can help both patients and doctors decide whether a particular treatment should be implemented. See page 37 for computational instructions.
- Is this diagnostic procedure really necessary?

    Serious concerns have been raised about the overuse of mammography screening, CT scans, and MRIs. Prostate-specific antigen (PSA) screening may detect an abnormality that meets the definition of cancer but never progresses to cause symptoms.

- If I undergo this procedure, what is the absolute risk reduction?
    Information is often presented as relative risk reduction. Presenting it as absolute risk gives a much clearer picture.

LOOKING AHEAD

In this chapter we've discussed how various sources of medical information might be biased, incomplete, or otherwise provide inaccurate and misleading information. In the next chapter, we look at decision making. Obviously, information of low quality will have a negative impact on the process, so we hope this chapter will help people make better decisions.

(3)

DECISIONS

Overview

An executive is a man who can make quick decisions and is sometimes right.

—Elbert Hubbard (1859–1915), American author, publisher

We make countless decisions daily, although some are so inconsequential that they barely reach the level of consciousness. Some people make the first decision before opening their eyes. "Should I get up now or stay in bed another ten minutes?" Then, while still half asleep, "Which socks? Eggs or cereal? Do I start on the front page or go right to the sports section?" Yet a huge body of literature shows that decisions are often far from optimal. When the issue is breakfast choices or color of socks, little harm is done. But doctors and their patients frequently make suboptimal choices even when the decisions have life-or-death consequences.

Crosskerry asked thirty physicians how important they thought decision making was in their practice. All of them answered, "very important." He also asked the last time they had read a journal article or book explicitly on decision making. None had done so within the previous year and only six within the previous five years.[1]

This chapter examines strategies for becoming a decision-making expert. We look at the value of intuition, the benefits of making decisions when in a good mood, the impact of stress on decision making, how subconscious factors can affect decisions, and the consequences of having multiple options from which to choose. We discuss how free drug samples impact prescription decisions, and we close by emphasizing that decisions should reflect the uniqueness of each patient.

OVERVIEW: DECISION TYPES

Some decisions are one time: Which specialty should I pursue? Should I have surgery immediately or wait to see whether I can heal without it? Should I marry that person? (A friend has already made that one-time decision six times.) Other decision types are frequently repeated: A manager hires people, a doctor makes diagnoses based on a certain test, a parole board decides whether to grant parole. The decision situation may be constantly evolving or static. Some decisions can be delayed, but at other times they must be made immediately. In some cases, most of the relevant information is available: Should I marry that person? Chocolate or vanilla? In other cases, there is considerable uncertainty: She tested positive for ___. Does she have the disease? Despite the differences, certain general principles apply to all decision types.

THE IMPORTANCE OF INTUITION

A classic decision-making strategy is to identify options, evaluate and rate them, then pick the option with the highest rating. Edward de Bono offers several variations on the classic strategy.[2] For example, the PMI involves drawing a table headed with "Plus," "Minus," and "Implications." To use the strategy, write down all the positive results of taking the action in the column underneath "Plus." Underneath "Minus," write down all the negative effects. In the "Implications" column, write down the implications, whether positive or negative. Then assign a positive or negative score to each point, and add up the score. A strongly positive score shows that an action should be taken, and a strongly negative score that it should be avoided.

De Bono's innovative and valuable techniques are used by corporate executives at some of the world's largest organizations, but many people resist using such a mechanical approach. They see little sense in listing the pros and cons of chocolate versus vanilla ice cream. A key part of deciding well is to draw on tacit knowledge and experience, which cannot be made wholly conscious or mapped on a decision tree. A cartoon in *New Yorker* magazine illustrated the point with a couple looking over a pile of papers.[3] The caption reads, "I've done the numbers, and I will marry you." Peer Soelberg taught the classic, structured decision-making techniques in a course. Then he asked his students whether they had used the strategies to determine which job offer they should accept. They hadn't.[4]

Intuitive judgments are often better than carefully reasoned ones. Wilson and Schooler asked college students to taste several brands of strawberry jams and indicate their preferences.[5] Compared with students who didn't analyze their choices, the students who were asked to analyze why they felt the way they did agreed *less* with expert ratings. Wilson and Schooler also compared college students' preferences for courses with expert opinion of the courses. Some students were asked to analyze reasons, others to evaluate all attributes of each course. Both groups made choices that, compared with those of control subjects, corresponded less with expert opinion.

Halberstadt and Levine had participants predict the outcomes of college basketball games. Some were asked to think about reasons, others to base their predictions on intuition. The intuition group made more accurate predictions.[6]

IMMEDIATE DECISION NEEDED

Klein studied experts who must make immediate, often life-or-death, decisions: emergency-rescue crews, fighter pilots, intensive-care unit workers, firefighters. He also studied others, such as chess players and businesspeople, who sometimes must make immediate, although less crucial, decisions. He found that experts do several things better than novices, which allows them to decide without performing extensive analyses. Experts

- recognize relevant cues more quickly and completely.
- ignore less relevant cues.
- frame problems so that their underlying structure can be easily detected.
- recognize problems that they have previously encountered and for which they already know solutions.

Instead of analyzing each problem as though it were brand new, experts use their experience to form mental simulations of the current problem and use the simulations to suggest appropriate solutions. This saves time. Novices often ignore a crucial type of cue—absence of a key event. Experts have the experience to form expectancies, so they don't miss such cues. Novices generate and compare options, but experts evaluate each option as they think of it. Generating options would slow them down. By imagining the option being carried out, they spot weaknesses and find ways to avoid these. They don't seek the best solution—just one that works.

Expert firefighters recognize when a typical or atypical situation is developing. Then they race through their memories for a fire that resembles the fire they are confronting. They consider a possible solution, evaluate it by rapidly running a mental simulation, and then imagine how it will probably unfold and play out. If everything works, they stick with their choice. Otherwise, they look for another one.

Expert nurses were able to tell from looking at premature babies when the babies were developing infections.[7] The nurses were reacting to subtle patterns of cues, including some that led to different conclusions from what was in the medical literature. For example, although the literature indicates that adults with infections become more irritable, premature babies become less irritable.

Klein wrote that technical training has been dominated by efforts to teach rules, facts, and procedures—a strategy that makes sense for simple, procedural tasks in high-turnover jobs with minimally educated workers. But experts must learn perceptual skills, and standard training has neglected that aspect. Nor are perceptual skills learned from reading about or taking courses on decision making. Most experts have done neither. The experts told Klein that they had learned through their experiences, and experience per se was what distinguished them from novices. An obvious implication is that novices should be given many and varied experiences so that they can accumulate the memories that will enable them to make better decisions. Simulations can be very useful in this regard.

EMOTIONS

Popular textbooks say that decision making would improve if emotions were removed. Neurophysiologist Antonio Damasio emphatically disagrees. He treats people with damage to the brain areas where emotions are generated. Some of his patients, although they show no deterioration of intellectual abilities, are incapable of making even trivial decisions. Damasio gave an example of a patient who listed the pros, cons, and maybes of each alternative day for their next appointment. But the patient never decided. After a half hour, Damasio finally picked one of the dates. "That's fine," the patient said, as though there had never been any problem.[8]

Emotion can, however, lead us to choices that fly in the face of logic. Students were willing to pay twice as much to insure a hypothetical beloved antique clock against loss in shipment than to insure a similar clock for which "one does not have any special feeling." In the event of loss, the insurance paid $100 in both cases. Other students were more willing to buy a warranty on a newly purchased used car if it was a beautiful convertible than if it was an ordinary-looking station wagon, even if the expected repair expenses and cost of the warranty were held constant.[9]

People tend to make better decisions when in good rather than bad moods.[10] Positive affect generally increases the efficiency, thoroughness, flexibility, and innovativeness of thinking about a wide range of ideas related to the issue at hand. It improves diagnostic skills. For example, Isen and colleagues induced positive affect in medical students by telling them they had succeeded on an anagram task; those students were more efficient than controls in deciding which of six hypothetical patients was most likely to have lung cancer.[11] Furthermore, they were more likely to go beyond the assigned task and attempt to diagnose additional cases and suggest treatments, showed less confusion in their decision process, and integrated information more efficiently.

Estrada and colleagues randomly assigned physicians to one of three groups: a no-treatment control group; a group that read phrases reflecting humanistic satisfactions from medicine (example: "By establishing rapport with patients, I enhance my human understanding"); and a group that received a small bag of wrapped candy in a large envelope.[12] (They were asked not to eat any candy right then so that they would not be given a sugar boost.)

All the participants read a brief description of a patient and were given folders containing information regarding the patient's history, physical exam, laboratory tests, and so forth. The seemingly trivial induction of positive affect by giving candy had several important effects: The candy recipients outperformed the other two groups on a standard test of creative problem solving. Although no quicker in reaching a final diagnosis, they more rapidly (and correctly) realized that the symptoms suggested liver disease. And they were less likely to hold onto an incorrect hypothesis by distorting or ignoring disconfirming evidence. This was assessed by two raters unaware of the experimental condition of the protocol when scoring it. Smart patients will bring their doctors a chocolate bar.

STRESS

Under certain circumstances, stress can improve some aspects of cognitive functioning. Alexander and Beversdorf gave medical students a battery of tests when they were highly stressed—one to two days before a big exam—and then again after the exam. They did better prior to the exam on a memory test; however, they did less well on tests requiring flexible thinking.[13] Among nurses, situations that elicited moderate levels of stress resulted in the best quality of thinking. But the long-term effects of functioning within highly stressful environments include unimaginative thinking and overgeneralizing.[14]

Liston and colleagues used fMRIs to scan the brains of subjects performing thinking tasks critical to decision making.[15] Medical students who said they were highly stressed because of an upcoming exam were compared with similar adults who claimed to be unstressed. The highly stressed subjects showed diminished activity in the prefrontal cortex, a brain region implicated in planning complex cognitive behaviors and decision making. They fared much worse than controls on an attention-shifting task (looking at two discs of different colors, one moving up and the other down, and being prompted to choose a disc according to motion or color). The good news is that the effects were reversible: after one month of reduced stress, the same subjects showed no significant differences from controls.

Stressful emergencies impaired decision making even in proven, efficient medical teams. Teams that encountered stressful emergencies became less vigilant, had poorer memories, and prematurely stopped evaluating alternative options.[16]

Stress can come from many sources. Merely watching a graphically violent or emotional scene in a movie can cause enough stress to interfere with problem-solving abilities. Beversdorf and colleagues asked volunteers to watch clips from the stress-inducing war film *Saving Private Ryan* or from the animated comedy film *Shrek*.[17] Then the subjects were tested for verbal mental flexibility. Performance was significantly impaired after the *Saving Private Ryan* clip compared to after the *Shrek* clip.

WE ARE OFTEN UNAWARE
OF THE BASIS FOR OUR DECISIONS

We often make decisions for reasons that, if we were made aware of them, would surprise us. On alternating days over a two-week period, North and colleagues played traditional French or traditional German music in a supermarket and tracked the sales of wine.[18] The wine shelves held French and German wines matched for price and flavor, with national flags attached to the display. When French music played, consumers bought forty bottles of French wine and eight bottles of German wine. When German music played, they bought twenty-two bottles of German wine and twelve bottles of French. Only one out of forty-four customers questioned at the checkout spontaneously mentioned the music as the reason they bought the wine. When asked specifically whether they thought that the music affected their choice, 86 percent said no.

Nisbett and Wilson asked women to judge which of four pairs of nylon stockings was the best quality. The stockings were hanging on racks spaced equal distances apart. Twelve percent of the subjects chose the leftmost pair, and 40 percent chose the rightmost pair. In fact, all the stockings were identical. When asked to explain their choices, the women gave a total of eighty different reasons such as knit, weave, sheerness, elasticity, and workmanship. Not a single woman mentioned the position of the stockings. When asked whether the position could have influenced their judgments, only one subject acknowledged the possibility.[19]

Several nonmedical factors, which may or may not reach the level of consciousness, affect the treatment decisions of doctors. McKinlay and colleagues videotaped actors playing the role of patients with two common types of complaints: chest pain and shortness of breath. They showed the videotapes to volunteer physicians and evaluated their treatment decisions. Nonmedical factors that made a difference included the patient's age, race, and gender, the doctor's age, race, gender, medical specialty, and level of training, and the organization of the practice (fee-for-service, HMO, PPO).[20] The researchers concluded that "medical decision making can be as much a function of who the patient is as what the patient has."

NUMBER OF ALTERNATIVES

Whether a decision involves trivial or consequential matters, as the number of options grows the likelihood that people will reject all of them also increases. Exploring more options heightens the burden of information gathering, which adds costs to the decision process and increases the likelihood that choosers will anticipate regretting their decision.

Doctors must often choose among several options. For example, Redelmeier and Shafir noted in 1995 that thirteen medicines were available for treating Parkinson's disease, thirty-one for chronic bronchitis, and ninety-one for hypertension. Confronted with so many options, doctors may choose one they would otherwise have rejected—or they may not choose at all. Redelmeier and Shafir asked family doctors to decide whether to start a patient with chronic hip pain on a new drug. For half the doctors, only one drug was available. For the other half, two similar drugs were available. Whereas 72 percent prescribed when given only the one-drug option, only 53 percent prescribed when they had to choose between two.[21]

The problem is not restricted to drug alternatives. As part of the same study, Redelmeier and Shafir asked neurologists and neurosurgeons to consider a hypothetical scenario in which patients A and B (group 1) or patients A, B, and C (group 2) awaited major surgery. Patients A and C were very similar. Participants had to decide which one to operate on first. In group 1, 38 percent of respondents decided on patient B. Logic suggests that, with the added option, no more than 38 percent in group 2 would choose patient B. In fact, 58 percent did so. The authors inferred that participants found it difficult to choose between the two similar patients, A and C, so they avoided the decision and chose patient B.

Ganiats listed the pros and cons of five options for colorectal cancer screening. Then he noted that having so many options might confuse patients and perhaps even physicians and would increase the likelihood that a patient will decline to have any screening.[22]

Imagine that two drugs are available to treat a certain condition, and the greater effectiveness of drug A is offset by the cheaper cost plus greater ease of use of drug B. As a result, doctors are evenly divided as to which one they would choose. See table 3.1.

If a new group of doctors is asked to choose between the same two drugs plus a third—see table 3.2—how do you think their choices will be distributed? Note that drug C is inferior to B in both effectiveness and cost plus ease of use.

Table 3.1. Two Fictional Drugs Given Properties So That Each Is Preferred by 50 Percent of Surveyed Physicians

Drug	Effectiveness	Cost Plus Ease of Use
A	8	5
B	6	9

Table 3.2.   Three Fictional Drugs: In Previous Survey, Physicians Chose A and B Equally—C Is Clearly Inferior to B

Drug	Effectiveness	Cost Plus Ease of Use
A	8	5
B	6	9
C	5	8

Schwartz and Chapman and Schwartz and colleagues devised two studies to test scenarios very similar to the one just described. In the first study, they asked medical residents to review patient cases and then choose the most appropriate drug for each patient. In some versions, two drugs were available. Other versions included a third drug (the decoy) that was inferior in every way to one of the original options (the target) but not to the other. The participants were told that the drugs shown were the only options available. Nobody chose the decoy, just as nobody should choose drug C in table 3.2. But adding the decoy increased the likelihood of choosing the target drug. The authors noted that the *Physicians' Desk Reference* often reports the effectiveness of drugs in a format similar to the one used in their experiment. Physicians might avoid making difficult trade-offs by choosing a drug that is clearly superior to one of the alternatives, and drug companies might try to increase sales of one of their products by positioning it near a clearly inferior one.[23]

In the second study, they asked physicians in one group to either prescribe a drug and make a referral to an orthopedic specialist or make a referral only. Physicians in a second group had the same two options plus the option of prescribing a different drug. In addition, half of the participants were asked to defend their choices for discussion at a later time. In keeping with the results of the previous study, physicians in group 2 chose the referral-only option significantly more than physicians in group 1. Importantly, the ones who had to defend their choices did so to a much greater extent. The authors inferred that critical decisions in patient care may not always result from judgments about what is best for the patient, but rather from what is most defensible for the practitioner. Physicians must frequently justify their decisions, so they may be particularly prone to seek out easily defensible options.

FREE SAMPLES AFFECT DECISIONS

Adair and Holmgren observed 390 drug decisions of twenty-nine physicians over a six-month period.[24] Highly advertised drugs were matched with drugs used for the same indication that were less expensive or available over the counter or as generics. Half of the physicians (chosen randomly) agreed not to use free drug samples. None of them had contact with drug company representatives—all samples were stocked in a cabinet in the clinic. Physicians with access to samples of the heavily advertised drugs wrote more new prescriptions for them, recommended fewer OTC drugs, and prescribed fewer inexpensive drugs. Adair noted that physicians have a strong tendency to continue to prescribe what a patient is already taking rather than switch to a drug they would normally prefer; and patients quickly develop brand loyalty.[25] So, their finding contradicts the widespread beliefs that drug samples are inherently different from other forms of marketing and that samples help patients manage drug costs in the long run.

CONTEXTUAL DECISION-MAKING ERRORS

To be effective, medical care plans must be tailored to a patient's individual circumstances. Weiner and colleagues imagined a patient with poorly controlled asthma who cannot afford her current medications; increasing the drug dose would ordinarily be appropriate, but not under the circumstances. To do so would be a decision-making error. Such errors, which occur because of inattention to patient context, can be called contextual errors, in contrast to all other medical decision-making errors, called biomedical errors.[26]

Weiner and colleagues asked trained actors to present as real patients to experienced volunteer physicians. The physicians were told that up to four actor patients would visit them over the next eighteen months. The actors followed scripts that contained hints of clinically significant biomedical or contextual issues that, if confirmed, would be essential to address in order to avoid error. The researchers used four different cases, each with four variants: uncomplicated, biomedically complex, contextually complex, or both biomedically and contextually complex.

At the beginning of each case, the actor presented a story suggesting a common condition for which a standard evaluation or treatment is usually appropriate. For example, one case involved a forty-two-year-old man with long-standing asthma that had recently worsened despite the prescription of a low-dose inhaled glucocorticoid. With no other clinically relevant information, appropriate care would include prescribing a higher dose of the drug or adding a second one.

In addition to the baseline story, on different occasions the actor also mentioned a biomedical red flag, a contextual red flag, or both. Each suggested the need for an alternative approach to care. For the biomedical red flag in the asthma case, the actor said, "Sometimes I wake up wheezing or coughing at night." This suggests the onset of gastroesophageal reflux symptoms. A diligent physician would investigate to see whether confirmatory symptoms of reflux are present. For the contextual red flag, the actor said, "Things have been tough since I lost my job." This raised the possibility that his worsening symptoms were due to inability to pay for the prescribed drugs. A diligent physician would probe to find out.

Physicians provided error-free care in 73 percent of the uncomplicated baseline encounters but did much more poorly in the variants. They failed to probe in 38 percent of the biomedically complicated encounters, 22 percent of the contextually complicated encounters, and 9 percent of the combined biomedically and contextually complicated encounters. Weiner and colleagues called failure to probe inappropriate care—medical decision-making error.

TIPS ESPECIALLY FOR PATIENTS

- Medical decisions often engender strong emotions. Popular textbooks say that decision making would improve if emotions were ignored. Neurophysiologist Antonio Damasio, among others, emphatically disagrees.
- Intuitive judgments are often better than carefully reasoned ones.
- People tend to make better decisions when in good rather than bad moods.

- Patients should consult with their doctors to ensure that any treatment plan is tailored to their specific circumstances.

LOOKING AHEAD

In this chapter we've discussed various factors that affect decision making. We've shown that both trivial decisions and critical medical ones are often suboptimal. In the next chapter, we look at specific types of biases, mostly unconscious ones, that impair decision making. By calling attention to the biases, we hope that their impact on future decisions will be minimized.

DECISIONS

Biases

Psychologist Daniel Kahneman received the 2003 Nobel Prize for his work showing that people use unconscious shortcuts, termed *heuristics*, to cope with complex decisions. The shortcuts usually produce the desired results with a minimum of delay, cost, and anxiety. But under certain circumstances, heuristics result in less-than-optimal decisions—biases. Clinicians should learn to recognize the potential errors that arise from reliance on specific shortcuts and override them when appropriate.

In this chapter, we describe the availability, representative, and anchoring heuristics and then look at the impact of how a decision is framed. We next discuss an array of other biases and close with suggestions for combating biases and making smart decisions.

AVAILABILITY HEURISTIC

Please look at lists A and B, one list at a time, for several seconds each, and then cover the lists and read the instructions immediately following before going on to the next paragraph.

List A	List B
Albert Einstein	Madonna
Robinson Crusoe	Queen Elizabeth
Jodi Rinke	Art Smith
Trina Miller	Jose Rivero
Raquel Welch	Frank Sinatra
Barack Obama	Serena Williams
Roger Federer	Cleopatra
Benjamin Franklin	Queen Latifah
Risa Mol	Martin Jasper
Zoe Letterman	Robert Sherman
Adolf Hitler	Emily Dickinson
Sarah Orville	Joe Sirota
Al Gore	Hillary Clinton
Dorothy Roberts	William Henriksen
Lorraine Wilson	Art Sanders
Marvin Carr	Susan Carr
Alicia Kagawa	Arnold Smith
Tiger Woods	Golda Meir
Melody Montoya	Steven Leshinski
Frankenstein	Jane Eyre

Instructions: *Are there more men's or women's names on List A? On list B? Or are there an equal number of women's and men's names on both lists?*

Although there are ten of each gender on each list, most people given similar tasks under carefully controlled conditions say that List A has more men's names and List B more women's names. The reason is that most of the men's names on List A and the women's names on List B are of famous people, whereas the women's names on A and the men's names on B are not. The names of famous people come to mind most easily, so they are better recalled. Usually, the ease with which we can recall something correlates with the frequency of that thing. The unconscious strategy is called the availability heuristic and, in most circumstances, leads to a correct answer.

The availability heuristic occurs when a person estimates the frequency of a class or the probability of an event by the ease with which instances or occurrences can be brought to mind. While generally helpful, it can also lead to errors. For example, when subjects were asked,

"Which causes more deaths in the United States: stomach cancer or motor vehicle accidents?" most selected motor vehicle accidents. In fact, stomach cancer causes twice as many deaths. Media stories about motor vehicle deaths increase their vividness and thus bias perceptions. Vivid events become especially available, and memorable cases may shape future diagnostic conclusions. Galanter and Patel speculated that widespread media coverage of bipolar disorder and Asperger's disorder has probably led to their overdiagnosis.[1] The availability heuristic can influence many types of medical decisions:

- Doctors are more likely to make a particular diagnosis if they have recently diagnosed a similar case.[2]
- The easier the search for a disease in medical journals, the more articles that a doctor is likely to read about it. If a disease has been featured in a recent conference, a doctor is more likely to think the disease dangerous and that a patient has it.
- Package inserts included with prescription drugs list every side effect reported during the drug's clinical testing and, when appropriate, the side effects of other drugs in the same class. Being made aware of a side effect, even a rare one, may increase a patient's perceived sense of risk. Similarly, when a doctor explains the risks of a particular procedure, the patient may give them undue weight.

REPRESENTATIVE HEURISTIC

The representative heuristic occurs when people classify something according to how similar it seems to a typical case—how representative it is of a given category. For example, when subjects guessed the occupation of a man with unusual tastes, married to a performer, and with multiple tattoos, they were more likely to choose the option trapeze artist rather than librarian or lawyer. The reason is that the description more closely matches the prototype of a trapeze artist than the prototype of either of the other two occupations. But just because something is similar to things in a certain category does not ensure that it is a member of that category. The subjects failed to consider that librarians and lawyers greatly outnumber trapeze artists.[3]

If symptoms are equally consistent with two different diseases, and one disease is much more common than the other, then the case is more likely to be the more common disease. But a doctor may diagnose based on how representative a case is of a particular category while ignoring other possibilities. Knowing that a patient smokes, the doctor may diagnose a smoking-related illness even if the symptoms also fit a more common illness. Although major depression is much more common among children than is bipolar affective disorder, the representative heuristic may lead a clinician to incorrectly diagnose bipolar disorder in an irritable child with sleeping and concentration problems. Berner and Graber imagined a patient presenting with chest pain radiating to the back, varying with posture, and associated with a cardiac friction rub.[4] The symptoms fit pericarditis, an extremely uncommon reason for chest pain, but a condition with a characteristic clinical presentation. By matching the clinical presentation only to the prototypical case, the clinician may ignore other much more common diseases that sometimes present similarly.

ANCHORING AND ADJUSTMENT HEURISTIC

Most people, when asked to give a numerical estimate of something, start with a number that easily comes to mind and then adjust. But they typically rely too heavily on the initial anchor, so their adjustments are too small. Highly available information is likely to serve as an anchor, and so may irrelevant numbers. In a classic study, Tversky and Kahneman[5] asked some subjects, "Is the percentage of African nations in the UN greater or less than 65%?" Others were asked, "Is the percentage of African nations in the UN greater or less than 10%?" Then they were all asked, "What is your best estimate of the actual percentage of African nations in the UN?" The mean estimate of the 65 percent anchor group was 45 percent; the mean estimate of the 10 percent anchor group was 25 percent.

Anchoring occurs even with ridiculous anchors. Subjects were asked, "Did Einstein first visit the U.S. before the year 1215?" Others were asked, "Did Einstein first visit the U.S. before the year 1992?" Then all were asked, "When did Einstein first visit the U.S.?"[6] Those in the first group guessed earlier dates. Doing five pages of computations on large numbers increased a later judgment about cancer incidence (relative to a no-anchor control condition).[7]

When a patient presents with symptoms, the physician often promptly starts thinking of possible diagnoses. It is generally a good strategy for physicians to develop hypotheses early in the diagnostic procedure—see pp. 106–7—but these should be revised as new information becomes available. Often, however, final judgments are biased in the direction of the initial one. When clinicians had to evaluate disability claims, their final decisions were heavily influenced by whichever case information was reviewed first.[8]

Brewer and colleagues sent physicians surveys with a vignette that introduced a case of possible pulmonary embolism. After reading the vignette, participants were asked whether the chance of a pulmonary embolism was greater or less than 1 percent (or 90 percent). Then they gave their precise estimate. Estimates of the likelihood of pulmonary embolism averaged 23 percent in the low-anchor group and 53 percent in the high-anchor group.[9] (Surprisingly, however, the irrelevant anchor numbers had little impact on treatment choices.)

Pothier gave fourth-year medical students ten questions, reproduced in table 4.1, about their views on surgical training.[10] First, the students were asked to write down the last two digits of their telephone numbers. Then, for each question, they were asked whether the answer was larger

Table 4.1.   Questions Asked of Participants

1. What proportion of surgeons decide on surgery as a career while in medical school?
2. What proportion of clinical time should be spent in a surgical discipline?
3. What proportion of time spent by students in a surgical discipline should be spent in the operating theater?
4. What proportion of time spent by students in the operating theater should be spent scrubbed into the surgery?
5. What proportion of medical student surgical training should be spent obtaining basic surgical skills?
6. What proportion of consultant surgeons are student friendly?
7. What proportion of surgical lists should be dedicated to training?
8. What proportion of surgeons should be allowed to have part-time training?
9. What proportion of surgical placements were encouraging about medical students becoming surgeons?
10. What proportion of surgeons do you think are happy in their jobs?

or smaller than the two digits, taken in the form of a percentage. Then they were asked the actual answer to the question. There was a significant correlation between the last two digits of the telephone numbers and the mean responses to the questions.

FRAMING

The way information is presented may affect a decision. For example, people saw a video describing angioplasty as either 99 percent safe or with a one in one hundred likelihood of complication. The two are arithmetically equivalent, but more who heard "99 percent safe" said they would have the operation to relieve chest pain.[11]

Framing choices in terms of survival rate or mortality rate makes a difference to decision makers. Doctors were told that a specific treatment option has either a mortality rate of 20 percent after five years or a survival rate of 80 percent after five years. More of the second group said they'd recommend the operation to their patients.[12] In another study, subjects chose between surgery and radiation for cancer treatment. One group was told the percentage of people likely to die from each treatment. The other group was told the percentage likely to survive. Otherwise, both groups received identical information. Decisions to choose surgery increased from 58 percent to 75 percent when the information was framed in survival rather than mortality terms.[13]

Decisions are influenced by whether they are made on the basis of relative risk reduction, disease response rate, or overall survival. Martin and colleagues asked three groups of medical students to read a scenario describing the effectiveness of chemotherapy in colorectal cancer. For one group, the results were presented as relative risk reduction (see pp. 38–39); for a second group, tumor response rate; and for a third group, overall survival. Then they were asked whether they would choose chemotherapy. Eighty-five percent of the first group and 88 percent of the second chose chemotherapy; but only 35 percent of the overall survival group did so.[14]

Decisions often differ depending on whether they are made on the basis of probability estimates or frequency estimates. Psychiatrists read an expert's assessment of the likelihood that a mental patient would commit a future violent act.[15] One group read, "Of every 100 patients similar to Mr. Jones, 20 are estimated to commit a future act of violence." The others read, "Patients similar to Mr. Jones are estimated to have a 20 percent chance of committing a future act of violence." The first group labeled Mr. Jones as more dangerous—41 percent would refuse to discharge the patient—compared with 21 percent in the second group. The authors suggested that representing risk in the form of frequency created violent images: "Some guy going crazy and killing someone." Representing in the form of probabilities led to images of the typical person, unlikely to harm anyone.

Another framing difference that matters is whether choices are presented in terms of their benefits or their harms. Detweiler and colleagues gave beachgoers one of two messages regarding sunscreen use. The messages promoted the same behavior and were similar in length and structure. They differed in that one message was framed in terms of benefits: "Using sunscreen increases your chances of maintaining healthy, young-looking skin." The other message was framed in terms of loss: "Not using sunscreen decreases your chances of maintaining healthy, young-looking skin." The subjects who received the benefit message were more likely to say that they would use sunscreen in the future; and they were more likely to redeem a coupon for sunscreen.[16] The matter is complicated. Women presented with a message emphasizing the costs of not receiving a vaccine were more willing to be vaccinated than women presented with a message emphasizing the benefits, but only among women who engaged in risky sexual behavior and with a tendency to avoid negative outcomes.[17] The important point is that the way an issue is framed can have a powerful impact on responses of others.

Another example in the benefit versus harm category involved subjects told to imagine the United States preparing for the outbreak of a disease expected to kill six hundred people.[18] Their task was to choose between two alternative programs to combat the disease. They were told, "Assume that the exact scientific estimates of the consequences of the program are as follows:"

(A) If program A is adopted, two hundred people will be saved.
(B) If program B is adopted, there is a one-in-three probability that six hundred people will be saved and a two in three probability that no people will be saved.

Seventy-two percent of subjects chose A, and 28 percent, B. Other subjects were given the same instructions, but the choices were phrased as C and D below. Note that A and C are equivalent, as are B and D. But 22 percent chose C, and 78 percent, D. Framing made all the difference.

(C) If program C is adopted, four hundred people will die.
(D) If program D is adopted, there is a one in three probability that nobody will die and a two in three probability that six hundred people will die.

Many other researchers have reported framing effects. Nevertheless, concerns about this phenomenon may be overblown. In the above examples, the decisions did not have consequences for the subjects of the studies—none had cancer or were preparing for the outbreak of a deadly disease. Studies on people who would be directly affected by their decisions found either no or greatly attenuated framing effects.[19]

BIAS TOWARD CERTAINTY

Exercise: Imagine a cancer that affects about 5 percent of the population and is caused by any of several viruses. Six vaccines have been developed to prevent these virus infections. Please rate them.

   Vaccine Descriptions:
(A) 70 percent effective against 100 percent of all virus strains that cause cancer
(B) 74 percent effective against 95 percent of all virus strains that cause cancer
(C) 82 percent effective against 85 percent of all virus strains that cause cancer
(D) 68 percent effective against 68 percent of all virus strains that cause cancer
(E) 95 percent effective against 74 percent of all virus strains that cause cancer
(F) 100 percent effective against 70 percent of all virus strains that cause cancer

Ubel and colleagues showed that people tend to overweight outcomes considered certain relative to merely possible outcomes.[20] Li and Chapman explored the phenomenon further by giving college students the above rating task.[21] The net effectiveness is .70 for all vaccines except for D. (Li and Chapman included D as a comprehension check because it is inferior to the others and nobody should choose it. Forty-four of the 180 subjects chose D.) All the other vaccines are equivalent in net effectiveness. Yet the ratings were highest for vaccine F. People were attracted by a vaccine that was 100 percent effective against 70 percent of virus strains causing a certain cancer, in comparison with a vaccine that was 70 percent effective toward 100 percent of virus strains causing this cancer. People overweight certainty. The authors argued that this has important implications for health promotion and public policy. It is a bias that can intentionally or unintentionally sway decisions.

ACTIONS AND NONACTIONS ARE TREATED DIFFERENTLY

Imagine preparing for a flu epidemic that is fatal to ten of every ten thousand children. A vaccine eliminates any chance of getting the flu but causes side effects that are also sometimes fatal. Suppose that the overall death rate for vaccinated children is five out of ten thousand. Would you vaccinate your child? Given that hypothetical situation, most respondents said they would not vaccinate their child.[22] They said they would feel responsible if anything happened because of the vaccine but not if anything happened because of the failure to vaccinate. Many people feel responsible for a bad outcome that occurs following their action—but not if the bad outcome occurs and they could have done something to make that occurrence far less likely.

SELECTION BIAS

Selection bias occurs when the procedures used to select subjects result in systematic differences between participants and nonparticipants in the factor under study. Selection bias can cause errors of inference that lead to poor decisions. For example, Dawn and colleagues wrote about cervical manipulation, a common treatment performed by chiropractors for neck pain and headaches. Some patients have developed stroke after cervical manipulation, and neurologists have then been called in to evaluate and treat them. The occurrence of stroke after cervical manipulation is extremely rare, so most chiropractors never see it. But neurologists see stroke in nearly every patient presenting to them after cervical manipulation. So chiropractors and neurologists are likely to have strikingly different perceptions of that particular risk of cervical manipulation.[23]

Dawn and colleagues gave other examples. Dermatologists rarely observe patients for a skin disease that has been effectively managed by a primary care physician. There is no reason for a patient to visit a dermatologist for a resolved problem. So a dermatologist might assume that primary care physicians rarely manage skin problems effectively. Similarly, people who have achieved satisfactory outcomes from over-the-counter products to treat acne or warts are unlikely to visit a dermatologist. Dermatologists see only the refractory cases and thus may conclude that such products are rarely helpful.

Gehr and colleagues wrote that new medical interventions are generally studied in severely ill patients, where significant benefits can be expected. Once a therapy is established, physicians prescribe it to many less-sick patients, who experience smaller improvements. So over time, the effectiveness of the therapy seems to diminish.[24]

Consumer groups, the media, patients, families, physicians, insurers, and health-care policy makers often rate hospitals by computing a statistic called the mortality index. The index indicates whether a hospital had more or fewer deaths than expected within a given specialty. But the mortality index can be misleading because of selection bias. The index fails to take into account whether a hospital treats complex cases transferred from other hospitals, low-risk elective cases, or high-risk nonelective cases. Hammers and colleagues examined neurosurgical mortality data from 103 academic medical centers.[25] Hospitals with the worst mortality index tended to be level 1 trauma centers with busy emergency rooms that treat large numbers of severe cases such as head and spinal injuries from car accidents, injuries from falls, and gunshot wounds. They also treat a high percentage of Medicaid patients who have poor access to medical care, are poorly educated in health, are uninsured, and present only if their symptoms have become severe. In hospitals with the lowest mortality index, at least 87 percent of the neurosurgeries were elective. Patients in poor health do not have such surgeries.

SUNK-COST BIAS: NOT A SERIOUS PROBLEM

Sunk costs are costs that have already been incurred and cannot be recovered. They should not affect a subsequent decision but often do. For example, a poker player who has put a lot of money into a pot may waste more money to see another player's raise, even though she has only a very slight chance of winning. A doctor who has invested a lot of time and effort in a particular treatment might be reluctant to change it, even though it is not working. Bornstein and colleagues gave medical residents hypothetical situations in which a person was portrayed as having to decide whether to persist with an original plan of action or switch to a better alternative. The results were encouraging. Although subjects showed the sunk-cost bias with nonmedical examples, their judgments about the optimal course of treatment were not influenced by previous treatment decisions. The authors suggested that some aspect of medical training made them immune to the bias within their domain of expertise.[26]

SELECT VERSUS REJECT BIAS

When people decide which alternative to *accept*, they search for good qualities. When deciding which to *reject*, they search for bad. Shafir asked subjects to imagine a custody battle and gave them the following information about each parent.[27]

Parent A: average income, health, and working hours, reasonable rapport with child, relatively stable social life

Parent B: above-average income, very close relationship with child, extremely active social life, lots of work-related travel, minor health problems

When asked who should be awarded custody, most respondents said B. But when asked who should be denied custody, most also said B. The explanation is that when they were asked who should get custody, they looked for positive qualities, and B has more than A. But when asked who should be denied custody, they looked for negative qualities, and again, B has more than A.

PEAK-END RULE

The peak-end rule causes us to bias our judgments of experiences based almost entirely on how they were at their peak (pleasant or unpleasant) and how they ended. Virtually all other information is discarded. Consider two sequences of painful stimuli, where "1" means very low pain and "10" means extremely intense pain. Suppose you had experienced both sequences at different times. Now you've got to have one of the sequences repeated. Which would you prefer?

- Sequence A: 5, 6, 7, 10, 10, 10
- Sequence B: 5, 6, 7, 10, 10, 10, 9, 8, 7, 6, 5, 5, 5, 5, 5, 4, 3, 1

Although sequence B is the same as sequence A with several more painful moments tacked on, subjects exposed to sequence B tend to rate it as less aversive than subjects exposed to sequence A. Two groups of people were subjected to loud, painful noises. Group 2 was then exposed to additional, somewhat less painful noises. Group 2 subjects rated the experience as much less unpleasant than those in Group 1, despite having been subjected to more discomfort. They had experienced the same initial duration plus an extended duration of reduced unpleasantness.

Subjects received two aversive experiences: in the short trial, they immersed one hand in water at 14°C for sixty seconds; in the long trial, they immersed the other hand at 14°C for sixty seconds and then kept the hand in the water thirty seconds longer as the temperature of the water was gradually raised to 15°C, still painful but distinctly less so for most subjects. Subjects were later given a choice of which trial to repeat. A significant majority chose to repeat the long trial.

Patients undergoing colonoscopy rated their moment-to-moment pain. Days later, they reported their judgments of how painful the procedures had been. Their remembered judgments correlated strongly with both the peak intensity of the pain and the pain experienced during the last few minutes. The duration had almost no effect.[28]

OPTIMISM BIAS

When asked about risk of having a stroke or heart attack in the next ten years, 57 percent of survey respondents rated their risk as lower than average and only 13 percent higher than average. They underestimated their risk of food poisoning, influenza, and asthma. Because they underestimate personal risks, they feel safe engaging in risky behaviors.[29]

BIAS AGAINST ADOPTING BENEFICIAL THERAPIES

Doctors read one of two versions of results of a hypothetical trial of a treatment for a critical illness.[30] An independent sample of doctors read results of one of two versions of a different hypothetical clinical trial. For both samples, one version showed that a treatment in common use is harmful; and the other version showed that the same treatment, not in common use, is beneficial.

The studies were described as well designed, with statistically significant results, large reductions in mortality, and published in respected journals. The main outcome was respondents' willingness to change the current practice based on the new information.

After reading the harm version of the first hypothetical study, 76.5 percent of respondents reported that they would apply the results to patient care. After reading the benefit version, only 33.3 percent said they would apply the results. The figures for the second hypothetical study were 95.3 percent for the harm version and 37.1 percent for the benefit version. The authors concluded that the rate of adoption of beneficial therapies is too low, the rate of abandonment of harmful therapies is too high, or there is some combination of these two effects.

They also considered a possible rebuttal: avoidance of harmful therapies ought to be assigned higher priority than provision of beneficial ones. They also offered the maxim that all medical students learn: "First, do no harm." They responded that if evidence of harm and benefit should be appraised differently, then the design of clinical trials should vary, depending on whether intended to show harm or benefit.

PROJECTION BIAS

The impact of many decisions is not felt until long afterward. In the interim, many circumstances that affected the decision may have changed. This is particularly true of health-relevant decisions. For example, a patient in a state of extreme fear or anxiety due to receiving an adverse test result might need to make important treatment decisions with long-term consequences. The patient's current preferences may differ substantially from future ones, when he or she has calmed down. Unfortunately, however, people tend to exaggerate the degree to which their preferences will remain constant. Loewenstein called the phenomenon projection bias and wrote that it "may cause people making summer vacation plans in the winter to choose overly warm destinations, diners to order too much food at the beginning of meals, and people unaddicted to cigarettes to underestimate the power of and drawbacks of addiction."[31]

Decisions to end one's life by refusing treatment are likely to be made when a patient is in a state of acute pain, misery, and depression. People in this situation tend to exaggerate both how long they have felt bad and how long they are likely to continue to feel bad. Thus, they are likely to have a much more negative view of their own situation than warranted.

A different form of projection bias occurs when a decision maker is not the person impacted by the decision, as when a pain-free physician prescribes for a patient in pain. In such cases, the physician is likely to underprescribe pain medication.

Loewenstein offered to pay volunteers to endure the pain of having their hands submerged in cold water. Some subjects were given a sample of the pain and then immediately asked how much money they would require to repeat the experience one week later. Others were asked one week after being given a sample of the pain. The first group demanded more compensation. The study suggests that people can't remember their own pain when they aren't in pain. So, Loewenstein asked, how likely is it that they can empathize with others' pain? Loewenstein asserted that projection bias is likely to pose problems for:

- people testing for or taking preventative measures to avoid conditions that don't cause immediate fear.
- patients needing to adhere to a drug regimen for a condition with intermittent symptoms. People not currently experiencing symptoms may underappreciate the benefits of treatment.
- manic-depressive patients who may not remember what it was like to be depressed and so stop taking the medication.
- end-of-life care.
  - Loewenstein cited a study in which no radiotherapists, 6 percent of oncologists, and 10 percent of healthy persons said that they would accept a grueling course of chemotherapy for three extra months of life. When current cancer patients were asked the same question, 42 percent stated that they would accept the chemotherapy.
  - People predicted whether a close other would want treatment such as cardiopulmonary resuscitation in various hypothetical end-of-life medical scenarios. They also stated their own preferences. The authors concluded: "Surrogate predictions more closely resembled surrogates' own treatment wishes than they did the wishes of the individual they were trying to predict."

There is no general solution to the problem of projection bias, but Ubel and colleagues developed a strategy for helping healthy people improve some of their projections.[32] They noted that people with any of a wide range of health conditions typically report greater happiness and quality of life than do healthy people who guess how they would feel under similar circumstances. Real patients may change their physical surroundings and expectations and find meaning in new aspects of their lives. Healthy people tend to underestimate this adaptive ability of patients. So Ubel and colleagues asked healthy people to imagine what their life would be like if they experienced a chronic disability, such as paraplegia. Then they asked the subjects to think back on powerful emotional experiences they'd had and to reflect on whether the emotions became stronger or weaker over time. The exercise helped people realize that adaptation occurs, and it promoted an increase in predictions of the quality of life they would experience if they developed paraplegia.

HINDSIGHT BIAS

Both laypersons and experts tend to evaluate decisions by their consequences.[33] For example, Caplan and colleagues asked experts to evaluate surgical cases that involved an adverse outcome.[34] Some read that the outcome was permanent, others that it was temporary. In all other respects, the information was identical. More reviewers who read the permanent version rated the quality of care as "less than appropriate." They showed hindsight bias.

When physicians in medical malpractice lawsuits are asked how they would have diagnosed a patient's symptoms, they already know that the outcome was bad. They respond that they would have predicted it. Their hindsight bias is relevant to the education of physicians. In clinicopathologic conferences, one person presents a medical case, offers a diagnosis, and awaits the announcement of the actual cause of death, presented later by a pathologist. Medical students are supposed to learn about treating people with the same symptoms. But hindsight bias reduces the effectiveness of these forums. Dawson and colleagues studied 160 doctors and medical students.[35] Group 1 completed a questionnaire after the case was presented but before the cause of death was revealed. They were given a list of five possible diagnoses and asked to assign a probability that each was the correct answer. Group 2 filled out the same questionnaire after the pathologist revealed the actual diagnosis, listing the probability they would have assigned to each item had they not known the correct answer.

People in group 1 acknowledged that the cases were difficult and wouldn't have been easy to diagnose. They were less likely to select the correct diagnosis. Members of the hindsight group were more likely to choose correctly. They felt they knew the right answer all along. Younger physicians—who need the training the most—were most likely to be overconfident. Dawson and colleagues concluded that teaching hospitals should have physicians and students list probable diagnoses before the actual diagnosis is offered. They'll make more mistakes initially but become better diagnosticians.

BIAS TOWARD NORMALIZATION

A doctor whose patient's lab results include an abnormal value is likely to initiate a treatment to bring the value within the normal range. The doctor assumes that replacing a missing quantity or normalizing a biochemical or physiological abnormality is beneficial. The doctor uses a rule of thumb: if it's abnormal, make it normal. Aberegg and O'Brien called this the normalization heuristic and argued that it is a misguided strategy.[36] They might have chosen a better term, since a heuristic is typically defined as an unconscious shortcut, whereas doctors make conscious decisions to normalize. But the concern is an important one. They point out that normalization of abnormal values is often the proper strategy, as when type I diabetics have low blood sugar or other patients have underactive thyroid glands. In certain situations, however, normalization may be ineffective or even harmful.

Throughout the 1970s and 1980s antiarrhythmic drugs were routinely administered to patients who had premature ventricular contractions after a heart attack. The goal, to normalize the cardiac rhythm, was usually achieved. But people who took the drugs were more likely to die.

For a second example, the authors cited a 2001 study that demonstrated a large reduction in mortality among critically ill surgical patients given intensive insulin therapy; the purpose was to normalize blood glucose levels to within a narrow range. Intensive insulin therapy was then widely adopted by critical care physicians for all types of critically ill patients, even though the preponderance of evidence does not favor its routine use. Aberegg and O'Brien gave many more examples of normalization practices that have not been shown to be beneficial and probably confer net harm.

BIAS AGAINST LOSSES

Kahneman and Tversky reported a variety of studies showing that people experience greater pain from a loss than pleasure from an equal-sized gain.[37] The bias against loss is relevant to many clinical situations. For example, chloramphenicol, the first antibiotic to be manufactured synthetically on a large scale, is effective against a wide variety of dangerous bacteria. However, approximately one in twenty-five thousand recipients suffers a fatal reaction. Although the gains greatly outweigh the risk, many patients were reluctant to take chloramphenicol.[38] For a similar reason, many healthy people refuse to be vaccinated against hepatitis, even though getting vaccinated would save lives.[39]

STRATEGIES FOR IMPROVING DECISION MAKING

The many and varied biases, most operating outside of conscious awareness, complicate decision making. But the situation is not as bleak as it might seem. Researchers have identified several strategies that help considerably. Perhaps the most useful strategy is to read about and become aware of all the potential biases.

Benefit from Smart Heuristics

Wegwarth and colleagues noted that research on heuristics has focused largely on errors and bias.[40] They challenged this perspective, arguing that using less-than-complete information sometimes improves the quality of decisions. They gave an example: a man is rushed to the hospital with serious chest pain, and the doctor must quickly decide whether he should be assigned to the coronary care unit or a regular nursing bed for monitoring. In some hospitals, doctors sent 90 percent of such patients to the coronary care unit. Yet only 25 percent of the patients actually had myocardial infarction. The errors were expensive, so researchers trained doctors to use a decision support tool, the Heart Disease Predictive Instrument. The HDPI presents all relevant information in a chart. To determine a patient's probability of having acute heart disease based on the chart, doctors had to check the presence and absence of combinations of seven symptoms and insert the relevant probabilities into a calculator. Although the HDPI improved their decision making, many doctors disliked its complexity and lack of transparency. But after using the HDPI for awhile, the doctors no longer needed it. They had learned the important variables and, even without doing the quantitative computations, their decisions remained at the improved level. So Green and Mehr developed a shortcut that asks only a few yes/no questions instead of the complete HDPI.

The sensitivity of a diagnostic procedure is the proportion of patients with disease who test positive. The specificity is the proportion of patients without disease who test negative. Green and Mehr's shortcut had greater sensitivity (identified more patients who had a serious heart disease) and specificity (sent fewer patients into the coronary care unit unnecessarily) than both doctors' intuitive judgment and the HDPI. Furthermore, because it used only limited information, the shortcut enabled rapid decisions in these life-threatening situations.

Wegwarth and colleagues gave additional examples to show that the quality of decisions does not invariably improve—and sometimes even diminishes—with increasing information. When uncertainty is high, as in many medical situations, the decision maker is often better off ignoring part of the available information.

Consult with Colleagues and Identify Thresholds

Woolever encouraged physicians to use their colleagues as resources when confronted with difficult medical decisions.[41] He wrote, "No textbook can help you with the probabilities and epidemiology of your unique patient population, but your colleagues certainly can." He also advised physicians to establish thresholds that must be crossed before initiating a particular treatment. "When the treatment has marked benefit for the diseased person and low risk for the non-diseased person, the threshold is low. When the treatment has only limited benefit for those with the disease and a moderate risk for those without the disease, the threshold is higher."

Be Mindful of Framing Effects

Some researchers have been able to weaken framing effects by asking subjects to provide rationales for their decisions.[42] Almashat and colleagues developed a method for reducing or even eliminating framing effects.[43] They presented volunteers with three vignettes, each consisting of a scenario depicting a diagnosis of cancer followed by two treatment options, surgery or radiation. The outcomes of each were framed as the probability of either surviving or dying following each treatment. Treatment outcomes were presented in three different ways: the cumulative number of people who have died/survived up to a certain time period, the number of people who die/survive during each specified time period, and the long-term survival rate.

After presentation of the vignettes and before they were asked to choose a treatment, the participants were given a questionnaire. The experimental group received questions requiring them to list the advantages and disadvantages of each option as well as the rationale for their choices. The control group answered unrelated questions. The framing effect occurred for two of the vignettes, but only in the control group. The debiasing procedure eliminated framing effects in the experimental group.

Simulation Training

Simulation training has been used to teach medical residents strategies to avoid common cognitive pitfalls.[44] Simulation training is discussed further on page 112.

Use Decision Aids

An important strategy for reducing biased reasoning is called decision analysis. Decision analysts collect data on cases with known outcomes that are relevant to the types of decisions to be made. Then they use computers to determine which information is crucial. For example, Swets and colleagues asked experienced radiologists to interpret a set of mammograms that included both normal images and benign and malignant lesions. The radiologists read each image and estimated the probability of malignancy. Then they used two decision aids: a checklist that guided them in assigning a scale value to the relevant features and a computer program that used the scale values to estimate the probability of malignancy. Then they re-estimated. Training in use of the aids took only about two hours yet improved diagnostic accuracy substantially.[45]

TIPS ESPECIALLY FOR PATIENTS

- Patients should become aware of all the potential biases and recognize that biases can affect decisions of both doctors and patients.
- Framing effects can be substantial, so patients should see whether the choices that doctors give them can be framed in more than one way.
- Most people are more optimistic than justified about their future health. Although optimism is generally good, an overly optimistic attitude may cause people to discount the necessity of practicing simple strategies for preventing or forestalling disease.
- People tend to exaggerate the degree to which their preferences will remain constant over time. Patients should be aware of this when confronted with difficult decisions. They should ask whether they can be put in contact with other patients who had to make similar decisions.

LOOKING AHEAD

In this chapter we've discussed various types of biases that impair decision making. The biases can affect decisions of both doctors and patients. Although most biases operate below the level of consciousness, people can be made aware of them and thereby diminish their impact. In the next chapter, we turn to decisions leading to medical diagnoses—often among the most important decisions of all.

(5)

MEDICAL DIAGNOSIS

The Problems

The treatment of many medical conditions is largely standardized. The difficult task for the physician is figuring out which condition to treat. There are about twenty thousand known human diseases, many with several subtypes, so it's understandable why making a correct diagnosis is no easy task. Yet although more than one million animal species and more than 1,500,000 plant species are known, competent zoologists and botanists are able to classify new specimens with great accuracy. The key difference between biological classification and medical diagnosis is this: all species within a biological grouping share some unique characteristic(s). For example, all mammals are warm-blooded vertebrates with a covering of hair on the skin and, in the female, milk-producing mammary glands for nourishing the young. The unique characteristic(s) may vary considerably among different species, as they do among mammals, but they can usually be easily identified. By contrast, a single disease may present itself in a dozen or more ways.

In addition, there is considerable overlap among symptoms for various diseases. For example, the signs and symptoms of influenza include abrupt onset of fever, severe muscular pain or tenderness, loss of appetite, sore throat, headache, cough, and a feeling of general discomfort or uneasiness. Patients may have other symptoms such as stuffy nose, sneezing, cough, or sore throat, and all of these can be caused by many different respiratory viruses or bacterial pathogens. Sonnenberg and Gogel noted that textbooks and review articles list more than fifty differential diagnoses for jaundice, abdominal pain, diarrhea, and constipation.[1]

Several factors compound the difficulties with diagnosis: a patient may have more than one disease, each with its own symptoms. Some tests for one disease will be inaccurate if the patient has an additional disease. General practitioners frequently lack access to the specialized equipment needed to diagnose certain serious conditions. And patients may neglect to tell their doctors about some symptoms that have crucial diagnostic value.

DIAGNOSTIC TESTS

Many diagnostic tests are available to help physicians, but test results provide only one piece of information. They must be used in conjunction with the patient's history and physical examination. For example, consider the prevalence of breast cancer in women of different ages, according to the National Cancer Institute.

from age thirty through age thirty-nine	0.43 percent
from age forty through age forty-nine	1.44 percent
from age fifty through age fifty-nine	2.63 percent
from age sixty through age sixty-nine	3.65 percent

Assume that a mammography test correctly identifies 90 percent of women who have breast cancer and also correctly identifies 90 percent of women who do not. Then, for every one hundred 30-year-old women who have a mammography, 0.43 × 90% = 0.387 will test positive and have breast cancer. Of the 99.57 who do not have breast cancer, 99.57 × 10% = 9.957 will also test positive. So, the likelihood that a thirty-year-old woman who tests positive has breast cancer is 0.387 / 9.957 = about 3.9 percent. See pp. 112–14 for further discussion on the computations.

The outlook for a sixty-year-old woman with a positive mammography is grimmer. For every one hundred 60-year-old women, 3.65 × 90% = 3.285 will test positive and have breast cancer. Of the 96.35 who do not have breast cancer, 96.35 × 10% = 9.635 will also test positive. So the likelihood that a sixty-year-old woman who tests positive has breast cancer is 3.285 / 9.635 = about 34 percent. The conclusion from a positive mammography is much different for a thirty- and a sixty-year-old, and for every age in between. And age is only one factor that must be considered when making a diagnosis. The patient's race, gender, and location may all be relevant. A person living in sub-Saharan Africa who complains of fever, chills, headache, sweats, and fatigue may receive a tentative diagnosis of malaria. The diagnosis will almost certainly be different for someone with the same symptoms who has never left Minnesota.

Two more points should be taken from the breast cancer example. First, about 20 percent of women with breast cancer have negative mammograms,[2] so a woman with a palpable lump should be closely watched no matter what the test indicates. Second, although additional tests can be ordered to increase the likelihood of making a correct diagnosis, absolute certainty is often not achievable. Whatever criteria a doctor uses to make her diagnosis, some healthy people may meet the criteria (false positives), and some unhealthy ones may not (false negatives). Making the criteria more stringent would reduce the number of false positives, but at the cost of increasing the number of false negatives. The two types of errors entail different costs: false negatives will not be treated for their condition, and false positives are likely to experience substantial anxiety and needless medical procedures. Doctors, patients, hospital administrators, and insurance companies may all weigh the factors differently. The next four paragraphs describe a personal example that illustrates some of the difficulties of diagnosis.

Diagnosis Difficulties: A Case History

Shortly after completing the first draft of this chapter, I (FL) developed a hacking, nonproductive cough, chills, loss of appetite, and extreme fatigue. My doctor, James Simons of Oakland Kaiser, said that he was pretty certain I had the flu, and he recommended that I rest and drink lots of fluids. I followed his orders but didn't improve and was losing about one pound per day from my already skinny frame. So I went back to his office a few days later, and he tentatively diagnosed pneumonia. He sent me for a chest x-ray, which confirmed it.

Pneumonia is a disease characterized by inflammation of the lung with fluid which has escaped from blood vessels and become solidified. Pneumonia may be caused by either bacteria or viruses, by inhalation of poisonous gases, accidental inhalation of food or liquids while unconscious, a blow or injury to the chest that interferes with normal respiration, or, in bedridden patients, merely by lying on one's back for a long period of time. Different causes require different treatments. After conferring with an infectious disease specialist and taking into account my age, symptoms, and medical history, Dr. Simons concluded that the most likely cause of my pneumonia was the bacterium Mycoplasma pneumonia. *However, he recognized other possibilities, especially the bacterium* pneumococcus. *We had a choice: he could start me immediately on an antibiotic to treat* Mycoplasma pneumonia, *or he could order some blood tests. The latter would have entailed having me wait in a crowded laboratory for at least thirty minutes while delaying the start of the antibiotic. He was willing to defer to my wishes, but we both opted for starting the antibiotic immediately. Two days later, I hadn't gotten any better. It was time for the blood tests. My white blood cell count was greatly elevated, and the responsible bacterium was* pneumococcus. *So he started me on a different antibiotic, and I quickly responded.*

Did Dr. Simons misdiagnose me? Twice? His initial diagnosis of flu was almost certainly correct. Anyone with a weakened immune system is especially vulnerable to the bacteria that cause pneumonia. My flu had prepared the way for an invasion of the pneumonia bacteria. But the Mycoplasma *diagnosis was incorrect. Had Dr. Simons ordered the blood tests immediately, I might have been saved two days of extreme discomfort. On the other hand, he had properly evaluated the probabilities and, in my view, made the correct choice. Many other examples of seeming misdiagnosis are probably of a similar nature.*

Two further points illustrate the incredible complexity of medical diagnosis. First, Dr. Simons considers it likely that, if the blood tests had been given early on, they would not have shown a greatly elevated white blood cell count. Second, common symptoms of pneumonia are cough that produces rust-colored or bloody sputum, shortness of breath at rest, and high fever. I had none of those symptoms.

CULTURAL FACTORS INFLUENCING DIAGNOSIS

What is by agreement recognized as diagnosis or therapy in one
country, is regarded in another country quite often as malpractice.

—Lynn Payer

Another important difference between biological classification and
medical diagnosis is that the former is not affected by cultural factors—a
rose is a rose is a rose, whether in the United States, Turkey, or Kenya—
but cultural values profoundly influence medical practices. American
medical journalist Lynn Payer's groundbreaking book *Medicine and
Culture* compares and contrasts the practice of medicine in the United
States, Britain, West Germany, and France.[3] The four Western nations
are similar in many ways, including average life span, but their doctors differ considerably in how they diagnose and treat.[4] For example,
surgeries per capita are much more common in the United States than
in England. French doctors prescribe drugs in suppository form much
more often than do their American counterparts. Uterine fibroids affect 30 percent of women and may cause abnormal uterine bleeding,
pressure, pain, or other symptoms. French doctors consider surgical
removal of the fibroids from the uterus, a procedure that preserves fer-
tility, as the treatment of choice. U.S. doctors generally favor the more
aggressive total hysterectomy.

In 1999, task forces in both the United States and France issued
recommendations for treating patients who have a mutation in genes
BRCA1 or BRCA2. Women (and men) who inherit the mutation are at
greatly increased risk of breast cancer. Both task forces concluded that
removal of the breasts reduces the disease risk for people with the gene
mutation, but the American panel was much more favorable to the procedure. The French advised doctors to remove a patient's breasts only
when the risk of breast cancer is more than 60 percent and to generally
oppose the surgery in patients younger than thirty.

Diagnoses of premenstrual syndrome (PMS) and premenstrual dys-
phoric disorder are made three to five times more often in the United
States than in France or Germany. The conditions are also treated differently in the different countries.[5]

Following are some quotes from the 1995 edition of Payer's book.

Patients and doctors in England and America . . . tend to see disease as something that comes from the outside. By contrast, Continental doctors and patients are more likely to emphasize weaknesses of particular organs or imbalances between various organs and/or systems.

French doctors diagnose vague symptoms as something to do with the liver; German doctors explain it as due to the heart, low blood pressure, or vasovegetative dystonia; the British see it as a mood disorder such as depression; and Americans are likely to search for a viral or allergic cause. What doctors don't know, they attribute to a virus, or when a condition doesn't respond to treatment, they attribute it to a virus. . . . America has an overall virus mentality.

When psychiatrists from six countries tried to agree on who was dangerous, the overall level of agreement was under 50 percent for three-quarters of the cases considered.

[F]ewer invasive procedures are used in intensive care units in France than in the United States—with patients doing equally well in both countries.

While Americans assume that if it's clean it must be healthy, the French point out the health advantages of tolerating dirt.

West Germans use about six times the amount of heart drugs, per capita, as do the French and English.

Poor circulation is held in West Germany to be the underlying cause of many diseases of specific organs.

The British doctor is much less likely to do routine examinations.

British doctors prescribe fewer drugs than French or West German doctors.

PATIENT AND DOCTOR DEMOGRAPHICS

Even within a single culture, both diagnoses and treatments are influenced by a patient's age, race, and gender. Graduate students in clinical psychology rated videotaped interviews of clients. There were significant differences as a function of race of client and race of therapist.[6] Blow and colleagues examined records from the 1999 National Psychosis Registry of 134,523 veterans diagnosed with schizophrenia, schizoaffective disorder, or bipolar disorder. They found pronounced ethnic disparities in diagnostic patterns. African Americans and Hispanics were much more likely than Caucasians to be classified as psychotic, even after controlling for relevant patient factors.[7]

Doctors are more likely to interpret men's symptoms as organic and women's as emotional.[8] They order more diagnostic testing for lung cancer in men than women patients with similar risk factors.[9] Women are more likely than men to die during an initial heart attack and during coronary bypass surgery because cardiovascular disease is further advanced in women at those times. The most likely explanation is that doctors are slower to diagnose and refer women at risk.[10] Of patients with abnormal exercise results, 40 percent of the men and only 4 percent of the women were referred for further testing.[11] For the same reason, women have worse functional status than men when undergoing major orthopedic surgery for degenerative arthritis.[12]

THE ISSUE OF RACE

Many medical textbooks and professors say that a patient's race should influence doctors' thinking about possible diagnoses. Garcia disagreed.[13] He wrote that, although Tay-Sachs disease is most likely to occur in Ashkenazic Jews, sickle cell anemia in blacks, and thalassemia in Southeast Asians, "the only infant I ever saw with Tay-Sachs was a Mexican child." He argued that doctors too easily assume the patient's race by defining ancestry in a single word: Asian, Hispanic, Caucasian, African American. But a "black" immigrant from Ethiopia does not have the same genetic disease risk factors as a Brazilian immigrant or a descendant of nineteenth-century U.S. slaves from West Africa. An Asian American man in Seattle who was born in the far eastern portion of the former Soviet Union differs in risk factors from a Korean woman living in Toronto or a child in California with maternal grandparents who immigrated from China and a father whose ancestors came to New Jersey from Europe.

Garcia, a Mexican pediatric urgent care physician, asked, "Do all Hispanics have the same genetic risk for asthma? Do Mexicans and Puerto Ricans eat the same diet? What about a patient from Spain—is he Hispanic in the same way that I am?"

Garcia is concerned that doctors who focus on race may ignore key factors in the patient's symptoms, geographic ancestry, diet, and general lifestyle. He gives an example: My childhood friend Lela wasn't diagnosed with cystic fibrosis until she was eight years old. Over the years, her doctors had described her as a "2-year-old black female with fever and cough . . . 4-year-old black girl with pneumonia." Lela is black. Had she been a white child or had no visible "race" at all, she would probably have gotten the correct diagnosis and treatment much earlier. Only when she was eight did a radiologist, who had never seen her face to face, notice her chest radiograph and ask, "Who's the kid with CF?"

Categorizing patients by race creates another problem. Although rating of physicians through publicly available report cards is intended to improve health care, Werner and colleagues noted an unintended consequence—physicians might avoid high-risk patients to improve their ratings.[14] "If physicians believe that racial and ethnic minorities are at higher risk for poor outcomes, report cards could worsen existing racial and ethnic disparities in health care." Their analysis supported their concern: "The racial and ethnic disparity in coronary artery bypass graft (CABG) use significantly increased in New York immediately after New York's CABG report card was released, whereas disparities did not change significantly in the comparison states." A substantial proportion of patients whom surgeons avoided were of racial and ethnic minorities whose initial problems may have derived in part from limited access to quality cardiovascular care.

DOCTOR IDIOSYNCRASIES

Trokel and colleagues examined 2,253 cases of children admitted to U.S. hospitals for treatment of traumatic brain injury or femur fracture. The proportion given a diagnosis of child abuse varied widely between hospital types: 29 percent of the cases were diagnosed as abuse at children's hospitals, compared with 13 percent at general hospitals. The variation was not related to observed differences in the patients or their injuries. The more likely explanation is underdiagnosis in general hospitals.[15]

Individual doctors and dentists have idiosyncratic biases and tendencies. When physicians are tested with standardized patients or scenarios, their diagnoses vary substantially. University physicians differed in diagnosing jaundice.[16] Podiatrists differed in diagnosing common foot and leg conditions.[17] Examiners differed substantially in diagnosing radiographic caries.[18] Lanning and colleagues asked periodontists, general dentists, dental hygienists, and first- and second-year periodontal graduate students to interpret, diagnose, and plan a treatment for three cases.[19] Ratings of percentage of bone loss varied among three categories for the same tooth. Diagnoses for one patient ranged from gingivitis to chronic and aggressive periodontitis. Six to nineteen different treatment plans were submitted for each of the cases.

John Glick of the Abramson Cancer Center at the University of Pennsylvania sees many patients seeking a second opinion or transferring their care to his center. Glick estimated that he and his colleagues concur completely with the original doctor in about 30 percent of cases. But in another 30 to 40 percent, they recommend major changes in the treatment plan and sometimes make a completely different diagnosis. "We interpret things differently, maybe because we have more experience," he said. "We see hundreds of patients with Hodgkin's disease. A community oncologist may see only a couple."[20]

Hashem and colleagues studied whether physicians tend to assign ambiguous cases to their own specialty.[21] They noted that Franklin Yee's abdominal pain was diagnosed as viral gastroenteritis by a gastroenterologist, resulted in his admission to a coronary care unit by a cardiologist, was suspected by a nephrologist to be the result of kidney stones, and was eventually found to be the result of a ruptured appendix. To investigate the matter further, Hashem and colleagues presented abstracts of four difficult but not misleading patient cases to eight board-certified physicians from each of cardiology, hematology, and infectious diseases, and eight general practitioners who did not subspecialize. They found that specialists tended to be biased toward their own specialty and that generalists were better diagnosticians.

Kalf and Spruijt-Metz also studied differences in diagnoses between specialists.[22] They asked geriatricians, geriatric psychiatrists, and internists to read and evaluate four paper cases concerning elderly patients and then to answer a questionnaire. The information was presented as coming from the patient's history and a physical examination. The subjects wrote down a maximum of seven "facts" from each case, ranked in order of importance for making a preliminary diagnosis. They reported a maximum of seven diagnoses, ranked in order of importance.

Psychiatrists focused most on cognitive and other psychiatric facts. Internists focused on facts from the somatic category more frequently, and geriatricians selected more facts from the function category. Age was mentioned significantly more often by internists. The three types of specialists formulated different diagnoses. The authors note that their findings have implications for choice of specialist, obtaining second opinions, and health policy.

Given the substantial variability in diagnoses, it follows that doctors make many errors. In the United States, an estimated forty thousand to eighty thousand hospital deaths result annually from misdiagnosis.[23] Errors that resulted in harm were more frequently diagnostic than drug related (14 percent versus 9 percent). The diagnostic errors more frequently resulted in serious disability than did drug-related errors (47 percent versus 14 percent).[24]

DIAGNOSTIC ERRORS

Elstein estimated a diagnostic error rate in clinical medicine of about 15 percent.[25] Amy and colleagues estimated that diagnosis-related errors account for up to 76 percent of medical errors.[26] Graber and Berner's literature review concluded that the diagnostic error rate ranges from 5 percent in pathology and dermatology up to 10 percent to 15 percent in most other fields.[27] Diagnostic error rates in radiology ranged from 4 percent to 30 percent.[28] In 80 percent of these cases, abnormal details were not perceived, and in 20 percent, abnormal details were identified but misinterpreted.[29] Radiologists had an error rate of 30 percent in interpreting chest radiographs, bone studies, gastrointestinal series, and special procedures. They disagreed on the interpretation of chest radiographs as much as 56 percent of the time, and they had a 35 percent error rate in interpreting results from patients who had undergone trauma. Gastrointestinal examinations failed to detect as many as 20 percent of colonic tumors. An estimated 10 percent to 30 percent of breast cancers are missed on mammography.[30] Harvey and colleagues reviewed the most recent previous mammograms of women with breast cancer.[31] For 75 percent of them that had initially been interpreted as having normal findings, at least one of three radiologists found signs of cancer.

In an emergency department study, unscheduled return visits within seventy-two hours were associated with diagnostic errors in 20 percent of cases.[32] About 6 percent of the admitting diagnoses in British hospitals were incorrect.[33] Diagnostic errors were the second largest cause of adverse events in New York State hospitals[34] and the second leading cause for malpractice suits against hospitals.[35] Between the years 1985 and 2000, more than one-third of the 49,345 malpractice claims were caused by diagnostic error.[36] A large-scale study indicated that diagnostic errors contributed to 6.9 percent of adverse events in Colorado and Utah.[37]

Autopsy findings identified diagnostic discrepancies in 20 percent of cases, and the authors estimated that in almost half of these cases, knowledge of the correct diagnosis would have changed the treatment plan.[38] About 25 percent of lung cancer patients were not diagnosed as such while alive.[39] Roosen and colleagues compared clinical diagnoses with postmortem diagnoses for intensive care unit patients.[40] In 26 percent of cases, the correct diagnosis was missed. Had it been known, in most of the cases treatment might have been different and survival prolonged.

In light of the facts and figures above, it's interesting that Scott claimed that no more than 10 percent of clinicians admit, when asked, to any error in diagnosis over the past year.[41] A major reason is that clinicians often do not receive feedback about their incorrect diagnoses. See pp. 110–12.

COMMONLY MISDIAGNOSED DISEASES

More malpractice suits are initiated for diagnostic than drug errors, and they result in the largest payouts.[42] Davenport listed the top five malpractice-risk conditions in order of prevalence as myocardial in-farction, breast cancer, appendicitis, lung cancer, and colon cancer.[43] He noted that almost all malpractice suits are cases of misdiagnosis or mismanaged diagnostic tests leading to delayed treatment. Ghandi and colleagues reported that nearly 60 percent of the lawsuits were for missed or delayed cancer diagnoses, especially breast cancer, followed by misdiagnosis of infection, fracture, and myocardial infarction.[44]

Schiff and colleagues analyzed diagnostic errors over a three-year period and reported that the most common missed or delayed diag-noses were pulmonary embolism, drug reactions or overdose, lung cancer, colorectal cancer, acute coronary syndrome, breast cancer, and stroke.[45] (They noted that many adverse outcomes associated with misdiagnosis or delay do not result from error—some cancers are un-diagnosable at an early stage, and some illness presentations are too atypical, rare, or unlikely for even the best of clinicians to diagnose early.) Scott[46] wrote that common clinical scenarios associated with a big risk of diagnostic error include back pain in the presence of known malignancy (osteoarthritis and other common causes of mechanical back pain may be considered over metastatic spinal disease) and pa-tients with dyspnea, raised jugular venous pressure, and hypotension, for whom systolic heart failure is diagnosed even though pulmonary thromboembolism and cardiac tamponade can present with similar features. McAbee and colleagues reported that the pediatric missed diagnoses that most commonly led to malpractice suits were of menin-gitis, appendicitis, and pneumonia.[47] Signs of appendicitis are difficult to assess in young children and elderly adults, so surgeons unneces-sarily remove a healthy appendix in 10–20 percent of appendectomies in the United States.[48]

FREQUENTLY OVERDIAGNOSED DISEASES

Some diseases are frequently overdiagnosed—the doctor gives the dis-ease as the diagnosis, although the symptoms are caused by something else. The following examples have been adapted from the health-care ratings organization HealthGrades.[49]

Attention deficit hyperactivity disorder (ADHD): Many doctors diagnose children with ADHD when their behavioral problems stem from other causes or they are normal, boisterous children.

Irritable Bowel Syndrome (IBS): IBS, particularly in the United States, is frequently the diagnosis for chronic digestive disorders. Other possible causes, such as celiac disease and Crohn's disease, tend to be overlooked.

Middle ear infection (acute otitis media) in children: Middle ear infection is often overdiagnosed in infants and young children. There are various other causes of redness of the ear membranes besides otitis media.

Sinusitis: Various conditions other than sinusitis, such as common cold, flu, and asthma, can lead to sinus passage inflammation.

Lyme disease: Lyme disease is difficult to confirm because of nonspecific symptoms and a lack of definitive tests.

Alzheimer's disease: Various other alternatives to mental deterioration in older people are overlooked.

DIAGNOSTIC TESTS THAT SHOULD BE USED JUDICIOUSLY

In the examples above, overdiagnosis is synonymous with misdiagnosis. An expanded definition of overdiagnosis includes the identification of disease that would not have produced signs or symptoms before death. For example, recent studies have called into question the value of the prostate-specific antigen screening (PSA) test. The reason is that, even if the test is positive, many more men die of alternative causes before developing symptoms due to prostate cancer; their tumors do not become clinically meaningful before they die.[50] From 1993 through 2001, 76,693 men at ten U.S. study centers were randomly assigned to receive either an offer of annual PSA testing for six years and digital rectal examination for four years, or usual care.[51] (Usual care sometimes included screening.) The subjects and health-care providers received the results and decided on the type of follow-up evaluation. After seven years of follow-up, the incidence of prostate cancer per ten thousand person-years was

116 in the screening group and 95 in the control group. The incidence of death per ten thousand person-years was 2.0 in the screening group and 1.7 in the control group. That is, although screenings identified prostate cancers, they did not influence the rate of death from the disease.

In a more recent study, men aged fifty to sixty-nine were randomly allocated to be either screened by digital rectal examination and PSA testing or not screened. After twenty years, the death rates in the two groups did not differ significantly.[52]

Widespread breast cancer screening programs may also fail to save lives. Jørgensen and Gøtzsche reported that one in every three women diagnosed with invasive breast cancers would have had no symptoms before she died of other causes.[53] Overdiagnosis leads to needless distress and overtreatment which, in the authors' words, "may increase a woman's overall risk of death (all-cause mortality). Indeed, once a woman is overdiagnosed with breast cancer, she might be subjected to cancer-specific treatments (surgery, systemic therapy, radiotherapy), all of which are associated with a very small risk of death."[54]

Welch and Black estimated that about 25 percent of breast cancers detected on mammograms, about 60 percent of prostate cancers detected with prostate-specific antigen (PSA) tests, and 50 percent of lung cancers detected by chest x-rays and sputum tests represent overdiagnosis.[55] They noted that data from the past thirty years show an increasing number of new cases of thyroid, prostate, kidney and breast cancer, and melanoma, but there has been no corresponding increase in deaths from those cancers.

An additional reason for limiting certain diagnostic screening tests has surfaced during the past few years—they may *cause* illness. Computed tomography (CT) scans provide detailed images of organs, bones, and other tissues, and the information they provide can help considerably in making a diagnosis. As a result, their use has increased from three million scans in 1980 to more than seventy million in 2009. But CT scans produce high levels of radiation. Smith-Bindman and colleagues reported that a single full-body CT scan can deliver a radiation dose comparable to what low-dose atom bomb blast survivors at Nagasaki and Hiroshima endured.[56] A companion study in the same journal estimated that CT scans from the year 2007 in the United States will ultimately cause about 29,000 cases of cancer and 15,000 deaths.[57] Children, younger adults, and women are especially susceptible. The authors projected that two-thirds of the excess cancers will occur in women.

Mammographies also require high levels of radiation, and they pose significant cumulative risks of initiating and promoting breast cancer. Premenopausal women undergoing annual screening over a ten-year period are exposed to a total of about ten rads for each breast. The premenopausal breast is highly sensitive to radiation; each rad of exposure increases breast cancer risk by 1 percent, resulting in a cumulative 10 percent increased risk over ten years of premenopausal screening.[58] Risks are even greater for screening at younger ages.

Welch and Black encouraged physicians to educate patients about the risks and benefits involved with early detection. They wrote, "Whereas early detection may well help some, it undoubtedly hurts others. Often the decision about whether or not to pursue early cancer detection involves a delicate balance between benefits and harms . . . different individuals, even in the same situation, might reasonably make different choices." They also suggested raising the threshold at which a screening test result is labeled abnormal or at which further steps are taken.

FREQUENTLY UNDERDIAGNOSED DISEASES

Some diseases are underdiagnosed. Crosskerry noted several factors that contribute to the underdiagnosis of rare diseases.[59] First, the diagnostic lab tests may be expensive. Second, doctors who hunt for rare diagnoses may be considered showoffs. Third, because the diseases are rare, most doctors have little experience with them and are uncertain how far to press the hunt. Other diseases are underdiagnosed primarily because they produce no (or only vague) symptoms. The following examples have been adapted from the health-care ratings organization HealthGrades.[60]

Type 2 diabetes and impaired glucose tolerance: Type 2 (adult-onset) diabetes often has a gradual onset of mild symptoms over years, often starting out as the milder impaired glucose tolerance. Many patients are unaware anything is wrong and never seek medical attention.

High cholesterol: This risk factor for artery and heart disease often has no symptoms.

Hypertension: High blood pressure has no early symptoms.

Osteoporosis: Many women and men suffer from thin bones and osteoporosis but are not diagnosed until they suffer a fracture.

Sexually transmitted diseases: Many people with genital herpes, chlamydia, HPV, trichomoniasis, bacterial vaginosis, or gonorrhea have no major symptoms, if any. Even HIV has a long latent phase, typically many years, before the early symptoms of AIDS begin.

Hemochromatosis: This genetic disease, affecting around one in two hundred to three hundred, causes iron overload that gradually damages various body organs. Because it has no early symptoms, it is often undiagnosed until serious organ damage causes other conditions or symptoms.

Chronic kidney disease: The onset of kidney disease may produce no noticeable symptoms.

Hypothyroidism, including Hashimoto's thyroiditis: The early symptoms of hypothyroidism or other thyroid disorders are often mild and vague, such as fatigue, weakness, and some symptoms of depression. So hypothyroidism is often underdiagnosed, particularly in women. As many as 10 percent of Americans may have undetected hypothyroidism.

Glaucoma: The early stages of glaucoma do not cause symptoms, so it is often undiagnosed.

Depression: Certain groups such as the elderly often have overlooked depression.

Infectious diarrhea: Severe digestive symptoms such as diarrhea, nausea, and vomiting may be caused by food poisoning but may also be due to a contagious viral or parasitic infection of the digestive tract. Viral digestive infections often go unreported and underdiagnosed.

Fecal incontinence: Many people with this condition are unaware that it is a treatable condition.

Lactose intolerance: Lactose intolerance usually causes digestive symptoms, but many people blame the symptoms on other digestive problems such as indigestion. Lactose intolerance is particularly common in Americans of African, Hispanic, or Asian descent and less common in Caucasians.

Polycystic ovary syndrome (PCOS): This condition causes hormonal and menstrual symptoms and can lead to infertility. Although it is common, many women are unaware that they have PCOS.

Flat feet: Many people are unaware that they have a treatable level of flatness of the arch.

Attention deficit hyperactivity disorder and hyperactivity: Although ADHD is overdiagnosed in children and adolescents, it is underdiagnosed in adults.

Sleep disorders such as sleep apnea and narcolepsy: Sleep apnea occurs while the person is asleep, and affected people may be unaware they have interrupted sleep patterns.

Asthma: Asthma is underdiagnosed in some populations, possibly in children who have episodes of wheezing. It is probably also underdiagnosed in the elderly. In one study of asthmatic men and women ages sixty-five and older, about 50 percent of them had previously had their respiratory symptoms either ignored or incorrectly attributed to chronic pulmonary obstructive disease.

Celiac disease: Celiac disease is a chronic digestive disorder that is often misdiagnosed as irritable bowel syndrome or another chronic digestive disease.

Whooping cough (pertussis): Although uncommon in children due to vaccination programs, protection wears off after about ten years. Because of this, whooping cough is making a worldwide comeback and is a common cause of persistent cough in teens, adults, and the elderly.

Of the 1.7 million patients admitted to U.S. hospitals each year with heart attacks or warning chest pains, about twenty-six thousand are incorrectly sent home. Women under the age of fifty-five are the least likely to be hospitalized. A major reason is that symptoms differ for men and women. A man having a heart attack is likely to experience pains in the chest and down the left arm. A woman is more likely to report neck, jaw, shoulder, or upper back pain or discomfort; unusual fatigue; indigestion, abdominal pain, or heartburn; shortness of breath; nausea or vomiting; lightheadedness or dizziness; and sweating. If she is brought to an emergency room with these symptoms, she may not receive an electrocardiogram or blood tests. Instead, she is likely to be diagnosed with indigestion. Nonwhite patients are also frequently misdiagnosed and sent home.[61]

Ely and colleagues surveyed family physicians about their most memorable diagnostic errors.[62] Most involved cancers, heart attack, trauma, bowel obstruction, and meningitis.

AGAINST DIAGNOSIS

For certain medical conditions, such as HIV, syphilis, and a torn aorta, patients can be placed in one of two groups: those who have the condition and those who don't. For patients in the first group, the course of treatment is often straightforward: antibiotics for syphilis, surgery for a torn aorta. But the medical conditions that most plague industrialized countries, including cardiovascular disease, type 2 diabetes, obesity, depression, autism, hyperactivity, back pain, arthritis, and even cancer occur with varying degrees of severity. Categorizing patients as either having or not having the conditions requires arbitrary cutoff points. For example, despite the inconsequential difference between systolic blood pressures of 140 and 139 mm Hg, only a person with the first reading would, according to the current standard, be diagnosed with hypertension. So Vickers and colleagues encouraged doctors to think differently about disease. They should use prediction models except for conditions for which diagnosis leads to unambiguous treatment. A doctor would estimate the likelihood of a patient having a clinically important event, such as a heart attack, within a certain time period.[63] Blood pressure would be one factor among many, including cholesterol level, diabetes, age, sex, and smoking history. A young man with few risk factors other than a systolic blood pressure of 145 mm Hg is unlikely to have a heart attack, and lowering his blood pressure would make little difference. But an elderly male smoker with high cholesterol and a similar blood pressure is at high risk; lowering his blood pressure would substantially reduce the risk.

Vickers and colleagues wrote that prediction modeling can be implemented readily with available data and technology, and modeling has two advantages over making traditional diagnoses. First, it gives doctors explicit information to share with patients, such as the risk for heart attack with or without treatment. This enables patients to make meaningful choices, for example, whether to accept an expensive or painful treatment that reduces the risk for a clinically important event by 2 percent. Second, prediction models can incorporate all of a patient's relevant characteristics. "A patient with high blood pressure benefits more from control of cholesterol than does a patient with normal blood pressure. For prostate cancer, the situation is reversed, with the patient at high risk for cardiovascular death less likely to benefit from prostatectomy, because he is more likely to die before his cancer progresses sufficiently to affect his survival or quality of life." Of course, risk predictions can be used only if good prediction models are available.

Patrick, while not disputing the value of a prediction approach, pointed to a serious obstacle toward implementing it: the medical/insurance/employment/military fields all require diagnoses. Diagnoses are entered into medical records, affect insurance premiums, and may disqualify people from various jobs.[64]

TIPS ESPECIALLY FOR PATIENTS

In many instances, medical diagnosis is straightforward, and patients can identify their condition before seeing a doctor. A patient who has recently come into contact with poison oak and developed a rash does not need a doctor to tell her what the problem is. But diagnosis is sometimes extremely difficult, and patients should realize that some errors are unavoidable. A doctor may occasionally do everything right and still diagnose incorrectly. Furthermore, doctors must often decide whether the value of additional diagnostic tests offsets the costs of those tests. The costs can be both financial and health related—many screening tests cause patients pain, discomfort, and potential harm, for example, by exposing them to high doses of radiation.

Diagnosis is a collaborative effort between doctor and patient. Patients can improve their chances of getting a correct diagnosis by describing all their symptoms, even if some seem trivial or are embarrassing. They should tell the doctor if they have any other diseases. After a diagnosis has been made, they should contact the doctor if treatment isn't working or symptoms occur that don't seem to fit the diagnosis.

Proper diagnosis is so important that a patient should not allow his shyness or a doctor's forcefulness to deter him from asking for a second opinion.

LOOKING AHEAD

In this chapter we've shown that doctors face great difficulties when making medical diagnoses. Diagnostic tests are imperfect, and doctors must often make diagnoses despite having incomplete information. As a result, diagnostic errors are common. Many commentators have offered strategies for reducing errors, and these are discussed in the next chapter.

(6)

REDUCING DIAGNOSTIC ERRORS

Advances in the medical sciences enable us to recognize and diagnose new diseases. Innovation in the imaging and laboratory sciences provides reliable new tests to identify these entities and distinguish one from another.[1] Despite these advances, however, for the reasons listed in the previous chapter, diagnosis will probably never be error-free. Even more disconcerting, recent research indicates that diagnostic accuracy in some fields has not improved appreciably over the past half century.[2] (An alternative view is that accuracy has improved but is measured against autopsy results, and only the most baffling cases are chosen for autopsy.)[3]

One useful strategy doctors can employ to improve their diagnostic skills is to cheer up. Fredrickson hypothesized that positive emotions facilitate the development of various intellectual skills.[4] Whereas negative emotions narrow attention to specific details of potential problems, positive emotions motivate a broadened focus on global patterns. Positive emotions foster the capacity to integrate diverse material, to consider unconventional possibilities, and to adapt behavior to accommodate changes in the environment. See pp. 47–48 for examples.

This chapter first addresses types of diagnostic errors and then suggests ways to improve the often-neglected diagnostic tools of history taking and physical exams. We follow with a discussion of decision aids and strategies for becoming an expert. Finally, we offer suggestions for interpreting results of diagnostic tests, including a discussion of probabilistic thinking and likelihood ratios.

TYPES OF DIAGNOSTIC ERRORS

Graber and colleagues described three types of diagnostic errors: no-fault errors, system errors, and cognitive errors.[5]

No-Fault Errors

No-fault errors occur when information from the patient is misleading, absent, or mimics a more common condition. Such errors can never be eliminated because new diseases emerge, tests are never perfect, and patients do not always describe their symptoms accurately. Even if the doctor identifies the most likely diagnosis, it may not be the correct one. For example, see the case study on pp. 81–82. Graber and colleagues analyzed one hundred cases of diagnostic error involving internists and reported that seven were due to no-fault errors alone.

System Errors

System errors arise because of imperfections in the health-care system. They contributed to the diagnostic error in sixty-five of the one hundred cases analyzed by Graber and colleagues. The most common system-related factors involved problems with policies and procedures, including inefficient teamwork and communication. Although system errors also can never be completely eliminated, they can be drastically reduced because improvements degrade over time and new fixes create the opportunity for novel errors. Graber offered several suggestions to combat this type of error:

- Diagnostic tests should be performed and results given to the patients and their doctors on a timely basis. Abnormal test results and trends should be visually obvious in test result information.

- Patient data should be available to all providers and shared in a timely fashion. This is not always the case: one study showed that almost 70 percent of specialists did not receive patient information from a primary care physician prior to a referral visit, and 25 percent of primary care doctors had not received information from a specialist even one month after a referral visit.[6]
- Doctors should have access to the Internet, electronic medical reference texts and journals, and decision-making aids at the point of care.
- Doctors and patients should be able to access second opinion and specialist consultation easily. One specific example: emergency room physicians are not usually experts at interpreting radiographs and cranial tomographic studies. Trained radiologists should be available to help.
- Distractions and production pressures should be reduced so that staff members have time to think about what they're doing.
- Patients should be informed of their diagnosis, told what to expect, and asked to inform their doctor of any discrepancies. ("Doc, my cholesterol level has always been below 200 and I'm shocked that it's now 420. Can I please be retested?")
- Doctors should get feedback as quickly as possible on the accuracy of their diagnoses. British radiologists receive more feedback than their American counterparts and make fewer diagnostic errors.[7]
- Diagnostic errors should be constantly reviewed, and types of adverse events that appear repeatedly should be identified.

Schiff encouraged doctors to seek feedback by calling patients soon after office visits to ask how they are. Doing so demonstrates caring and gives the patient an important role to play in testing the diagnostic hypothesis. Schiff gave examples from his own practice of data that emerged through follow-up:

- Schiff attributed a patient's rash to a drug. During follow-up, the patient said he had checked and found that the rash had started before he first took the drug.

- A patient reported that leaning forward relieved his chest pain. This clue for possible pericarditis had not been mentioned during the initial visit.
- A patient reported that the treatment helped at first but was no longer helping. This suggested that the diagnosis or treatment was incorrect.
- A patient elaborated on the comment of a specialist: "The cardiologist you sent me to didn't think the chest pain was related to the mitral valve problem but she wasn't sure."
- Diagnosticians may get valuable clues if they encourage patients to think about life events that may be relevant to their current symptoms. For example, "After I went home and thought about it, I remembered that as a teenager I once had an injury to my left side and peed blood for a week," stated a patient with an otherwise inexplicable nonfunctioning left kidney. "I remembered that I once did work in a factory that made batteries," offered a patient with an elevated lead level.

Cognitive Errors

Graber and colleagues found that cognitive errors—errors due to the physician—contributed to the diagnostic error in seventy-four of the one hundred cases. Groopman agreed about the importance of cognitive error. He wrote, "Why do we as physicians miss the correct diagnosis? It turns out that the mistakes are rarely due to technical factors, like the laboratory mixing up the blood specimen of one patient and reporting another's result. Nor is misdiagnosis usually due to a doctor's lack of knowledge about what later is found to be the underlying disease. Rather, most errors in diagnosis arise because of mistakes in thinking."[8]

Berner and Graber contended that the overconfidence of physicians is a major cause of cognitive error.[9] They wrote, "The remarkable discrepancy between the known prevalence of error and physician perception of their own error rate lies at the crux of the diagnostic error puzzle." They cited many studies to support their position. A few examples follow:

- Physicians diagnosed 126 patients who had died and undergone autopsy. They also indicated their level of certainty. Clinicians who claimed to be completely certain of the diagnosis were wrong 40 percent of the time, according to the autopsy results.[10]
- The confidence level of physicians was uncorrelated with their ability to predict the accuracy of their diagnoses.[11]
- Diagnostic accuracy varied among ninety-five board-certified radiologists: the confidence level of the worst performers was higher than that of the top performers.[12]
- Medical trainees overestimated their skills in communicating with patients.[13] There was a very low correlation between physicians' self-assessment of competence and an external measure of competence. The least expert physicians tended to be the most overconfident.[14]

Friedman and colleagues created detailed synopses of challenging medical cases, each with a definitive correct diagnosis.[15] They asked their subjects, senior medical students, senior medical residents, and faculty internists, to generate a diagnostic hypothesis set. To assess their subjects' confidence, they asked, "How likely is it that you would seek assistance in establishing a diagnosis for this case?" They considered four possible outcomes for each case: a highly confident subject making the correct diagnosis; a highly confident subject making an incorrect diagnosis; and subjects with low confidence making correct or incorrect diagnoses.

Medical residents were overconfident in 41 percent of cases where their confidence and correctness were not aligned, faculty in 36 percent of such cases, and students in 25 percent. The authors concluded that even experienced clinicians may be unaware of the correctness of their diagnoses at the time they make them.

Baumann and colleagues examined decisions of nurses working in intensive care units and physicians treating breast cancer.[16] For both groups, individual respondents were highly confident they had made the right choice, but there was no consensus across respondents as to what that choice was. The conclusion is that many were overconfident, and it helps explain the persistence of practice variation.

Berner and Graber cited inadequate feedback as a major reason for overconfidence. Most cases are diagnosed correctly. Physicians are likely to devote extra time and attention to puzzling cases and to seek the advice of specialists. But they may never be made aware of many of their incorrect diagnoses, either because the patient doesn't return for follow-up or gets better despite the error.

In addition to overconfidence, causes of cognitive diagnostic error include faulty data collection, flawed reasoning, or incomplete knowledge. These areas offer the most opportunity for improvement. Graber and colleagues, Crosskerry and Norman,[17] Sanders,[18] and Trowbridge[19] offered several suggestions for reducing cognitive errors, although Graber and colleagues warned that implementing their suggestions might in some cases *worsen* medical outcomes. The extra time required might delay a diagnosis or reduce time spent with other patients. Expanded diagnostic possibilities might lead to additional tests that pose risks, cause discomfort, and increase costs. And patients may question the competence of doctors who give less than authoritative diagnoses.

Be aware of order effects. Chapman and colleagues asked doctors to read a case vignette describing a patient with a history of lung cancer, weakness of the right arm and leg, and a negative CT scan of the head.[20] The doctors were more likely to diagnose the problem as a brain tumor rather than warning signs of a stroke when the patient's history of lung cancer was presented last. In a similar study, subjects were more likely to diagnose lung cancer if the patient's history of lung cancer was given late.[21] Cunnington and colleagues found that information presented first about simulated cases exerted a disproportionately large effect on judgments.[22] Completely eliminating order effects may be impossible, but making clinicians aware of them is likely to help.

Avoid premature closure. Initial information often suggests a diagnosis or establishes a framework for further analysis. Clinicians may then stop searching or search harder for confirmatory rather than disconfirmatory evidence.[23] They may also remember confirmatory information better.[24] Premature closure was the single most common cause of diagnostic error in the Graber and colleagues cases. So they encourage doctors to continue to consider reasonable alternatives even after an initial diagnosis is reached. They should search for information contrary to the initial diagnosis while asking themselves, "Could it be anything else?"

and "What's the diagnosis that I don't want to miss?" Interestingly, the risk of premature closure *increases* with years of experience.[25]

Pretend your initial diagnosis is incorrect. Poses and colleagues asked physicians to estimate the probability of survival of patients who had just been admitted to a medical-surgical intensive care unit.[26] When two physicians gave estimates for the same patient, they often disagreed widely. During the next two days, despite receiving additional information, they adjusted their estimates only slightly. Their initial disagreements were not substantially reduced. (See the discussion on anchoring, pp. 60–62) Several authors have suggested that physicians pretend that their diagnosis is incorrect while actively examining flaws and searching for alternatives. The strategy should help them keep in mind that several diseases may underlie a particular clinical picture. Graber also encouraged medical school teachers to emphasize that the signs and symptoms of many diseases are quite variable.

Get second opinions. Routinely seek a second opinion. When Kronz implemented a procedure requiring a second opinion on every surgical pathology diagnosis, clinically relevant changes were made in 1.4 percent of 6,171 cases.[27]

Get enough sleep. In one study, sleep-deprived interns had a fivefold increase in diagnostic errors.[28]

As mentioned above, each of the preceding suggestions entails costs. Scott[29] noted that several of them may have unintended consequences: decisional delays, constant second-guessing, increase in unnecessary investigations (and expense) in response to expanded lists of differential diagnoses, patient anxiety arising from clinicians' expressions of uncertainty, and more errors as more investigative and treatment options are considered.

HISTORY TAKING AND THE PHYSICAL EXAMINATION

Physicians should not rely solely on diagnostic tests but instead consider all data as components of a comprehensive evaluation. Despite advances in diagnostic technology, the clinical examination, including history and physical, remains crucial to the evaluation of most patients. Bordage argued that history taking and physical examination of patients is more important than laboratory tests and imaging techniques for di-agnostic accuracy.[30] The patient history helps lead to the final diagnosis about 75 percent of the time.[31] In the case of chest pain, 90 percent of diagnoses are made on the basis of the history alone.[32] Ghandi and col-leagues analyzed closed malpractice claims; failure to obtain a thorough medical history or perform a thorough physical examination had been a contributing factor in 42 percent of the cases.[33] Sanders wrote that one of the most reliable diagnostic tools is what the patient has to say.[34] (She added that doctors should not necessarily believe patients' versions of their symptoms; the patient may be embarrassed or think key symptoms inconsequential.)

In clinical practice, however, the history and physical examination are being superseded by laboratory tests and biomedical technology. Many students do not improve their interviewing techniques through medical school, and senior students have the same deficiencies as less advanced students. Stillman and colleagues studied residents in nineteen internal-medicine residency training programs.[35] Slightly over 12 percent had never been observed for the purpose of assessment by faculty members, and 55 percent had been observed only once or twice taking a history and doing a physical. Although several studies have shown that the phys-ical examination skills of most medical residents are unsatisfactory, they also show that substantial improvement is possible.[36] Two paths for im-provement are discussed below: first, doctors should have diagnoses in mind to guide their history taking and examination; second, they should create an ongoing history-taking relationship with patients that ensures that patients communicate new and relevant information. At the end of this section, we discuss the concept of "misleading one detail" (MODE) and how to counteract the confusion a MODE may create.

Elstein observed that thoroughness of data gathering is not a good predictor of diagnostic accuracy.[37] Instead of gathering data blindly, medical students should be taught to pause to look things up and select a limited set of plausible diagnoses to compare and contrast. Diagnostic accuracy is maximized by having clinical signs and diagnostic hypotheses in mind during the physical examination (PE). This approach contrasts with the rote, hypothesis-free screening PE learned by many medical students; because the physician's procedures are not linked to patient complaints, students do not learn to appreciate how an abnormal finding would appear or what it might mean. This may help explain why students have difficulty in selecting relevant procedures and interpreting findings to reach a diagnosis.

Yudkowsky and colleagues developed a hypothesis-driven procedure to provide medical students with practice in anticipating, eliciting, and interpreting critical aspects of the PE.[38] They developed nineteen presenting complaints chosen to include all anatomical regions of the body, covering 160 PE procedures. For each case, students listed anticipated positive PE findings for two plausible diagnoses. Then they examined a standardized patient (SP) simulating one of the diagnoses and received immediate feedback from the SP. Their diagnostic accuracy was substantially better than that of typical students. When they encountered some of the scenarios during their year 4 clinical skills examination, they performed better on cases on which they had received feedback as year 3 students.

Schiff disputed the idea that most physicians are overconfident.[39] He wrote that they are more likely to feel beleaguered and distracted; and he argued that "good medicine is less about brilliant diagnoses being made or missed and more about mundane mechanisms to ensure adequate follow-up." He contended that many misdiagnoses occur not because of failure to consider a particular diagnosis, but because physicians have no reliable systems for obtaining feedback. He gave as examples a patient with chest pain being sent home from the emergency room (ER) with a missed heart attack or a radiologist missing an abnormality on a mammogram. The problem is not that the physician has failed to consider the correct diagnosis—ER physicians invariably consider heart attack in chest-pain patients, and mammograms are performed specifically to test for breast cancer—but that the results are not definitive, so the patient is sent home with no automatic follow-up.

Misleading One Detail

Arzy and colleagues presented doctors in internal medicine with ten clinical vignettes, each of which included a single misleading detail (MODE).[40] In clinical practice, a MODE might originate from false information (incorrect history or physical examination, misinterpretation or misreporting of imaging or laboratory results) or findings unrelated to the present problem. The cases were based on real emergency room cases in which a misleading detail caused misdiagnosis. The doctors were randomly assigned to one of three groups: received no special notification to be aware of MODEs; instructed to be aware of possible MODE; or had a trivial detail substituted for the MODE.

Being made aware of a possible MODE did not have an effect. The average number of correct initial diagnoses in the first two groups was equivalent and significantly less than in the third group. However, when the doctors were asked to identify a leading diagnostic detail and then to formulate an alternative diagnosis after omission of the detail, their diagnostic error rate was reduced by nearly 50 percent. The authors note that doctors in practice who try to reduce diagnostic errors by deliberately omitting leading details would increase errors in correctly diagnosed patients. However, in troublesome cases such as repeated referral to medical assistance or unanticipated complications, systematic reexamination and verification of leading diagnostic clues may help reduce diagnostic mistakes.

DIAGNOSTIC AIDS

As noted on pp. 24–25, the medical literature is enormous, and beleaguered physicians cannot possibly keep up to date with all the most recent findings. They need help, some of which comes in the form of clinical practice guidelines—statements about appropriate health care for specific clinical circumstances. The guidelines contain diagnostic recommendations based on evidence from rigorous reviews of the medical literature. The National Institutes of Health website, http://www.nhlbi.nih.gov/guidelines/archive.htm, has guidelines for diagnosing and managing many diseases.

Help is also available in the form of computer-based decision support systems (DSSs). Programmers upload descriptions of thousands of possible diseases into computers along with all the possible signs and symptoms for each disease. The computer DSS uses what is known about the patient plus any other available information to develop a small list of diagnostic possibilities, typically by body system, such as cardiology. The computer may list rare medical conditions that the diagnostician had not considered.[41] Some programs then offer nothing further unless specifically requested to do so. Others give information and advice and may pose questions to the physician. Each answer stimulates additional analysis that narrows the number of diagnostic possibilities. DSSs can generate alerts and reminders and critique treatment plans.

Some DSSs are available for free to anyone with Internet access. Tang and Ng, a rheumatologist and a respiratory and sleep trainee, selected twenty-six diagnostic cases from the case records of the *New England Journal of Medicine*.[42] They picked three to five search terms from each and then did a Google search, recording the three most prominent diagnoses that seemed to fit the symptoms and signs. Then they compared the results with the correct diagnoses as published in the case records. Google searches found the correct diagnosis in fifteen cases. Tang and Ng noted that the efficiency of such searches and the usefulness of the retrieved information depend on the searchers' knowledge base. Google searches are less likely to be successful for laypeople and for complex diseases with nonspecific symptoms and/or rare presentations. Conditions with unique symptoms and signs are more likely to be diagnosed correctly. A related strategy is to go to specific diagnosis websites.[43]

The use of DSSs creates some problems. Because DSSs suggest possible but unlikely diagnoses, they increase clinician cost and workload and patient uncertainty. Berner and Graber wrote, "A patient who is reassured that he or she most likely has constipation will probably sleep a lot better than the one who is told that the abdominal CT scan is needed to rule out more serious concerns." A surprising additional concern is that DSSs may reduce diagnostic accuracy. When medical residents read electrocardiograms and the computer advice was correct, their accuracy increased from 53.1 percent to 68.1 percent correctly interpreted findings. But when the advice was incorrect, as it often is, accuracy dropped from 56.7 percent to 48.3 percent.[44] Thus, although potentially useful, DSSs have not been widely accepted, and several commercial ventures were discontinued. Another computer-aided approach, fuzzy medical diagnosis, holds promise but is beyond the scope of this book.[45]

Telemedicine is a rapidly developing field that links more than 3,500 medical centers in all fifty U.S. states and many other countries. Telemedicine uses satellite technology, video-conferencing equipment, and other data-gathering and communication devices to enable specialists to provide services to nonspecialist health professionals. A specialist can view patients' histories, order diagnostic tests, examine test results, and consult with doctors in distant locations. Specialists can rapidly diagnose patients and give second opinions. They can sometimes definitively rule out serious diseases, thereby eliminating the need for expensive and invasive procedures. For certain medical conditions, such as stroke, speedy treatment is essential in order to prevent brain cells from dying. So if a possible stroke victim shows up at a hospital that does not have an appropriate specialist, a telemedicine diagnostician can be invaluable.

BECOMING AN EXPERT

Experienced clinicians are better decision makers than are novices, but not because they have read more journal articles or books on decision making. Crosskerry concluded that the most reasonable explanation is experience per se.[46]

Ericsson investigated the qualities that distinguish experts from other people.[47] He wrote that even the most talented chess masters, creative artists, and scientists are not usually more intelligent than less proficient individuals of comparable education. The experts' superiority is limited to their particular domain of expertise, and they typically require at least ten years of experience to achieve their status. Most people reach an acceptable level of job performance after about two years and are satisfied—they don't strive to get to the next level. So beyond those first two years, length of experience correlates weakly with performance.[48] In fact, according to Ericsson, the correlation between experience and proficiency in the medical field is often negative. That is, most doctors perform worse the longer they are out of medical school. Their accuracy in diagnosing mammograms declines steadily. The reason is that doctors who read mammograms don't know for certain whether there is breast cancer. They will learn only weeks later, from a biopsy, or years later, when no cancer develops. Delays between initial diagnosis and conclusive findings may also occur when they diagnose other x-rays or heart sounds. Without meaningful feedback, their abilities deteriorate over time.

Ericsson wrote that people entering a new field typically focus initially on understanding it and acting appropriately. With experience, their behaviors become increasingly automatic, and they lose conscious control over their actions. They stop making adjustments, and their development stops. The experts, by contrast, undergo lengthy and specific training. They practice every day, including weekends. They force themselves to seek out tasks that stretch their performance by correcting specific weaknesses. Even professional athletes, despite their considerable natural abilities, must engage in such practices to become stars. *Sports Illustrated* magazine had a feature on Idan Ravin, who trains such basketball luminaries as LeBron James, Carmelo Anthony, and Chris Paul. Ravin believed that James's weakness was his dribbling, so he ran James through a series of intricate ball-handling exercises.[49] He develops other specific exercises for each person he trains.

Compared with their less-skilled counterparts, elite-level soccer players spent significantly longer per week in deliberate practice. Similar findings were obtained for tennis, dart throwing, ice skating, singing, playing a musical instrument, typing, and insurance salesmanship. The amount of solitary chess study was the best predictor of chess skill, with only a very small benefit from the number of games played in chess tournaments.

The core assumption of deliberate practice is that expert performance is acquired gradually. Improvement requires suitable training tasks that can be mastered sequentially. Performers are given tasks initially outside their current realm of reliable performance that they can master by concentrating on critical aspects and refining their performance through repetitions with feedback. This type of deliberate practice requires full attention and concentration, which is what sets deliberate practice apart from both mindless, routine performance and playful engagement. Still, some kind of failure is likely to arise, so corrections and repetitions are necessary.

In light of the above, Ericsson wrote a prescription for doctors who want to become expert diagnosticians. They should diagnose radiographic information from old cases and get immediate feedback of the correct diagnosis. They might see more different cancers in one day than in years of normal practice. They should check up on their patients, taking extensive notes on what they were thinking at the time of diagnosis and checking back to determine their accuracy. This will help them understand how and when they are improving. He noted that surgeons are an exception to the finding that most doctors perform worse the longer they are out of medical school. The reason, he explained, is that surgeons are constantly exposed to two key elements of deliberate practice: immediate feedback and specific goal setting. Graber suggested that physicians seek out feedback by asking for autopsies and attending morbidity and mortality conferences.[50]

Pilots should never have to pull out of a spin or fly with a damaged engine without having practiced. So, much of their training is done with simulators. They get immediate feedback and are shown how to correct their mistakes. The same is true of nuclear power plant operators, military officers, and, increasingly, medical personnel. Doctors, nurses, and paramedics are shown controlled medical events so that they can match their diagnostic skills with those of experts. Simulators have been developed for both basic practices such as blood draw and complex surgical and trauma care procedures. Participants evaluate the patient, either a trained actor or virtual patient, or they simply read a set of symptoms. Then they order whichever tests they deem appropriate and make a diagnosis. They can rehearse dealing with common as well as rare medical emergencies, and they receive rapid feedback. Mistakes—and mistakes in the early going are likely—do not harm patients. Simulation training has been used to teach residents strategies to help them avoid common cognitive pitfalls.[51]

Simulations can re-create entire clinical situations, helping participants develop skills in teamwork and communication. For example, Stanford University requires anesthesia residents to go through a simulation in which a mannequin "patient" dies from a severe, unexpected allergic reaction. The residents must provide and coordinate medical care with other members of the team and then break the news to a live actor playing the role of a shocked and then grieving widow. Many simulations are available on the Internet.[52]

INTERPRETING THE RESULTS OF DIAGNOSTIC TESTS

In 1982, Eddy described a study in which he gave medical doctors the following hypothetical information:[53]

The probability that a woman at age forty has breast cancer is 1 percent.

The probability that the disease is detected by a mammography is 80 percent.

The probability that a woman tests positive although she does not have the disease is 9.6 percent.

Then he asked the doctors, "If a woman at age forty tests positive, what is the probability that she has breast cancer?" The results were remarkable and frightening. Eddy reported that ninety-five out of one hundred doctors estimated the probability to be about 75 percent. The correct answer is 7.8 percent.

Eddy's finding has been extensively replicated, with most doctors estimating the probability between 70 percent and 80 percent and only around 15 percent getting close to the right answer. Gigerenzer and Hoffrage gave German doctors the same problem, and their estimates ranged from 1 percent to 90 percent, the most frequent estimate being 90 percent.[54] Gynecologists gave similar results. Doctors evaluating a colorectal cancer screening test estimated the probability of cancer given positive results with the maximum variability possible—their answers ranged between 1 percent and 99 percent. AIDS counselors mistakenly took a positive HIV test to indicate certain infection. (According to Gigerenzer, a reasonable estimate is about 50 percent.)

Eddy concluded that medical personnel make major errors in statistical thinking that threaten the quality of medical care. Millions of people each year become terrified and despondent because they have been incorrectly diagnosed with a serious disease.

Gigerenzer and Hoffrage sought ways to help doctors interpret the results of diagnostic tests, and they demonstrated that numbers presented as counts of occurrences instead of probabilities are much easier to understand. Sedlmeier and Gigerenzer developed a brief and effective tutorial program for calculating probabilities of disease based on diagnostic test results.[55] Rather than saying that 1 percent of women have breast cancer, say that one out of one hundred women has breast cancer. Say that eighty out of one hundred women with breast cancer get a positive mammography, and so on. The different phrasing helps promote correct reasoning. The problem above would be given as follows:

Suppose that:

- One hundred out of 10,000 women at age forty who participate in routine screening have breast cancer.
- Eighty of every one hundred women with breast cancer will get a positive mammography. (The probability that the disease is detected by a mammography is 80 percent.)
- Nine hundred fifty out of 9,900 women without breast cancer will also get a positive mammography. (The probability that a woman tests positive although she does not have the disease is 9.6 percent.)

If women in this age group undergo a routine screening, about what fraction with positive mammographies will actually have breast cancer?

The answer is straightforward. The total number with positive mammographies is 80 + 950, or 1,030. Of those 1,030, 80 have cancer. Expressed as a proportion, this is 80/1,030, or 0.07767, or 7.8 percent.

Laypersons, too, if they are to make informed choices regarding their medical options, must often evaluate the results of screening tests. So Galesic and colleagues presented information about two medical screening tests to older and younger laypersons with varying degrees of competence in mathematical skills.[56] When the information was presented as counts of occurrences rather than probabilities, subjects evaluated the results much more accurately. They did so even without having received any explicit training.

PROBABILISTIC THINKING

Andereck wrote about a doctor whose patient was suffering from an easily diagnosed sinus infection.[57] The doctor ordered a series of tests that cost the patient $10,000. In trying to explain why so many doctors order expensive and unnecessary tests, Andereck rejected the notions that they do so for financial gain or as defense against malpractice suits.

He wrote that they rarely receive financial compensation from tests or procedures performed by others, and most have never been successfully sued for malpractice. His explanation is that doctors as a group have little tolerance for ambiguity and uncertainty. He wrote that if a doctor is 90 percent sure of a diagnosis and there is a $10,000 test that can make her 95 percent certain, she is likely to order the test. She might say that the reason is to give her patient the best possible care, but the underlying motivation is her need for certainty.

But many medical disorders cannot be diagnosed with certainty, so diagnosticians must rely on probabilities. Unfortunately, many are poorly trained in probability assessment. Following are some suggestions for improvement.

Skilled diagnosticians collect the relevant evidence about their patients' signs and symptoms and develop tentative hypotheses about disorders that could plausibly be responsible. They may order one or more diagnostic tests, many of which have well-documented sensitivity and specificity (see the next section for definitions). The tests can help them revise their probability estimates. Regrettably, as Richardson and colleagues pointed out, the probability estimates are often incorrect.[58] For example, physicians know that certain risk factors, such as family history of premature coronary artery disease, age, male gender, smoking, diabetes mellitus, increased serum cholesterol, and hypertension are powerful predictors of long-term coronary artery disease. But when patients are brought into emergency department settings, the classical risk factors add little or no useful information to that derived from the patients' specific symptoms, history of heart disease, and electrocardiographic findings. Nevertheless, the classic factors strongly influenced the decision making of board-certified, highly experienced emergency physicians.[59]

Unless pretest probabilities are accurate, revising them on the basis of diagnostic test results is a meaningless exercise. So Richardson and colleagues surveyed the literature to see whether credible research evidence was available to inform estimates of pretest probabilities. For a large majority of medical conditions of their newly admitted patients, the answer was yes. They urged doctors to seek and make use of such evidence.

LIKELIHOOD RATIOS

Many diagnostic tests give inconclusive results. For example, Croswell and colleagues reviewed data from a large-scale study in which patients received screening tests for several cancers, including prostate cancer for men and endometrial and ovarian cancer for women.[60] For 60 percent of the men and 49 percent of the women, at least one positive test was not associated with cancer. Still, tests provide one piece of evidence that doctors can use in conjunction with other pieces to estimate whether or not a patient has a particular disease. Likelihood ratios are helpful in this regard. The likelihood ratio for a positive result (LR+) tells how much the odds of the disease increase when a test is positive. The likelihood ratio for a negative result (LR−) tells how much the odds of the disease decrease when a test is negative.

To compute LRs, it is necessary to know the sensitivity and specificity of the diagnostic test. These are typically provided by the test's manufacturer. The Cochrane Collaboration (a group of more than ten thousand volunteers in more than ninety countries who review the effects of health-care interventions) has begun publishing reviews of test accuracy.

Sensitivity: Sensitivity describes the degree to which a test gives false negative results. A test with 0.9 sensitivity will come back positive 90 percent of the time for patients who have the condition tested for. These patients are called true positives. Ten percent of patients who have the condition will get negative test results. They are called false negatives. A doctor who wishes to rule out the possibility that her patient has a particular disease should use a highly sensitive test—a patient with the disease is unlikely to have a negative result.

Specificity: Specificity describes the degree to which a test gives false positive results. A test with 0.8 specificity will come back negative 80 percent of the time for patients who do not have the condition. They are called true negatives. Twenty percent of patients who do not have the condition will get positive test results. They are called false positives. If a test has high specificity, a doctor can be confident that a patient who tests positive has the disease.

$$LR+ = \text{sensitivity} / (1 - \text{specificity})$$

$$LR- = (1 - \text{sensitivity}) / \text{specificity}$$

For a test with 0.9 sensitivity and 0.8 specificity,

$$LR+ = 0.9 / (1 - .0.8) = 4.5$$
and

$$LR- = (1 - 0.9) / 0.8 = .125$$

A likelihood ratio calculator is available on the Web.[61]

If test results are positive, the larger the LR+, the more likely it is that the patient has the disease. An LR+ greater than ten indicates that the patient very probably has the disease. For negative results, the smaller the LR−, the less likely that the patient has the disease. An LR− less than .1 indicates that the patient very probably does not.

The likelihood ratio plus whatever additional information is available can be used to compute the patient's odds of having the disease. This is done by multiplying the likelihood ratio by the doctor's pretest estimate of the odds of disease. The odds, given a positive test, = estimate of odds before testing × LR+; and the odds for negative test results = odds before testing × LR−.

Example: Computing LRs, Odds Ratios, and Likelihood Ratios

Suppose that after taking into account a person's age, gender, symptoms, and all other pertinent information, a doctor estimates that a patient has a probability of 40 percent of having a particular disease. Suppose, too, that a test for that disease has a sensitivity of 90 percent and specificity of 90 percent. Then LR+ = 0.9 / (1 − 0.9) = 9; and LR− = (1 − 0.9) / 0.9 = 0.11.

To find the odds that the patient has the disease, first convert the pretest probability to odds form. For a probability of 40 percent, the odds are 40: (100 − 40) = 4:6.

Next, if the test results were positive, multiply the odds by the LR+: (4:6) × 9 = 36:6.

Convert the answer back to a probability. The probability is the number before the colon divided by itself plus the number after the colon.

36:6 = 36 / (36 + 6) = 36 / 42 = 0.86 = 86 percent. The likelihood that the patient has the disease is 86 percent.

For negative test results, use LR–. First convert the pretest probability to odds form. The answer is 4:6, as before. Next, multiply by LR–: 4:6 × 0.1 = 0.4:6.

Then convert the posttest odds back to a probability: 0.4:6 = 0.4 / (0.4 + 6) = 0.4 / 6.4 = 0.06, or 6 percent. The likelihood that the patient has the disease is 6 percent.

One website contains a list of likelihood ratios for many tests and medical conditions.[62]

TIPS ESPECIALLY FOR PATIENTS

Patients should feel comfortable about seeking second opinions. The NYU Medical Center suggests that patients do so under any of the following circumstances:

- A medical condition or problem is considered serious.
- Surgery is one of the treatment options suggested.
- Numerous possible treatment options are available.
- After consulting with his or her doctor, the patient still has a number of unanswered questions.
- The patient is told by the doctor that a specific type of treatment cannot be used to treat his or her condition.
- The patient is told by the doctor that nothing, or nothing more, can be done to treat his or her condition.
- Following treatment, the condition recurs.
- A cause for the patient's symptoms is not found, but the symptoms continue.
- The patient feels that something is wrong with the diagnosis or suggested treatment.

LOOKING AHEAD

In this chapter we've discussed various strategies for improving diagnostic accuracy. Most errors occur because the health-care system is imperfect—teamwork and communication are inefficient—and because of cognitive errors on the part of individual physicians. Straightforward solutions have been proposed for many of the system errors. Many cognitive errors can also be easily corrected. Commentators have urged physicians to be open to alternative possibilities even after they have made a preliminary diagnosis; premature closure is a major cause of diagnostic error.

Once a diagnosis is made, treatment can be initiated. In the United States, treatment most often takes the form of drug prescription. In the next chapter, we cite evidence showing that drugs are often incorrectly prescribed, and we suggest ways to improve prescribing practices.

(7)

PRESCRIPTIONS FOR PRESCRIBING

The prescription of drugs plays a major role in medical practice. During 2006, drugs were prescribed in 70.6 percent of all office visits to a U.S. physician. About 1.9 billion drugs were mentioned in office visits that year, resulting in an average of more than two drug mentions per visit.[1] In 2009, consumers spent more than $300 billion on prescription drugs.

Doctors can choose from more than 13,200 approved drug products, and more are added each year. In the years 2005 through 2008, between 78 and 101 new drugs were approved annually. So it is important to ask where physicians get their drug information. In part, they learn by experience, especially if it is accompanied by feedback (see pp. 110–112). Conferences and discussions with colleagues also help. They read the medical literature—but see pp. 24–25 to appreciate why that is problematic. Several other sources also give reason for concern, because drug company marketing plays a role in all of them. We discuss medical schools, the *Physicians' Desk Reference*, continuing medical education courses, drug advertisements aimed at doctors, use of experts, drug company representatives, FDA committees, expert panels, and formularies.

Marketing

U.S. drug companies spend an average of about $10,000 per physi-
cian per year on marketing. The *New York Times* reported that "doctors
who have close relationships with drug makers tend to prescribe more,
newer and pricier drugs regardless of the drug's efficacy over less expensive brand name or generic medications."[8] When residents at one
teaching hospital were checked, 97 percent were found to have items
bearing drug company brand names in their pockets.[9]

The newest, most expensive brand-name drugs are marketed most
heavily because they have the highest profit margins. Consumers end
up paying higher prices. A greater problem is that many adverse effects of drugs do not show up until after the drugs have been approved,
so the first users are essentially test subjects. From a purely medical
standpoint, the best strategy would be to introduce new drugs gradually
to a limited number of patients. But drug companies want to market
the drugs while they are protected by patent. The painkiller Vioxx was
launched in 1999 and within five years had been prescribed to more
than eighty million patients. It was withdrawn from the market in 2004
due to safety issues. One FDA official estimated that Vioxx caused
88,000–139,000 heart attacks, 40 percent of which were fatal.

Medical Schools

Medical school students take at least one formal course in pharmacology. Several excellent textbooks are available, but much of the
information comes from lectures and other interactions with faculty.
Yet instructors often have strong conflicts of interest and present biased
information. A Harvard Medical School student became upset when
one of his professors promoted the benefits of cholesterol drugs and
belittled a student who asked about side effects.[2] The student searched
the Internet and learned that the professor was a paid consultant to ten
drug companies, including five makers of cholesterol treatments.

The American Medical Student Association (AMSA) urges both students and practicing physicians to refuse all personal gifts from drug
companies. In 2008, AMSA released the PharmFree Scorecard, which
evaluated medical colleges and colleges of osteopathic medicine according to the extent to which they interacted with drug companies. Only five

U.S. medical schools received an A grade, signifying that school policy restricts pharmaceutical representatives from access to both the medical school campus and its academic medical centers. Harvard's prestigious medical school received an F (signifying that a school either lacks policies or encourages students to get information from drug representatives). In the months following the report, almost 20 percent of Harvard faculty admitted that they or a family member had a financial interest in a business related to their teaching, research, or clinical care. As a result, Harvard changed its policies and in 2009 received a grade of B.[3]

Other schools lag behind. In the 2009 report, of participating U.S. medical schools, nine received As, thirty-six Bs, eighteen Cs, seventeen Ds, and thirty-five Fs. A survey of all 125 accredited medical schools and the fifteen largest teaching hospitals in the United States revealed that nearly two-thirds of department heads have financial ties to the drug or medical-device industry.[4]

New drugs have an effective patent life of about thirteen to fifteen years. After that, generic versions sold at substantially lower prices may come onto the market. Faced with reduced profit margins, drug companies typically try to develop new drugs—even if the old ones are effective. One consequence is that consumers end up paying more for drugs. A second is that older drugs are constantly being phased out. By the time that twenty-five-year-old medical students have matured into forty-year-old physicians, most of the drugs that they have learned about will no longer be in vogue.

The *Physicians' Desk Reference*

The *Physicians' Desk Reference* (*PDR*), a volume published annually, is a major source of post–medical school drug information. Although the list price of the 2010 *PDR* is $96.95, it is distributed free to most physicians. Drug companies share the cost of the free distribution. The *PDR* lists drugs by class and has information on dosages and contraindications. Ninety percent of doctors call it their most used reference book.[5] But there are problems:

- The information for the *PDR* is supplied by drug houses, and they push for high doses.[6]

- Data on dose-response relationships are regarded as internal working data of the company and hardly ever published. So doctors who rely on the *PDR* rarely learn what the lowest effective dosage is or how far a dose should be increased if the initial effect is insufficient.
- Drug company sales representatives may push a drug for many conditions, but the *PDR* typically lists it for only one, leading to problems with dosages.
- The standard dose may be the wrong one for at least some patients. Individuals may differ greatly in their sensitivity to both beneficial and harmful effects, but drug company marketing departments prefer a one-size-fits-all approach.

Mullen and colleagues compared *PDR* overdose treatment recommendations with those of five major textbook references.[7] Of the twenty *PDR* entries studied, sixteen had at least one deficiency, and five had two or more deficiencies. Thirteen omitted an indicated specific treatment, three recommended treatments that should never be used, and four recommended ineffective treatments with potential for harm. One entry had remained unchanged for twenty-four years.

Continuing Medical Education Courses

Most physicians must complete accredited continuing medical education (CME) programs to maintain their medical licenses, hospital privileges, and specialty board certifications. About half of CME funding comes from drug companies that pay experts to develop, review, and present content for CME programs. The Accreditation Council for CME (ACCME), which sets and enforces CME program standards within the United States, reported that commercial enterprises provided $1 billion in 2008.[10] Many accredited program providers violate standards set by ACCME. Davis wrote:

[I]ndustry funding can skew CME content in various ways to match the goals of industry. This skewing may be felt in the subtle influence of industry on the selection of topics (do medical-school CME curricula devote as much time to the *diagnosis* of hypertension as to its *treatment*?) or, at a more general level, in what receives support and what does not (courses on social pathologies are less common than those, say, on diseases with specifically "medical" management).[11]

Ten physicians were invited to attend an all-expenses-paid symposium at a popular vacation site. The company tracked the physicians' prescribing patterns for two drugs for twenty-two months before and seventeen months after the symposium. The physicians had predicted that their attendance would not affect their prescribing practices, but their prescriptions for one drug increased 87 percent and for the other, 272 percent.[12]

Drug Advertisements Aimed at Doctors

> Without pharmaceutical sponsorship many journals would not survive.
>
> —Abassi and Smith[13]

Advertisements are a major source of information about drugs for doctors, but the ads frequently cite medical research unsupported by the advertised claims. Drug companies often cite their own research, which is typically located in company files and off-limits to outsiders.

Villanueva and colleagues assessed all ads for antihypertensive and lipid-lowering drugs published in six Spanish medical journals that had at least one bibliographical reference. In 44.1 percent of cases, the promotional statement was not supported by the reference.[14] Following the introduction of tougher regulations for drug advertisements in Switzerland, Santiago and colleagues assessed drug claims published in major medical journals—53 percent either were not supported by the cited referenced studies or were based on potentially biased study information.[15] Othman and colleagues examined twenty-four articles that reviewed advertisements from twenty-six countries.[16] Less than 67 percent of the claims made in the advertisements were supported by a systematic review, a meta-analysis, or a randomized control trial. Othman and colleagues wrote that their results "suggest the need for a global pro-active and effective regulatory system to ensure that information provided in medical journal advertising is supporting the quality use of medicines."

Doctors typically report that advertising has minimal influence on their prescribing habits. They are either fooling themselves or lying. Despite the absence of scientific support, they tend to believe in the effectiveness of heavily promoted products.[17] Abt Associates randomly assigned doctors to receive low, medium, or high frequencies of exposure to advertisements for a specific cardiovascular drug.[18] The publishers of journals to which the doctors subscribed agreed to place the ads with the appropriate frequency. During the yearlong study, doctors in each of the three groups wrote more prescriptions for the drug than they had written previously. The ones exposed to the most ads increased the number of their prescriptions the most.

Reliance on Experts

When experts voice strong opinions, doctors listen—possibly unaware that the experts, often referred to as "key opinion leaders," may be receiving generous fees to peddle influence on behalf of drug companies. Moynihan[19] quoted Kimberly Elliott, a former drug company sales representative: "Key opinion leaders were salespeople for us, and we would routinely measure the return on our investment, by tracking prescriptions before and after their presentations. If that speaker didn't make the impact the company was looking for, then you wouldn't invite them back." Elliott said that she would pay these respected doctors $2,500 for a single lecture, which was based largely on slides supplied by the company.

As noted in a *New York Times* article, these experts typically claim that payments from drug companies have no effect on their medical practice.[20] The same article quoted two people with very different opinions:

- Harvard professor Max Bazerman: "When honest human beings have a vested stake in seeing the world in a particular way, they're incapable of objectivity and independence. A doctor who represents a pharmaceutical company will tend to see the data in a slightly more positive light and as a result will overprescribe that company's drugs."
- Kathleen Slattery-Moschkau, a former sales representative for Bristol-Myers Squibb and Johnson & Johnson: "The vast majority

of the time that we did any sort of paid relationship with a physician, they increased the use of our drug. I hate to say it out loud, but it all comes down to ways to manipulate the doctors."

Influential Harvard child psychiatrist Joseph Biederman's endorsement of the use of powerful antipsychotic drugs in young people helped fuel a huge increase in their use.[21] Whether or not the children benefited, Biederman certainly did—he received at least $1.4 million in income from drug companies. Ortho-McNeil-Janssen Pharmaceuticals, Inc., a subsidiary of Johnson & Johnson, drafted a scientific abstract on their drug Risperdal; Biederman signed it as the author and gave advice on how to handle the fact, not mentioned in the abstract, that children given placebos rather than Risperdal also improved. The abstract was presented at a professional meeting. Biederman persuaded Ortho-McNeil-Janssen to provide almost $1 million to fund a research center to focus on children and adolescents with bipolar disorders. One of the center's publicly stated missions was to "move forward the commercial goals of J & J."

In Minnesota, drug makers must disclose payments to doctors. Seven of the past eight presidents of the Minnesota Psychiatric Society have served as consultants to drug makers.

Influential psychiatrist Frederick Goodwin, a former director of the National Institute of Mental Health, received at least $1.3 million from drug companies from 2000 through 2007.[22] He said on radio that children with bipolar disorder face the risk of brain damage if not treated. He added that modern treatments "have proven both safe and effective in bipolar children." On the same day he received $2,500 from Glaxo-SmithKline to lecture on Lamictal—one of the drugs. He received more than $329,000 during that year for promoting Lamictal.

In 1999, Surgeon General C. Everett Koop testified before a U.S. Congress hearing on the health hazards of latex gloves.[23] He said that the reports of allergic reactions to these gloves by hospital nurses and other health-care workers were exaggerated. He called the complaints borderline hysteria. Koop's opinions were widely reported and had an important impact on Congress and the general public. At the time he testified, Koop had just completed a four-year business contract with a major latex-glove manufacturing corporation, WRP. He did not tell the committee of his involvement. Koop earned $656,250 in consulting fees from the company in the four-year period from 1994 to 1998.

Many of the apparently impartial researchers used by the World Health Organization are paid by the companies that produce vaccines, signing their names with other titles but actually representing the drug industry. They played a major role in persuading the public that the H1N1 swine flu is a pandemic—and that worldwide vaccination is necessary to defeat the disease. As of June 2009, one of the experts in the WHO H1N1-specific advisory group, Albert Ostenhaus, had economic interests in several drug companies. Frederick Hayden was part of a group that advises WHO on vaccines—and also a paid adviser for drug companies Roche, RW Johnson, SmithKline Beecham, and Glaxo Wellcome. Arnold Monto, also a member of the advisory group, was a paid consultant for MedImmune (which produces the intranasal flu vaccine), Glaxo Wellcome, and ViroPharma. Wolf Dieter Ludwig, head of the drug commission of the German Medical Association, said, "The authorities have succumbed to a campaign by pharmaceutical companies, which seeks to monetize a non-existent threat." [24]

Drug Company Representatives (Detailmen)

You'll never meet an ugly drug rep.

—Psychiatrist Thomas Carli

Drug companies hire young, attractive people to promote drugs to doctors. About one hundred thousand of them in the United States visit doctors' offices with drug samples, dinner invitations, tickets to ball games, and various other gifts. Drug companies spend about $5 billion annually on detailmen and their gifts. Detailmen try to build strong relationships and encourage their clients to increase prescriptions of their company's drug. They claim that they provide a service by keeping doctors updated on the newest and best drugs. But Gene Carbona, executive director of sales for *The Medical Letter*, wrote, "There's nothing of value with respect to drug information that comes from a pharmaceutical industry rep. There is absolutely no reason for any physician to enter into a clinical discussion about the care of his or her patients with somebody who's not a physician."[25] Carbona noted that each drug rep talks to five or ten physicians a day, causing the medical profession to be flooded with far more daily targeted messages than any other industry.

A meta-analysis of twenty-nine studies showed a strong relationship between gifts or meals given by drug representatives to doctors and the doctors' subsequent prescribing habits and requests for formulary additions.[26] The altered patterns were still evident two years later.

Drug manufacturers can legally promote drug use only for indications that have been FDA approved, but doctors can prescribe any approved drug for any condition. Nonapproved use, called off-label prescribing, is sometimes justified. For example, after carbamazepine was approved as an anticonvulsant, doctors observed that it is also effective in treating bipolar disorder; European physicians use it for this purpose. But U.S. drug companies did not do the research to get FDA approval for carbamazepine as a mood stabilizer until they developed a long-acting patentable form. Before that happened, it was prescribed off-label.

Although off-label prescribing is sometimes justified, more frequently it is not. Radley and colleagues examined off-label prescribing of 160 common drugs and found that it accounted for 21 percent of all prescriptions. Most off-label drug uses (73 percent) were shown to have little or no scientific support.[27] Walton and colleagues found that fourteen drugs commonly prescribed for off-label uses lack proof of safety and effectiveness for such uses.[28]

Drug companies use detailmen to try to indirectly promote off-label drug uses. Steinman and colleagues analyzed market research forms completed by physicians after they had received a detail visit for the drug gabapentin.[29] Physicians rated the visits (of median duration five minutes) to have high informational value and overall quality even though some of the off-label uses for which gabapentin was promoted were not well supported by clinical trial evidence. During this period, gabapentin was approved by the FDA only for the adjunctive treatment of partial seizures, but in 38 percent of visits the main message involved at least one off-label use. After receiving the visit, 46 percent of physicians reported the intention to increase their prescribing or recommending of gabapentin in the future. No physicians reported the intention to decrease their future use or recommendation of the drug.

Steinman and colleagues cited several studies that found positive associations between the frequency of interactions with sales representatives and prescribing behavior. In self-report studies, approximately one-third to two-thirds of physician respondents perceive themselves to be influenced by sales representatives; even more believe that other physicians are influenced.

Comparing Four Marketing Strategies

Neslin analyzed 391 drugs that each had annual revenues of at least $25 million between 1995 and 1999.[30] His purpose was to find out how spending on different forms of marketing affected the profitability (return on investment, ROI) of each drug. He examined the four principal methods used to market drugs: detailing, direct-to-consumer advertising, medical journal advertising, and physician meetings and events. For every dollar spent on detailing, the company's return on investment increased by $1.72 (72 percent rate of return). For drugs with $200 million or more in annual sales, the ROI for detailing was $10.92. Advertising in medical journals for the same class of drugs had a $5.42 ROI; direct-to-consumer advertising had a $1.37 ROI; and physician meetings and events had a $3.56 ROI. Marketing pays.

FDA Committees

Federal law forbids experts who vote on new drug approvals to have a direct financial interest in the drug they are evaluating. But most experts have ties to the drug industry. If FDA officials were to choose completely unbiased panelists, they would be leaving the treatment guidelines largely to non-experts. So the FDA grants waivers to the experts. Most drugs available today were evaluated by FDA committees packed with industry-funded scientists. At 92 percent of the 159 FDA advisory committee meetings between 1998 and 2000, at least one member had a financial conflict of interest. Many had contracts of more than $100,000 with the companies that produced the drugs under evaluation. At 55 percent of meetings, half or more of the FDA advisers had conflicts of interest. And at 102 meetings that dealt with approval of a specific drug,

33 percent of committee members had conflicts.[31] At least one committee member disclosed a conflict of interest in 73 percent of the 221
advisory committee meetings held from January 1, 2001, to December
31, 2004. Only 1 percent of committee members were recused over that
period.[32] (Compounding the problem, approximately one-fourth of researchers have industry affiliations, and roughly two-thirds of academic
institutions hold equity in start-ups that sponsor research performed at
the same institutions.)[33]

Lurie and Wolfe surveyed doctors who reviewed new drugs for the
FDA.[34] The doctors told of twenty-seven drugs that the FDA had approved in the previous three years even though the reviewer most
familiar with all the data on the drug opposed approval. The doctors
described inappropriate phone calls from sponsors and pressure from
Congress. In some instances, supervisors did not permit them to present
data critical of drugs to FDA advisory committees.

Expert Panels

Expert panels are selected by government agencies to write guidelines for doctors. Ezra Klein, an associate editor at *The American Prospect*, wrote about a survey of two hundred expert panels that issued
practice guidelines; one-third of the panelists acknowledged having
financial interest in the drugs they considered.[35] Ninety percent of the
psychiatrists on panels who wrote the 2009 clinical guidelines for treating depression, bipolar disorder, and schizophrenia had financial ties to
drug companies. The guidelines focus heavily on drugs and devote little
space to nondrug treatments or to removing mentally ill patients from
drugs. In 2004, a government-selected panel changed the definition of
high cholesterol level that reclassified more than 23 million people as
borderline at-risks who should begin taking cholesterol-lowering drugs.
Drug company sales and stock prices soared. Perhaps the increase reflects sound medical practice, but there is reason for doubt—eight of
nine members of the panel writing the recommendations had financial
ties to the makers of cholesterol-lowering drugs. A 2002 survey found
that more than 80 percent of the doctors on panels that write clinical
practice guidelines had financial ties to drug makers.[36]

Business Deals

Lists of drugs that can be used by HMO doctors are called formularies. The rationale behind formularies is a good one—experts within the HMO can pick the best drug for treating a particular condition, and all the prescribers can then share and learn from their experiences. (Doctors may prescribe drugs not on the formulary, but they have to justify their decisions and do considerable paperwork.) In many instances, however, drugs have been added to formularies for business rather than medical reasons. Drug manufacturers may give a discount to an HMO if their particular drug is used exclusively—or if another of their drugs is added to the formulary even though it is inferior to a competitor's drug.

ALL IS NOT LOST

Interventions

Several strategies have been developed for improving prescribing practices. Grindrod and colleagues[37] and Ostini and colleagues[38] reviewed the literature comparing different types of interventions. Ostini's group encouraged future researchers to identify ways to prevent inappropriate prescribing of new drugs rather than attempting to intervene once prescribing habits are entrenched.

The two types of interventions that most consistently showed a positive effect on prescribing were audit and feedback and educational outreach visits. Audit and feedback has been defined as "the provision of any summary of clinical performance over a specified period of time. The summary may include data on processes of care (e.g., number of diagnostic tests ordered), clinical endpoints (e.g., blood pressure readings), and clinical practice recommendations (proportion of patients managed in line with a recommendation)."[39] Jamtvedt and colleagues wrote, "It appears logical that healthcare professionals would be prompted to modify their practice if given feedback that their clinical practice was inconsistent with that of their peers or accepted guidelines."[40] Their review concluded that audit and feedback can improve professional practice, although the effects are generally small to moderate. Audit and feedback was most effective when baseline compliance with recommendations was low.

Educational outreach visits, also called academic detailing, are typically implemented in a medical school or school of pharmacy and operate independently of drug companies. The programs employ physicians, pharmacists, nurses, and other clinical professionals to provide unbiased information to prescribers. After thoroughly reviewing the literature on a topic, they distill the findings into key messages for presentation in training and educational materials. They focus on clinical topics where the gap between evidence-based prescribing and actual prescribing is large. They may recommend generic options in lieu of costly brand-name drugs. As they grow in number, their cost may come down through sharing of educational materials, training programs, and data management systems. Several states have developed academic detailing programs.

Encourage Comparative Effectiveness Studies

To gain FDA approval of a drug, the manufacturer must show only that the drug is both safe and more effective than a placebo for the condition it is designed to treat. So a safe drug that cures 60 percent of patients while a placebo cures only 40 percent will be approved—even if an already available and less expensive drug cures 90 percent.[41] Although a "me-too" drug may confer no medical benefits beyond those already available, it will probably increase company profits and may even outsell the more effective drug. Sales often depend less on medical effectiveness than on marketing department creativity. From the time it went on the market in 2001 until 2005, Nexium, a "me-too" drug for stomach acid, earned $3.9 billion for its maker, AstraZeneca. As another example, TNF inhibitors are used to treat diseases such as rheumatoid arthritis. The 2007 sales of three virtually identical ones were $5.3 billion for Enbrel, $3.3 billion for Remicade, and $3.1 billion for Humira. Research on completely new types of drugs is much riskier. From 1998 through 2003, 379 of the 487 drugs approved by the FDA were classified as having therapeutic qualities similar to those of one or more already marketed drugs. Only 67 of the 487 were new drugs considered likely improvements over older ones.[42]

Alexander and colleagues argued that the current method of testing new treatments (not just drug treatments) against placebo causes a variety of problems and should not be the sole mechanism for determining approval.[43] "A drug with no objective advantage over other available drugs can enter the market easily when the threshold is performance relative to placebo. This process may favor look-alike drugs and allow for market differentiation based on characteristics (e.g., capsule color) that obscure potential clinical comparison based on effectiveness."

Recent history offers several instances of enthusiastically adopted innovations that were later found wanting. Examples include short-acting calcium channel blockers for hypertension, troglitazone for diabetes, tegaserod for irritable bowel syndrome, and rofecoxib for mild to moderate pain. And, because there were no head-to-head comparisons of treatments, some outdated clinical strategies persisted while effective therapies were not broadly adopted. Therefore, Alexander and colleagues suggested that drug packages be labeled to indicate performance against competitors. For example, a package insert might state: "This drug has not been found to be superior to the other calcium channel blockers in the treatment of hypertension." Such statements would help prescribers make better decisions.

The health-care bill passed by Congress in March 2010 calls for increased funding for comparative effectiveness research: directly comparing different treatments and strategies against one another. Hochman and McCormick[44] mentioned, and then refuted, several criticisms of the proposed change.

The first potential criticism they address is that comparative effectiveness studies focus on analyses of older, previously completed studies and are therefore unlikely to help patients in 2010. In response, Hochman and McCormick state that "comparative effectiveness research differs from non-comparative studies only with respect to the types of questions they address. There is no reason to suspect these studies will focus on older data."

Next they address the concern that requiring drug companies to compare new therapies with alternative treatments rather than placebos might make drug research too expensive or risky. They acknowledge that the proposed change will require a shift in how companies study their drugs, but they argue that this will encourage rather than stifle innovation. "If companies were required to compare new therapies with existing ones, it might promote the development of novel classes of medications that offer real advantages."

They consider the criticism that comparative effectiveness studies, by denigrating therapies that prove inferior in large studies but are effective among certain patients, will dissuade doctors from using clinical judgment to tailor treatments to individual patients. They respond by noting that comparative effectiveness research will make personalized medicine more meaningful. It will lead to examination of therapies in different populations such as the elderly, children, and underrepresented minorities, as well as toward research that will help doctors tailor therapies using genetic information.

Finally, they answer the concern that comparative effectiveness studies could be used by insurers to deny coverage for expensive therapies that prove no better than cheaper alternatives. They acknowledge the possibility but point out that such denials will usually be in the patient's best interest. Many patients currently receive treatments that are less effective than alternatives, but without comparative effectiveness studies no one knows which treatments they are. "Furthermore, comparative effectiveness research may be used to justify therapies that are not effective in the population as a whole but work among a subset of patients."

Ban Direct-to-Consumer Advertising

The only two developed countries where direct-to-consumer advertising (DTCA) is currently legal are the United States and New Zealand. In 2007, drug companies spent more than $4.9 billion on DTCA of prescription drugs in the United States.[45] Proponents claim that ads educate people about health conditions and available treatments and empower them to become more active participants in their own care. Critics argue that DTCA leads to poor prescribing. Patients ask for the latest, most costly, and most heavily marketed drugs or devices. Physicians may try to dissuade them, but only by lengthening the office visit and straining the doctor-patient relationship.

Patients' drug requests are typically granted—even when more effective drugs or nondrug treatments would serve them better. Mintzes and colleagues asked 1,431 patients from the cities of Sacramento, California, and Vancouver, British Columbia, to fill out questionnaires regarding drug ads.[46] Of the Sacramento patients (who are presumably exposed to DTCA), 7.2 percent requested advertised drugs as opposed to 3.3 percent in Vancouver (where patients are not exposed to DTCA). Two-thirds of the patients requesting a specific drug received it.

The FDA requires that all DTCA contain both an accurate statement of a drug's effects and an evenhanded discussion of its benefits and risks/ adverse effects. But that does not happen. Frosch and colleagues analyzed ads shown on television during evening news and prime time hours.[47] They found that 82 percent made factual claims and 86 percent made rational arguments for product use. But few described causes of the medical condition (26 percent), risk factors (26 percent), or prevalence (25 percent). Ninety-five percent made emotional appeals, and 58 percent portrayed the product as a medical breakthrough. The authors concluded, "The ads have limited educational value and may oversell the benefits of drugs in ways that might conflict with promoting population health."

Abel analyzed thirty-nine advertisements for twelve products for bleeding disorders.[48] On average, approximately twice the amount of text was devoted to benefits as compared to risks/adverse effects, and the latter was more difficult to read. Only about two-thirds of the advertising claims were considered by a majority of the experts to be based on at least low-quality evidence.

Kusuma and colleagues cited literature showing that nearly 87 percent of television ads present the potential benefits of drugs in vague, qualitative terms not backed by scientific data and that only seven out of fifty claims made by implant manufacturers in print media ads were well supported by scientific data.[49] The authors expressed concern that DTCA for orthopedic surgery services and devices is rapidly increasing.

TIPS ESPECIALLY FOR PATIENTS

In this chapter, we have shown that even the brightest, most conscientious doctors cannot possibly know everything about the drug and non-drug alternatives available for each medical condition, so we encourage patients to take active roles in their treatments. We offer a few suggestions to patients to increase the likelihood that they will have favorable outcomes.

First, appreciate that medical experts who write guidelines for doctors often have strong incentives to encourage drug prescription as the treatment of choice. Patients should not be reluctant to ask their doctors whether nondrug treatments or general lifestyle changes are feasible alternatives. Second, if a drug is prescribed, they should ask whether it's for an approved condition or an off-label use; if the latter, they should ask about the evidence for its effectiveness for the unapproved condition. Patients should ask whether the prescribed drug is on the formulary and, if so, whether there might be a better drug that is not on the formulary.

Patients should not allow advertisers to encourage them to try to influence doctors about which drugs to prescribe. They should realize that advertising material rarely has sufficient information and is designed to sell, not to promote good prescribing habits. Patients should trust doctors who would rather prescribe a nonadvertised drug.

Patients who want to get seriously involved in their treatments should go to the Cochrane collaboration at http://www.cochrane.org. They can type in keywords and learn what volunteer (not-for-profit) experts have to say. PubMed (http://www.ncbi.nlm.nih.gov/sites/entrez) is another useful source.

Following are some additional dos and don'ts:

- Whenever you go to the doctor, tell her about all the drugs you take. Carry a written list that includes dosage and frequency.
- If your doctor prescribes a drug, ask about generics or alternatives.
- Don't be afraid to ask your doctor whether she has a sample of the drug; then you can try it out before committing to it.
- If you have any questions about the drug, first ask your doctor, and then ask your pharmacist.

LOOKING AHEAD

In this chapter we've discussed various factors that make it difficult for doctors to get reliable information about the drugs they prescribe.

Certain remedies were suggested, but, unfortunately, two important ones (requiring comparative effectiveness studies and banning direct-to-consumer advertising) cannot be implemented by individuals. The government must legislate the remedies. In the next chapter, we show that the specific properties of drugs and other treatments contribute only partially to their effectiveness. The expectations of patients concerning the treatments often play a major role.

(8)

EXPECTATION EFFECTS

Power to the Placebo

There is nothing either good or bad, but thinking makes it so.

—William Shakespeare, *Hamlet*, Act 2, Scene 2

The bard was prescient. Medical researchers have learned that people's beliefs play an enormous role in their general health and responses to treatment. Belief effects are pervasive, although often subtle. Seemingly trivial factors such as how doctors greet patients, diplomas they have hanging on the wall, and general office décor can profoundly affect patients' expectations and therefore treatment outcomes. First, we give a potpourri of examples outside the medical arena to show the range and power of belief effects. These are followed by many examples from within the field of medicine. Although subjective measures such as reported relief from pain have been used most frequently, many objective measures are strongly affected by expectations. Following the examples, we discuss suggested mechanisms to account for expectation effects. We conclude by suggesting strategies for maximizing positive expectations to improve patient health.

BELIEFS ABOUT INANIMATE OBJECTS AND NONHUMAN ANIMALS

In 1903, French physicist Andre Blondlot announced his discovery of a new kind of ray, which he called an N-ray, that intensified reflected light and was bent by aluminum. By 1906, at least forty people, including several eminent scientists, had reported observing N-rays, and more than three hundred scientific papers had described their properties. Then Blondlot gave a public demonstration. He placed an aluminum prism in the middle of several lenses and, with the room darkened (because N-rays are affected by light), he manipulated an apparatus to turn the prism. As the apparatus was moved, Blondlot's assistant reported changes in the intensity of the readings. But when the lights came back on, the audience saw physicist R. W. Wood in the front row with the prism in his hand. He had secretly removed it early in the demonstration. The observers' preconceptions had helped them "see" the nonexistent N-rays.[1]

People sampled wines while undergoing brain fMRIs. The subjects were told they were tasting five different cabernet sauvignons, but there were actually only three. Two wines were offered twice, marked with different prices. A $90 wine was marked with its real price and also marked $10, while another was presented at its real price of $5 and also marked $45. The medial orbitofrontal cortex, a brain area believed to encode for experienced pleasantness, became more active in the testers at the higher prices than at the lower ones. They also reported that the higher-priced wines had more pleasant flavor.[2]

Philosopher Bertrand Russell wrote about the effect of nationality of scientists on lab rats. "Animals studied by Americans rush about frantically, with an incredible display of hustle and pep, and at last achieve the desired result by chance. Animals observed by Germans sit still and think, and at last evolve the solution out of their inner consciousness."

BELIEFS ABOUT OTHER PEOPLE

Intellectual Performance

Rosenthal and Jacobson gave elementary-school students a test they called "The Harvard Test of Inflected Acquisition." They told the teachers—falsely—that the test could identify those students who would make especially rapid intellectual progress in the coming year, whether or not they were currently good students. Then they gave the teachers the names of students who, they said, had scored well on the test. In actuality, they had picked the names randomly from the class list. Any differences between these children and the rest of the class existed only in the minds of the teachers. When an intelligence test was administered at the end of the year, the selected children had greater IQ gains than the rest of the students. Their teachers gave them higher reading grades and reported that they were better behaved, friendlier, and more intellectually curious than their classmates, with greater promise of future success.[3]

Race

Subjects listened to a college basketball game and evaluated the performance of one of the players. All heard the same game, but some were led to believe that the player was black and others that the player was white. Those who believed him black thought he had exhibited greater athletic ability but less intelligence than did those who thought him white.[4]

Health

Patients with multiple sclerosis received either the drug cyclophosphamide or a placebo. After time intervals of six, twelve, and twenty-four months, they were examined by two neurologists. One neurologist knew which treatment each patient had received, and the other did not. Only the unblinded neurologist's scores demonstrated an apparent treatment benefit.[5]

BELIEFS ABOUT SELF

White golfers did better against black opponents if told that they were being judged on their "sport strategic intelligence" rather than on their "natural athletic ability."[6]

Steele argued that people whose social identity is attached to a negative stereotype tend to underperform in a manner consistent with the stereotype. They become anxious that they will conform to the negative stereotype, and the anxiety causes distraction that impairs performance. Steele noted that both genders and virtually every ethnic and racial group have had negative stereotypes applied to them.[7] Steele and Aronson matched black and white Stanford students in ability level and tested them on items from the Graduate Record Examination. They reasoned that the test would evoke in the black students the negative stereotype of blacks as having limited intellectual ability. And when the test was presented as a test of ability, whites outperformed blacks by a wide margin. But when the same test was presented as a laboratory task for studying how certain problems are generally solved, with no implications about level of intellectual ability, black and white students performed equally well.

In another study, Steele and Aronson asked one group of black and white students to list their race at the top of a difficult exam. The simple manipulation made race salient, and the black students performed more poorly than their SAT scores suggested they should. Another group was not asked to list race, and black students performed as well as their SAT scores suggested they should. White students were not affected by the manipulation.

Not all stereotyped beliefs are harmful. Two widely accepted stereotypes about mathematics ability are that men are superior to women and that Asians are superior to people of other races. Shih and colleagues asked some Asian American women subjects to indicate their gender and answer questions related to gender identity. Others were asked to indicate their ethnicity and answer questions related to their ethnic identity. Once prompted to think of themselves as either women or Asians, they were given a math test. Those reminded of their identity as Asians outperformed those reminded of their identity as women.[8] To get your highest possible score on a math test, pretend that you're an Asian man.

MEDICAL ISSUES

Mondloch and colleagues meta-analyzed studies that related patient expectations to health outcomes.[9] In fifteen of the sixteen studies, positive expectations were associated with better outcomes. The authors urged clinicians to clarify patients' expectations and assist them in having appropriate expectations of recovery. Patients who expect complications should be targeted for support and education prior to surgery. Following are representative examples that show effects of expectations on medical outcomes.

Psychotherapy

Southworth and Kirsch told some agoraphobics (people who fear open spaces) that they were to receive a proven treatment for agoraphobia. Then they received ten exposure sessions over a two- to three-week period. Others were given identical exposure sessions but told that the sessions were part of an assessment procedure and that actual treatment would begin at a later date. Those in the first group improved more rapidly and to a greater extent. Many other studies have shown that patients' expectations of psychotherapy treatment effectiveness are powerful predictors of outcome.[10]

Desharnais and colleagues had two groups of subjects participate in an aerobic exercise program. People in one group were told that the exercise would enhance their aerobic capacity. The others were told that the exercise would enhance both aerobic capacity and psychological well-being. Although both groups improved their aerobic capacity, only the second showed enhanced psychological well-being.[11]

Memory

Levy and Langer recruited mainland Chinese people and deaf Americans, because both groups tend to hold positive views of aging. They also recruited hearing Americans as a comparison group. As expected, the Chinese expressed the most positive views of aging, the deaf Americans the next most positive, and the hearing Americans the most negative views. Among the older participants, the pattern of memory performance mirrored the views of aging; the Chinese performed best, and the mainstream Americans worst. Among all the older participants, positivity of aging stereotypes and memory scores significantly correlated.[12]

Menopause

The relation between hormones and menopausal symptoms is complex and mediated to a great extent by expectations. There is substantial cross-cultural variation. Sievert and colleagues collected four-week recalls of twenty-five symptoms in women aged forty-five to fifty-five in the United States, Spain, Lebanon, and Morocco. The intercorrelation among symptoms differed in country-specific ways. For example, hot flashes grouped with vaginal dryness and sexual symptoms in Spain, grouped with general somatic symptoms in Morocco, and did not cluster with other symptoms in the United States or Lebanon. Vasomotor symptoms are the most frequently reported symptoms in Europe and North America, but in Asia, psychological complaints are more common. Yoruba women in Nigeria described joint pain most commonly.[13]

Warts

Talbot reported that doctors successfully eliminated warts by painting them with a brightly colored, inert dye and promising patients the warts would be gone when the color wore off.[14]

Whiplash

Carroll and colleagues surveyed individuals who had suffered traffic-related whiplash injury to the neck. After adjusting for several relevant factors, they found that those who expected to get better soon recovered and returned to work much more quickly than those who expected that they would never get better.[15]

Surgery

Mahomed and colleagues evaluated the relationship between patient expectations of total hip and knee arthroplasty (replacement of a joint or part of one by metal or plastic parts) and satisfaction six months after surgery. Patients filled out self-report questionnaires prior to surgery and six months postsurgery. Their expectations were not associated with preoperative health status. Yet people who expected complete pain relief showed better physical function and improvement in level of pain at six months postsurgery. Those who had had expectations of low risk of complications reported greater satisfaction.[16]

Yee and colleagues evaluated patients' expectations prior to spinal surgery and again postoperatively. Patients with high expectations reported greater postoperative improvements.[17]

Acupuncture

Patients who had just had dental surgery were given real acupuncture, in which a needle is inserted into the skin, or sham acupuncture, in which the needle does not enter the skin.[18] Then they were asked whether they believed they were in the placebo or treatment group. There was no significant difference between acupuncture and placebo groups in pain relief, but participants who believed they had received real acupuncture reported significantly less pain than patients who believed they had received a placebo.

Mass Hysteria

Mass psychogenic illness (MPI) has been described for more than six hundred years in a variety of cultures and settings. Jones gave an illustrative example. A high-school teacher noted a gasoline-like odor in her classroom one morning. She developed headache, nausea, shortness of breath, and dizziness. Students began complaining of similar symptoms. The school was evacuated, and emergency personnel from several counties responded. That day, one hundred people went to a local emergency department with symptoms reportedly related to exposure at the school. Five days later, the outbreak recurred. The school closed, and approximately seventy people sought emergency care. Physical examination and laboratory testing revealed no evidence of a toxic cause for the symptoms. A thorough multiagency environmental examination also failed to identify an explanation for the outbreak.[19]

Lorber and colleagues created a laboratory version of MPI.[20] They randomly assigned volunteers to inhale or not inhale a placebo described as a suspected environmental toxin that had been linked to four symptoms. The volunteers observed a confederate of the researchers inhale the substance and subsequently display the specified symptoms. Students who inhaled the placebo reported greater increases in symptoms, especially of the four specified ones.

Death

Women in the large-scale Framingham heart study who believed they were prone to heart disease were four times more likely to die than other women with similar risk factors.[21]

A dramatic proof that expectations can affect health comes from the 1940s work of physiologist Walter Cannon on so-called voodoo deaths. Cannon collected anecdotes from around the world of people who had died after being cursed, and he proposed a physiological explanation. He speculated that the fear caused by expectation of dying results in intense overactivity of the brain and nervous system, which causes severe malfunction and damage to other organs, especially the heart. Sternberg wrote that modern research shows that Cannon's explanation, although incomplete, was largely correct.[22]

ACTIVE DRUGS AND PLACEBOS

Whereas real drugs are designed to have direct effects on the conditions for which they are administered, placebos act by a variety of mechanisms. See pp. 156–61. Any substance, including sugar pills, saline injections, and even active drugs, can act as a placebo. In fact, as discussed below, procedures such as surgery, acupuncture, and chiropractic can also under certain conditions be considered placebos. The crucial criterion is that the substance or procedure does not directly affect the condition being treated.

Physicians from medieval times and even further into antiquity cured many of their patients. Their pharmacopeia of almost five thousand drugs and more than sixteen thousand prescriptions included remedies such as moss from the skulls of victims of violent death, saliva of a fasting man, crabs' eyes, and wood lice. Shapiro and Shapiro noted that none of those has a useful pharmacological effect. Therefore, they concluded, the history of medical treatment is essentially the history of the placebo effect.[23] In fact, even many fairly recently introduced medical treatments owed their effectiveness to the enthusiasm of advocates rather than any special treatment properties. An initial pattern of improvement of 70 percent to 90 percent declined to 30 percent to 40 percent as skeptical investigators tested the treatment under circumstances that minimized the placebo effect. The treatment was then abandoned, which validates Trousseau's 1833 warning to healers to hurry and use new drugs while they still work.

Henry Beecher, a pioneer in work on placebos, reported that about 30 percent of placebo recipients improve.[24] Levine reported a 39 percent improvement rate in analgesic response to postoperative dental pain,[25] Benedetti a 27 percent rate in analgesic response to arm pain,[26] and Petrovic a 46 percent analgesic response to pain from heating of the hand.[27] The placebo effect has been reported to be around 40 percent in disorders without apparent organic or structural cause[28] but lower in bipolar mania (31 percent)[29] and migraine (21 percent).[30]

Shapiro analyzed data from 1,006 patients who applied for outpatient psychiatric treatment and were given a placebo described as "a drug that would help determine how best to help you." Within an hour, placebo response was positive (decreased symptoms, feeling better) in 51 percent, negative (increased symptoms, feeling worse) in 12 percent, and no placebo response (no change) in 37 percent.[31]

Hoffman and colleagues considered two possibilities: (1) all individuals in the placebo group exhibit a moderate response or (2) a relatively small subset of individuals in that group exhibit a large magnitude response and others don't respond at all. The little bit of available evidence suggests that the second scenario is correct.[32]

Placebo effects can last a long time. Khan and colleagues identified eight placebo-controlled antidepressant trials with a total of 3,063 depressed patients in which, after acute phase placebo treatment, placebo was continued for more than twelve weeks.[33] Seventy-nine percent of placebo responders (and 93 percent of drug responders) remained well throughout the duration of the study.

Following are several examples of drug/ placebo effects:

Volunteers drank SoBe Adrenaline Rush, a drink that claims on its package to help increase mental acuity. Some were told that the drinks cost $1.89, others that the researchers had paid a bargain price of $0.89.

They then tried to solve a series of word-jumble puzzles (e.g., TUP-PIL—solution PULPIT). Fewer puzzles were solved in the reduced-price than the regular-price condition.[34]

Waber and colleagues administered electric shock to volunteers before and after giving them a placebo pill and a brochure. Half read that the pill was a newly approved painkiller that cost $2.50 per dose, the other half that it had been marked down to 10 cents, without saying why. More people in the full-price than in the low-price group reported reduced pain after taking the placebo.[35] The findings help explain why some high-cost drugs, such as cyclooxygenase-2 inhibitors, are more popular than inexpensive, widely available alternatives such as the over-the-counter drugs aspirin, ibuprofen, and naproxen and why patients switching from branded drugs often report that their generic equivalents are less effective. The authors suggested that generalizations about real-world effectiveness should take into account how drugs are sold in addition to how they are formulated. They added that clinicians should try to deemphasize potentially deleterious factors such as low price or generic manufacturer.

Several studies have shown that what alcoholics *think* the effects of alcohol are on their behavior influences that behavior substantially. For example, college students were told that they were drinking either vodka plus tonic water or tonic water alone. They actually all got plain tonic water. The ones who thought they had received vodka did worse on a memory test.[36]

The drugs naltrexone and acamprosate have been used to treat people addicted to alcohol. Alcohol-dependent patients received naltrexone, acamprosate, or placebo for twelve weeks. In addition to being assessed on various indices of alcohol dependence, they were asked whether they believed they had received active medication or placebo. There were no differences in outcomes between drug and placebo groups, but those who believed they had been taking an active drug consumed fewer alcoholic drinks and reported less alcohol dependence and cravings.[37]

Smokers were randomly assigned to receive nicotine replacement therapy or placebo. After six months, they guessed which they had received. Regardless of actual treatment, smokers who believed they had received nicotine were more likely to have quit than those who believed they had received placebo.[38]

Volkow administered the stimulant methylphenidate under one of four conditions: (1) expect placebo, receive placebo; (2) expect placebo, receive methylphenidate; (3) expect methylphenidate, receive methylphenidate; or (4) expect methylphenidate, receive placebo. When the methylphenidate was expected, it increased brain glucose metabolism by about 50 percent and in different brain areas than when it was unexpected. Increases in reports of feeling high were also about 50 percent greater when the methylphenidate was expected.[39]

Luparello and colleagues sprayed asthma patients with a harmless saline solution and told them they were inhaling an allergen. Several immediately developed breathing difficulties, and some had full-blown attacks. The attacks disappeared when they were sprayed with the same substance and told it was therapeutic.[40] The results support Eccles's assertion that the placebo response is the largest component of any allergy treatment.[41] BBC News reported that a biotech company found that an experimental vaccine for food allergies was effective in 75 percent of patients. But the news did not make shareholders happy—70 percent of patients who received placebos also reported getting rid of their food allergies.[42]

For decades until the 1970s, people with ulcers were encouraged to drink milk—and it eased their pain. Then studies showed that drinking milk increases gastric secretions, so doctors stopped prescribing it. In a study of patients with bleeding ulcers, some were given placebo and told by a doctor that they would receive a drug that would definitely help. Others were given the same placebo by a nurse and told that it was an experimental drug with uncertain effects. Seventy percent of the first group and only 25 percent of the second reported significant relief.[43]

Medical students received placebo psychotropics. Fifty percent had psychological changes, and 60 percent had physical effects.[44]

Volunteers were told they would receive a painful injection followed by a second shot—either a painkiller or a placebo. In actuality, everyone received a placebo. Half of the participants who believed they were receiving painkillers reported considerable pain relief. The participants who reported more pain relief had more dopamine activity in their nucleus accumbens than did the others, from the moment they were told they were receiving painkillers. (The nucleus accumbens is a collection of neurons that plays an important role in reward and pleasure.) And they had anticipated that the "painkiller" would give good relief before they even received it.[45]

Archer and Leier treated patients suffering from moderate to severe congestive heart failure with standard treatment alone or standard treatment plus a placebo. At the end of the trial period, those receiving the placebo treatment did substantially better on an exercise treadmill.[46]

Parkinson's disease is caused by the impairment or deterioration of neurons in brain areas including the substantia nigra, motor striatum, and subthalamic nucleus. Patients with Parkinson's disease received either human fetal mesencephalic transplantation or sham surgery treatment. For up to twelve months later, there were no differences between the transplant and sham surgery groups. But patients who believed they had received transplanted tissue improved significantly in both quality of life and motor outcomes, regardless of whether they received sham surgery or fetal tissue implantation.[47] Placebos given to Parkinson's patients induced a potent release of dopamine, and the degree of release was related to the degree of perceived clinical benefit. Placebos have modified both the rate and pattern of firing of neurons in these areas.[48]

Benedetti and colleagues devised a clever procedure that may cause nightmares to agencies that monitor athletes for performance-enhancing drugs. They administered morphine, which reduces pain and hence increases endurance, twice to athletes during their training. Then they gave the athletes a placebo on the day of competition. Performance was improved, just as it had been after morphine.[49]

As discussed below, placebos are not all alike. Drugs that produce discernible effects, but not specifically on the condition being treated, are called active placebos. Because recipients experience some effects from active placebos, they are particularly effective. For example, atropine causes dry mouth and has been used as an active placebo in studies of antidepressants. Forty of the sixty-eight antidepressant studies published between 1958 and 1972 using an inert placebo control reported the antidepressant more effective; only one of seven studies using atropine as an active placebo reported the antidepressant more effective.[50]

Even nonhuman animals show placebo effects. Rats given repeated scopolamine injections show the same behaviors when later injected with placebo.[51]

Is There a Placebo Effect?

Given everything preceding, the heading of this section may seem strange. However, in 2001 Hróbjartsson and Gøtzsche startled many in the scientific community by presenting their analysis of pooled data from 114 studies for a range of conditions. They found no significant difference between patients who had received placebos and those who had not. They attributed reduction of symptoms following placebo administration to spontaneous remission (the condition got better on its own) or regression to the mean (the tendency for people who get extreme scores on some measure to score closer to the mean when measured again). Hróbjartsson and Gøtzsche concluded, "There is no justification for the use of placebos in medical practice." In a 2004 update, they asserted that the only evidence of a placebo effect in medical interventions is a possible small effect for pain.[52]

Critics quickly responded.[53] They pointed out that the conditions analyzed by Hróbjartsson and Gøtzsche ranged from infertility and compulsive nail biting to marital discord, orgasmic difficulties, and fecal soiling. Those disparate studies were inappropriately lumped together. For each of them, the number of patients was very small and many of the outcome measures were unreliable. Most importantly, each of the studies assigned subjects to one of three groups: active drug, placebo, or no treatment. Hróbjartsson and Gøtzsche defined the placebo effect as the difference between placebo and no treatment groups. But the "no treatment groups" had arranged for treatment and received attention from a physician, both of which may have affected their expectations. So Hróbjartsson and Gøtzsche had really compared two placebo groups rather than evaluated the placebo effect.

Evolution

Humphrey addressed an obvious and puzzling question: if people can get better by their own efforts, why don't they do so as soon as they get sick?[54] His plausible answer requires considering the placebo effect in an evolutionary context. All animals respond to threats against health by mounting defenses such as pain and fever, actively attacking infections, repairing bone and tissue damage, indulging in sickness behaviors, and so on. All the defenses have a cost (pain is debilitating, immune resources are expensive, acting sick is time wasting, etc.). So an internal health management system evolved to optimize responses to threats. The system evaluates available information about what the future holds.

A sick individual should sometimes get well rapidly; at other times, prolonged illness conserves resources for later use. For most of human history, sick people with favorable prospects had reason to recover quickly. In the past, the health management system used many sources of information: the nature of the threat; costs of the defensive measure; prospects for spontaneous remission; evidence of how others were faring; and the social support network. Today, the best predictor of how things will turn out is the doctor. So today, the belief that doctors and their treatments have curative powers—has curative powers.

Humphrey cited a study by Breznitz that required subjects to keep a hand in ice-cold water until they could no longer stand the pain.[55] Breznitz told some subjects that the test would be over in four minutes but told others nothing. The test lasted a maximum of four minutes in both cases. Whereas 60 percent of those who knew when the test would end endured the full four minutes, only 30 percent of the others did so. Humphrey's interpretation was that when subjects knew that the threat posed by the cause of the pain was soon to be lifted, they had less need to feel the pain as a precautionary defense. Feeling less pain, they were able to last longer.

Mechanisms of the Placebo Effect

Several mechanisms have been proposed to explain placebo effects. They are not mutually exclusive and may complement or oppose one another.

Relief from Stress   Both stress and negative emotions increase pain.[56] Because people believe that doctors and their treatments have curative powers, visits to the doctor often relieve stress. Cummings and Vanden Bos estimated that 60–90 percent of visits to doctors are prompted by conditions related to stress or other psychological issues that are not effectively treated by drugs or surgery.[57] Over a three-year period, Kroenke and Mangelsdorff reviewed the records of more than a thousand patients with complaints such as chest pain, fatigue, dizziness, headache, edema, back pain, dyspnea, insomnia, abdominal pain, numbness, impotence, weight loss, cough, and constipation. Diagnostic tests uncovered an organic cause in only 16 percent of the cases.[58]

From a large study of patients at a psychiatric clinic, Shapiro and Shapiro concluded that positive placebo results are most likely to occur in people who have (a) high levels of symptom distress, especially anxiety, (b) a favorable attitude to the physician, and (c) a therapeutic situation that seems relevant and meets their expectations.[59]

Conditioning Many placebo responses are due to classical conditioning, a form of learning that has been demonstrated in every animal species tested and even in some plants. Classical conditioning requires a stimulus that invariably produces a specific response. The stimulus is called an unconditioned stimulus (UCS), and the response an unconditioned response (UCR). If a second stimulus, one that does not normally produce a similar response, is presented repeatedly just before the UCS, it will eventually come to elicit a response as well. The second stimulus is called a conditioned stimulus (CS), and the response a conditioned response (CR). For example, acetylcholine (UCS) causes hypotension (UCR). If a dog repeatedly hears a tone (CS) and is injected immediately afterward with acetylcholine, the dog becomes hypotensive (CR) after any injection following the tone. Some people who have allergic reactions (UCR) to flowers (UCS) show similar reactions (CRs) when presented with an artificial flower that contains no pollen (CS).[60]

The CR is often similar to the UCR, but not invariably so. Classical conditioning prepares the body for what is about to come, and in some cases the most appropriate CR is in the opposite direction from the UCR. For example, heroin (UCS) induces respiratory depression. All of the injection procedures—being in a specific room with specific people, preparing the heroin, preparing the injection site, filling a syringe, and injecting—become CSs. After repeated injections, a heroin addict's respiration is likely to increase (CR) just prior to injecting. Siegel presented evidence suggesting that deaths from heroin overdose in experienced users occur because the heroin is taken under different from normal circumstances; the conditioned stimuli are not experienced, so the compensatory increase in respiration does not occur.[61]

Prior experiences with effective medical treatments condition people to associate pills, syringes, and physicians' opinions with pain relief.

Every successful visit to the doctor strengthens the association. Evidence for the importance of classical conditioning is that placebo medication is more effective when it follows effective drug therapy, and an active drug is less effective when it follows an ineffective treatment.[62]

Ader and colleagues gave rats several pairings of saccharin-flavored drinking water followed immediately by injections of the immunosuppressive drug cyclophosphamide. When the conditioned rats were then given saccharin water alone, without the cyclophosphamide, their immune systems continued to function poorly, and many of them died.[63]

Humans can be conditioned as easily as rats. Goebel and colleagues administered the immunosuppressive drug cyclosporin A to healthy subjects in four sessions over three consecutive days. The cyclosporin A served as a UCS and was paired with a green, novel-tasting drink, the CS. In the next week, the subjects were re-exposed to the green drink but now paired with placebo capsules. Their immune functions were suppressed.[64]

A child with lupus received cyclophosphamide (UCS) paired with taste and smell stimuli (CS). Over a twelve-month period, the child received taste and smell stimuli alone on half the monthly chemotherapy sessions and responded favorably.[65] In another study, multiple sclerosis patients received cyclophosphamide (UCS) paired with anise-flavored syrup (CS), and eight out of ten patients displayed decreased peripheral leukocyte counts following the syrup alone.[66] An important implication is that, by taking advantage of classical conditioning, doctors can administer some drugs at lower doses or less frequently, thereby reducing expense and minimizing side effects.

Colloca and Benedetti exposed three groups of volunteers to painful stimuli (UCS).[67] The first group received standard classical conditioning: the stimulus intensity was secretly reduced each time a green light (CS) came on. Subjects in a second group first watched as a demonstrator showed pain relief when the stimuli were paired to a green light. Then they received a second round of painful stimuli, but this time preceded by the green light. Group 3 subjects were merely told to expect a benefit from a green light. Then they received the second round, preceded by the light. The first two groups experienced substantial placebo analgesic responses. The third group derived some, but smaller, benefit. The results show that learning can occur solely through observation, and they also support the view that expectations play a major role in the placebo effect.

Expectancy-Value Theory

According to expectancy-value theory, information alone can produce a conditioned response. Patients taking a placebo often report the same side effects as patients taking the active drug—the experiences of others create the expectancy of an effect. Walsh and colleagues analyzed fifty-seven studies and found that a higher percentage of depressed patients get better on placebos today than twenty years ago. The reason, they speculated, is that extensive media coverage has increased expectations about what drugs can do.[68] (Another likely reason is that subjects for studies on antidepressants used to come primarily from referrals of psychiatrists. Today, they are recruited largely through advertising, and their probably milder forms of depression are more responsive to both antidepressants and placebo.)

Responses of schizophrenic patients show a similar trend: antipsychotic drug/placebo differences became progressively smaller between 1991 and 2006. In fact, in recent years most tests of compounds designed to treat either schizophrenia or depression have not yielded statistically significant results. In 2007, the International Society for CNS Clinical Trials and Methodology and the International Society for CNS Drug Development held a collaborative session to explore possible reasons.[69] Changing expectations of the patients was suggested as a major reason. The speakers noted, as had Walsh, that continuously increasing media coverage and advertising are important factors. In addition, they speculated that a trend toward higher dosing frequency leads to enhanced placebo effects. Also, some people, especially in the United States, earn money by enrolling in as many drug studies as possible. They may believe that they enhance their chances of being invited for additional trials by claiming to respond to whatever they are given.

Alternative explanations for the reduced responsiveness to active drugs were considered: The recent studies may have been poorly designed or executed. The disease itself or its diagnosis may have changed. Perhaps the newer drugs are less effective than older ones. Or patients may have more trouble detecting newer than older drugs because the

newer ones cause fewer discernible side effects. (See p. 169 on the value
of letting patients know when they are getting a treatment.) The older
drugs may work well enough, so only the most refractory patients enroll
in research in hopes of finding better treatment.

Montgomery and Kirsch applied a painful electrical stimulus to volunteers and then administered a placebo cream analgesic and secretly
lowered the intensity for several trials.[70] When they reapplied the stimulus at its original intensity, the subjects reported less pain than they had
initially. Then some of them were told about the deception, and others were not. Although the conditioning aspect was the same for both
groups, when the stimulus was reapplied, only the subjects who had not
been told continued to have an analgesic response. The same researchers administered a placebo cream anesthetic to one index finger and
then applied shock to both index fingers; most subjects reported less
pain in the finger with the sham anesthetic. Their results fit better with
an expectancy than a conditioning explanation.[71]

Multiple Placebo Effects and Mechanisms

Stimuli may affect brain and body in many ways, so there are many
types of placebo effects, each with different mechanisms and in different systems and diseases. Following a series of elegant experiments,
Benedetti and colleagues wrote, "The study of the placebo effect, at its
core, is the study of how the context of beliefs and values shape brain
processes related to perception and emotion and, ultimately, mental and
physical health."[72] They suggested that expectation is important when
conscious functions, such as pain perception and motor performance,
are involved; whereas conditioning plays a role in unconscious physiological functions such as immune and hormonal responses. Below are
brief descriptions of some of their findings.[73]

- They told subjects that a drug—actually a placebo—would relieve
  pain and increase the production of growth hormone while inhibit-
  ing cortisol secretion. The expectations induced pain relief but did
  not change hormone secretion.
- A classical conditioning procedure did change hormone secretion.
  They administered sumatriptan, which stimulates growth hormone

(GH) and inhibits cortisol secretion, for two consecutive days. On the third day they administered a placebo; plasma concentrations increased for GH and decreased for cortisol.

- Conditioning also explains their results with buprenorphine, an opioid drug that induces mild respiratory depression. A placebo given after several buprenorphine administrations produced a similar depression even though the patients neither expected nor noticed the effect.

- Expectations can override conditioning. They gave two groups of subjects the analgesic ketorolac for two consecutive days. On the third day, both groups received a placebo. Subjects told that it was analgesic reported less pain, while subjects told that it was hyperalgesic reported more pain.

An emerging view is that expectancies mediate most placebo effects, and conditioning is one means by which people initially form and then activate expectancies. Expectations can be influenced by reading a book, the circumstances under which the drug is administered, and so forth. All such factors affect the meaning of the situation.

Meaning

Moerman and Jonas suggested a new perspective for understanding placebo and related phenomena.[74] They argued that the crucial feature is the meaning that treatment recipients attach to their experiences. They wrote:

> Insofar as medicine is meaningful, it can affect patients, and it can affect the outcome of treatment. Most elements of medicine *are* meaningful, even if practitioners do not intend them to be so. The physician's costume (the white coat with stethoscope hanging out of the pocket), manner (enthusiastic or not), style (therapeutic or experimental), and language are all meaningful and can be shown to affect the outcome; indeed, we argue that both diagnosis and prognosis can be important forms of treatment.

Whalley and colleagues treated one finger of volunteers' hands with one of two placebo creams, each with a different label, and left the matching finger on the other hand untreated.[75] Then they administered identical pain stimuli to fingers on both hands. They repeated the procedure between one and eight days later using one or the other of the creams. When placebos bore the same name, but not when they had different names, the pain sensations in the two trials were highly correlated. The authors concluded that accurate predictions of placebo response are possible as long as contexts (meanings) remain constant.

The significance of meaning explains the importance of verbal explanations of proposed treatments, the influence of physical characteristics of drugs and placebos, and effectiveness of various nondrug treatments such as chiropractic and acupuncture. It also explains the difficulty in identifying placebo responders—people's experiences determine the meanings they attach to situations, so a person may respond to placebo in one situation but not in another. In one study, men responded more than women to nocebo suggestions, but nocebo conditioning was more effective with women.[76] Many biological and psychosocial variables have been tested to see whether they accurately predict response to antidepressants. The results have been inconsistent.[77]

Schweinhardt and colleagues injected a pain-inducing saline solution into the legs of volunteers under the guise of testing an experimental analgesic cream.[78] The cream was actually inert. The researchers said they would test one leg with the treatment and one leg with a nonmedicated lotion. Then they asked the subjects to rate the pain. The placebo responders—those who reported less pain in the leg treated with the supposed analgesic—scored higher than the nonresponders on tests that measure sensation seeking (pursuit of novel and intense experiences). But sensation seekers do not respond more strongly to placebo than non–sensation seekers in all situations.

Considering meaning as the crucial mediating factor explains cultural differences in response to both placebos and active drugs—cultures differ in the meanings attached to the substances. Potter found that by the late 1990s, the antianxiety drug Valium did better than placebo in France and Belgium but not in the United States, whereas Prozac performed better in the United States than in Western Europe and South Africa.[79] Macedo and colleagues meta-analyzed the response rate of people given placebos to prevent migraine headaches. A higher percentage of patients improved in Europe than in North America, and a higher percentage of North Americans experienced adverse side effects.[80] Moerman compared 117 placebo-controlled ulcer studies from all over the world. Drugs were effective in 38–100 percent of cases, placebos in 0 to 100 percent. In countries where patients responded most to ulcer drugs, they also responded most to placebos for ulcer. Placebos for ulcers were effective in 59 percent of German patients, 22 percent of Danish and Dutch patients, and only 7 percent of Brazilians. But neither drug nor placebo responses generalized across diseases. Germans were among the lowest in responses to treatments for moderate hypertension, and they were middling for generalized anxiety disorder. Moerman attributed the differences among countries to cultural variations in the meanings attached to both diseases and treatments.[81]

Walach and colleagues also found a high correlation between placebo and treatment response rate.[82] The authors made an additional interesting point: although treated groups generally did better, which shows that the treatments were beneficial, the high correlation proves the importance of nonspecific treatment effects for most disease categories and across a wide variety of interventions.

Physiological Underpinnings

Placebo responses are not all generated by the same mechanism.[83] Many brain regions play a role in reduction of pain, whether the pain is due to a chronic medical condition or applied to volunteers in a laboratory. These include the anterior cingulate cortex, anterior insula, prefrontal cortex, and periaqueductal grey. Kong and colleagues speculated that placebos for pain may act on at least three stages of pain processing. They may influence prestimulus expectation of pain relief, modify pain perception, and distort poststimulus pain rating. Change in one stage may induce change in another.[84]

The endorphin system plays a crucial role. Endorphins are substances produced within the brain that attach to the same cell receptors as does the powerful analgesic morphine. Endorphins are released after severe injury and reduce the sensation of pain. Effective placebos also stimulate the release of endorphins. In chronic pain patients, placebo responders show higher concentration of endorphins in the cerebrospinal fluid than do placebo nonresponders.[85] Naloxone blocks the analgesic actions of both morphine and placebo-induced expectations of analgesia, which indicates the importance of endorphins in these responses. However, endorphins are not always required—and analgesia due to classical conditioning with agents unrelated to morphine is not naloxone reversible.

Endorphins are involved in both the respiratory centers and the cardiovascular system. The evidence is that naloxone blocks both the respiratory depressant response to placebo after repeated administrations of the opioid buprenorphine and the heart rate reduction that typically accompanies placebo analgesia. Endorphins also play a role in the regulation of reproductive and stress hormones.

The activation of endorphins by placebos can be counteracted by cholecystokinin (CCK), a hormone secreted by cells at the top of the small intestine. Colloca and Benedetti hypothesized that expectations of pain induce anxiety. Anxiety triggers the activation of CCK, which facilitates pain transmission. Proglumide antagonizes CCK and potentiates placebo analgesia. These data suggest that the endorphin and CCK systems have opposing actions on pain perception.[86]

The nucleus accumbens, a collection of neurons within the striatum, plays an important role in rewards, pleasure, and placebo responses to pain. Scott and colleagues exposed healthy volunteers to experimental pain and an analgesic placebo. Those who anticipated the most pain relief had the greatest increase of dopamine and endorphin activity in the nucleus accumbens—and the most relief. In a second part of the study, the subjects were led to expect monetary reward. There was a positive correlation between nucleus accumbens responses to monetary reward and to placebos.[87] This suggests that placebo responsiveness depends on the functioning of the reward system and that people with the most efficient dopaminergic reward systems are the best placebo responders. An implication is that the placebo response to painful stimuli can be accurately predicted.

The placebo effect for conditions originating in the central nervous system, such as pain and depression, can be traced in part to changes in the spine. Eippert and colleagues told healthy men that one of their arms was being treated with an anesthetic cream and the other with a placebo.[88] Both creams were actually placebos. They then applied painful heat to both arms. The men reported experiencing significantly less pain when treated with the cream they believed to be anesthetic. Furthermore, fMRI scans showed reduced activity of their spinal nerves, indicating that their bodies actually felt less pain.

Depressed patients treated with either the antidepressant drug fluoxetine or placebo showed changed activity in several of the same brain areas. Some areas changed only in response to fluoxetine, none only in response to placebo. Some changed well before any clinical benefits were observed and may have been due to the expectation of benefits. Placebo responders exhibited different brain changes from responders to active drug. That is, improvements of placebo and drug responders were achieved through different mechanisms of action. So there is no single antidepressant response pathway. In fact, effective psychotherapy induces still different brain changes. Since they act by different mechanisms, an implication is that placebos and other nonspecific conditions can augment or diminish the effects of active drugs.[89]

Placebos that relieve anxiety may act through similar brain pathways as those that mediate placebo analgesia. Petrovic and colleagues treated anxious subjects with the anti-anxiety drug midazolam and then showed them anxiety-provoking pictures. Midazolam reduced the unpleasantness. On the second day, the subjects were told they would receive the same drug but instead were given a placebo. They showed reduced unpleasantness, and changes in their brain activity were similar to those seen during placebo analgesia.[90]

NOCEBO

When expectations of sickness cause sickness, they are called nocebo effects. For example, headaches were reported by 70 percent of medical students told that a (nonexistent) electric current was passing through their heads.[91] Vomiting, a common side effect in women given placebo estrogen, is rare with other placebos. In a chemotherapy study, 30 percent of the placebo control group members lost their hair, and 56 percent experienced nausea or vomiting.[92]

Lynoe purposely misinformed patients that they had been infected by hazardous bacilli. He treated them with a placebo. Some subjects developed infection-like conditions that did not respond to the placebo.[93]

Rosenzweig and colleagues reviewed 109 double-blind placebo-controlled studies involving 1,228 volunteers. The overall incidence of adverse events in the healthy volunteers during placebo administration was 19 percent. Complaints were more frequent after repeated dosing (28 percent) and in elderly subjects (26 percent). The most frequent adverse events were headache (7 percent), drowsiness (5 percent), and loss of strength (4 percent).[94]

HARNESSING THE POWER OF THE PLACEBO

In the popular television series *House*, Hugh Laurie stars as the brilliant, antisocial, misanthropic Dr. Gregory House. Dr. House seems to think of patients as puzzles rather than people but, although devoid of bedside manner, he manages in each weekly episode to solve a challenging medical puzzle that has baffled all his colleagues. Almost always, he saves the patient. Yet despite his spectacular success rate, House is not a good role model for any aspiring or practicing doctor. George Bernard Shaw's doctor Ralph Bloomfield Bonington (in *The Doctor's Dilemma*) is a much better one. Bonington is "cheering, reassuring, healing by the mere incompatibility of disease or anxiety with his welcome presence. Even broken bones, it is said, have been known to unite at the sound of his voice."

Bedside manner is a vital part of medical practice. Caring, empathetic physicians maximize positive expectations and favorable medical outcomes. See chapter 1 for further discussion. Cold, emotionless, "House"-like physicians induce nocebo responses. Good caring and weak medicine can give a better outcome than poor caring and strong medicine. Almost a half-century ago, Wolf reported that one of two physicians who administered placebos increased his patients' gastric acid secretions consistently; the second consistently decreased secretions.[95] Little and colleagues analyzed outcomes for 579 patients who presented with sore throats and were randomly assigned to receive antibiotics or no antibiotics. About two-thirds in each group got better within five days. The factor most closely associated with rapid improvement was satisfaction with the visit with the doctor.[96] Di Blasi reviewed the outcome literature. Doctors who adopted a warm, friendly, and reassuring manner were more effective than those whose consultations were formal and did not offer reassurance.[97]

Inspire Confidence

Doctors should dress and speak appropriately and prominently display diplomas and awards. Of course, the factors that inspire confidence depend to some extent on the patient's background. A devout Catholic might be most impressed by a Notre Dame diploma, whereas a Mormon might feel better about one from Brigham Young University.

A simple doctor-patient consultation can be therapeutic and as effective as placebo or symptomatic medication. Thomas assigned patients who had symptoms but no clear-cut diagnosis to one of four groups: a placebo treatment with a positive expectancy ("No serious disease has been found and you will soon be well"); no treatment with a positive expectancy; placebo treatment with a negative expectancy ("I am not sure this treatment will have an effect"); or no treatment with a negative expectancy. There were no differences in outcome between placebo treatment and no treatment but a significant difference between positive and negative statements about prognosis.[98]

Doctors should listen and ask questions, even when the answers to those questions are not needed. "An internist may know immediately when a patient walks through the door that he has bronchitis. Nonetheless, the physician performs chest auscultation and has at least a brief conversation with that patient before discussing treatment. . . . Simple tests go a long way toward making people believe they are cared for. . . . Once you know the patient's point of view [of his or her problem], it is easier to work with it or attempt to persuade him to your point of view."[99]

Crow and colleagues did an extensive review of doctor-patient interactions.[100] They cited several studies showing that medical outcomes are improved when doctors or nurses explain to patients the procedures they are going to undergo. Informed patients typically require smaller doses of analgesic drugs and shortened hospital stays, and they experience less discomfort. Crow's group concluded that patients should be:

- given accurate expectations about medical procedures and how to cope with them and their effects;

- taught skills for self-management of their illness and their ability to communicate about their health problems with health-care providers;
- encouraged to believe in the benefits of effective medical treatments.

Be Enthusiastic

The effects of active drugs have depended on whether or not the administering nurse favored drug therapy for those patients and whether or not physicians acted enthusiastically while administering the drug.[101]

Patients about to have teeth extracted were injected with placebos but told that they were receiving a drug that would make their pain better. Their dentists were initially told that some of the patients would receive an analgesic but then that a supply problem meant that the analgesic was unavailable. Later, some dentists were told that the problem had been resolved. When the dentists thought their patients might receive an analgesic, the patients experienced much less pain than those whose dentists thought they definitely would not receive one.[102]

Enthusiasm may create positive outcomes even if based on faulty information. A therapy that seems rational imparts meaning and thus can be effective even if it has no physiological basis. And the stronger the healer's belief in the therapy, the more likely it is to work. For example, in 1986 a dental surgeon tried a new treatment for the painful swelling that follows wisdom teeth removal. The surgeon massaged patients' cheeks with an ultrasound probe, and the patients' jaws shrank by 35 percent compared with a control group. But unbeknownst to both the patients and the dental surgeon, the machine had been unplugged.[103]

Roberts and colleagues reviewed the literature on five medical and surgical procedures thought effective at the time administered. Physicians had used them to cure, not as part of an experiment, although subsequent research showed that they were no more effective than placebo. So the physicians were more optimistic about results than in the typical placebo study, and effects were maximized. Of 6,931 patients, 40 percent had excellent outcomes, 30 percent good outcomes, and 30 percent poor outcomes.[104]

Frank and Frank wrote about several features that promote healing of psychotherapy patients.[105] Their advice probably applies to most medical situations. The therapist should allow the patient to verbalize distress, carefully evaluate all of the patient's complaints, offer a plausible treatment plan that leads to the anticipation of improvement, and at all times act with enthusiasm and commitment.

Kaptchuk and colleagues randomly assigned patients suffering from irritable bowel syndrome to one of three groups: a waiting list, placebo acupuncture from a clinician who refrained from small talk, or placebo acupuncture with a clinician who treated them with warmth, attention, and confidence. (The clinician asked them questions about symptoms, outlined the causes of IBS, and displayed optimism about their condition.) Those in the third group improved most. They got as much relief as did people taking the two leading prescription drugs for IBS.[106]

Shape the Patient's Expectations or Go Along with Them

When patients suffering from anxiety consulted a medical practitioner, they obtained considerable relief from placebo—but only the ones who were seeking relief in the form of medicine. Those who had sought psychiatric help did not improve.[107]

Real acupuncture was compared with sham acupuncture for different painful conditions, such as migraine, tension-type headache, chronic low back pain, and osteoarthritis. Patients were asked what they expected from acupuncture treatment. Patients with higher expectations experienced larger clinical benefits than those with lower expectations, regardless of their allocation to real or sham acupuncture. All that mattered was whether they expected a benefit.[108]

Lutz and colleagues questioned patients about to undergo surgery for sciatica and again twelve months postoperational. Patients who had expected a shorter recovery time after surgery were more likely than those who had expected a longer recovery to be delighted, pleased, or mostly satisfied with their outcomes at the twelve-month mark. Also, compared with patients who had not preferred surgery, patients who had preferred it even after learning that sciatica could get better without surgery had better symptom scores twelve months postoperational. The researchers suggested that patients' expectations should be elicited to help physicians identify those most likely to benefit from surgery.[109]

Patients with chronic low back pain were asked their expectations concerning massage, acupuncture, or usual care. Then they were randomly assigned to treatments. Of those assigned to a treatment they thought would help, 86 percent showed significant improvement. Only 68 percent of those with lower expectations improved.[110]

Patients who visited a chiropractor's office and then received chiropractic care experienced greater benefits than patients who presented to physical therapy and were assigned to chiropractic care.[111]

Recognize That Even Subtle Cues Can Affect Patients' Self-Images and Thus Their Health

Crum and Langer studied hotel maids who spend long hours engaged in physical activity.[112] But even though the maids all far exceeded the surgeon general's recommendation for daily exercise, 67 percent of them answered a survey by saying they didn't exercise. Their body fat, waist-to-hip ratio, blood pressure, weight, and body mass index matched their perceived rather than actual amount of exercise. Crum and Langer divided them into two groups:

Group 1: Researchers went through each maid's daily tasks, explaining how many calories those tasks burned. They were told that the activity met the surgeon general's definition of an active lifestyle.
Group 2: Was given no information at all.

One month later, the women in group 2 hadn't changed. But those in group 1 had lowered systolic blood pressure, weight, and waist-to-hip ratio. Both the women and their managers claimed that they had not altered their daily routines. Changed beliefs had changed bodily responses—presumably by a mechanism similar to that which causes changed bodily responses to placebos.

In a series of studies, Levy and colleagues showed that other simple manipulations can have powerful effects on health.[113] Using elderly subjects, they flashed positive or negative age-stereotype words (wisdom, decrepit) on a screen at speeds that allowed perception without awareness. Then they measured various types of performance:

- Subjects primed with negative aging stereotypes performed worse than those exposed to positive stereotypes on memory tasks.
- A panel rated the handwriting of those exposed to negative aging stereotypes as older and more deteriorated, senile, and shaky than the handwriting of those exposed to the positive stereotypes.
- Before and after exposure to positive aging stereotypes, the subjects walked down a hallway with devices in their shoes that measured balance and gait speed. They improved substantially, with gains comparable to those observed when older individuals participate in rigorous exercise programs for several weeks.

Levy and colleagues asked people aged seventy and older, "When you think of an old person, what are the first words or phrases that come to mind?" The responses were judged on how negative or positive they were. Negative responses included words like *senile* and *feeble* and visual images such as gray hair, wrinkles, and stooped posture. Positive responses included terms like *wise* and *active*. Hearing was measured at the same time and again three years later, with adjustments for initial levels of hearing. The more negative the initial age stereotypes, the worse the subjects performed on hearing measures three years later.

A remarkable finding came from analysis of data on self-perceptions of aging collected as long ago as twenty-three years earlier. Older individuals who had had more positive views of aging lived an average of 7.5 years longer than those with less positive views. The difference was independent of age, gender, socioeconomic status, loneliness, and functional health. Levy's group noted that the effects of negative self-stereotypes of aging can be minimized by enhancing the influence of positive self-stereotypes.

Order Diagnostic Tests

Brody and Waters wrote that the diagnostic process not only paves the way for treatment but also functions as a type of treatment itself.[114] Performing a series of tests in patients with nonspecific chest pain reduced disability from 45 percent to 20 percent even if the tests were negative or unnecessary.[115] But there is a downside—diagnostic tests may encourage illness beliefs. A long delay before the test is taken allows time for negative illness beliefs to become established. By the time patients undergo tests, they have already developed negative beliefs about their symptoms, so posttest reassurance from doctors is less effective. Giving patients prior information about diagnostic tests can improve outcomes.

Patients with chest pain were split into three groups before they underwent diagnostic testing: (1) one group was given the normal information sheet on the test; (2) another group was given a pamphlet, which detailed the test and included an explanation of the meaning of negative test results; and (3) the third group was given the pamphlet plus a meeting with a health psychologist to discuss the test and the meaning of results. Patients who received a normal test result were then asked to complete a questionnaire and take part in a follow-up interview. At follow-up, patients in group 3 reported less chest pain, were more reassured by the test, and were taking fewer cardiac drugs compared with patients in the other groups. After a month, most patients in group 1 had still not been reassured by the results.[116]

Provide a Diagnosis: Give an Explanation for Symptoms

Patients expect their doctors to make diagnoses. These can provide meaning and emotional relief. But doctors need not always inform patients of unpleasant diagnoses, which can wreak havoc on self-perceptions and perpetuate or exacerbate symptoms. Huibers and Wessely analyzed the literature and concluded that patients diagnosed with chronic fatigue syndrome have a worse prognosis than patients without such a label.[117]

Tell Them It Won't Hurt

Sawamoto and colleagues exposed volunteers to one of two conditions: (1) a series of nonpainful stimuli or (2) the same nonpainful stimuli intermixed randomly with a few painful ones. On the nonpainful stimulus trials, the group that did not know what to expect had enhanced responses in brain areas that are sensitive to pain and greater subjective unpleasantness.[118] The anticipation of possible pain had created discomfort.

Keltner and colleagues conditioned volunteers to red or blue visual cues. One cue was always followed by a highly painful stimulus, the other cue by a somewhat less painful one. Once the subjects had been conditioned, they received twenty more of each stimulus, presented in random order. On half the occasions the stimulus was preceded by the high-intensity visual cue and on half the occasions by the low-intensity cue. The subjects reported greater pain when the noxious stimulus was preceded by the high-intensity cue. They showed significant differences in brain activity in several regions. Their expectations had affected their perception of pain.[119]

Make Sure That Patients Know When They Are Getting a Treatment and That It Has Worked for Others

Benedetti and colleagues did a series of experiments in which they eliminated the placebo component of various treatments while maintaining the treatments' specific effects. For example, a doctor administered morphine to some postoperative patients while telling them that the drug would relieve their pain within a few minutes. Other patients received the same dose of morphine from a preprogrammed infusion machine without any doctor or nurse present, so they were unaware that a painkilling medication was being given. Both groups rated their pain in a diary. At both thirty and sixty minutes after the morphine infusion, the pain decrease was larger in the open than in the hidden condition.[120]

Don't Be Afraid to Use Placebos

Nitzan and Lichtenberg surveyed physicians and reported that fifty-three of eighty-nine acknowledged using placebo as a therapy, thirty-three of them at least once a month. Most respondents reported placebos to be generally or occasionally effective.[121] More recently, 45 percent of physician respondents reported using placebos in clinical practice. The most common reasons were to calm the patient and as supplemental treatment.[122] Nurses routinely apply placebos.[123] Lichtenberg and colleagues argued that, in select cases, their use may be morally imperative.[124] And Brown wrote, "As physicians, we should respect the benefits of placebos—their safety, effectiveness and low cost—and bring the full advantage of these benefits into our everyday practices."[125]

Unfortunately, however, doctors have tended to give placebos to the least appropriate patients: neurotic patients, who are least likely to respond, demanding patients, who have an investment in not responding, and chronically ill patients, who have not responded to other treatments.[126]

Placebos Are Not All Alike

Placebo efficacy increased with increasing number of pills, pill size, and frequency of administration.[127] Placebos labeled as brand-name drugs were more effective than those labeled as generic for treating headaches. And yellow placebo pills were more stimulating than green, blue more sedating than pink.[128] However, the relationship between color and effectiveness for both active drugs and placebos depends at least to some extent on recipient characteristics. White and black subjects were appreciably different in their expectations of drug action based on color and size.[129]

Procedures Work Better Than Pills

Devices such as injections, surgery, and acupuncture have enhanced placebo effects. A sham acupuncture device had a greater placebo effect than an inert pill on self-reported pain and severity of symptoms. The types of side effects differed in the two groups and mimicked the information given at informed consent.[130] A pacemaker placebo was far superior to a placebo pill.[131]

Moerman noted that chiropractic patients typically express more satisfaction than patients of family doctors with treatment for lower back pain. Moerman contrasted the behaviors of the typical physician and chiropractor when confronted with a patient with low back pain. The physician is likely to advise the patient to "take aspirin, rest in bed, take it easy." By contrast, "the chiropractor carries out a focused, pointed, attentive examination and then explains the course of treatment, its goals and likelihood of success. The adjustment on an elaborate table is itself replete with satisfying pops and snaps, rolling over, and just enough pain to suggest that something good may come from it."

Recognize That Nocebo Effects Can Occur to Both Placebos and Legitimate Medical Procedures

Patients receiving active drugs or other medical procedures frequently experience adverse side effects that are best classified as nocebo phenomena. Barsky and colleagues identified several relevant factors: the patient's expectations of adverse effects, prior experiences that conditioned the patient to associate a procedure with bodily symptoms, psychological characteristics such as anxiety and depression, and situational and contextual factors.[132] Patients who blame their symptoms on a beneficial treatment may discontinue it. The authors cited a study of a commonly prescribed drug that led to many reports of adverse side effects; but researchers attributed only 11 percent of those effects directly to the drug—the rest, presumably, were nocebo effects. So the authors encouraged medical personnel to avoid generating self-defeating attitudes in patients and to be aware that nonspecific side effects of treatments may be nocebo effects. On the other hand, adverse effects, whether caused by a procedure, active drug, or placebo, may convince the patient that the treatment is having an impact. Thus, they may enhance therapeutic efficacy.

Take Advantage of Conditioning Phenomena

An implication of classical conditioning is that placebos are more effective when they follow effective drug therapy, and active drugs are less effective when they follow ineffective treatments. It follows that drug recipients should be started off on the highest reasonable dose so that they are conditioned to experiencing strong effects, and then lower doses should be prescribed without telling them. Laska and Sunshine gave hospitalized patients in pain either a placebo or varying doses of an analgesic. Twenty-four hours later, all patients who complained of pain received placebo. The mean analgesic effect correlated with the initial dose of the analgesic.[133]

Be Judicious about Terminating Treatment

After having received morphine for forty-eight hours, some patients were told that the morphine was about to be stopped. Others had the morphine stopped without being informed. The pain intensity had not differed between the two groups at the time of the interruption. When patients were aware that interventions were terminated, their symptoms recurred faster, they experienced more pain, and more of them requested further painkillers.[134]

Patients receiving eight weeks of placebo or antidepressants were improving equally until those taking placebo were told so. Most deteriorated and had to be put on active drugs.[135]

But it is possible to terminate a treatment without having patients regress. Chung and colleagues administered placebos to both healthy volunteers and patients with irritable bowel syndrome and then told responders that they had received placebo. Neither their attitudes nor their responses to subsequent placebo treatments changed.[136] Davison and colleagues speculated that changes attributed to self-effort are more long lasting than changes attributed to an external agent. They gave insomniac volunteers a treatment package of chloral hydrate plus relaxation and scheduling procedures. Following treatment, some subjects were told that they had received an optimal dosage of the sleep aid, and others that the dosage they had received was too weak to have had any meaningful effect. All subjects were instructed to discontinue the drug but to continue with the relaxation and scheduling procedures. Those who could not attribute their changes to the drug maintained greater therapeutic gain.[137]

AN ETHICAL DILEMMA

One of the authors (FL) has posed the following ethical dilemma to both college students and physicians. Almost to a person, the physicians have opted for telling patients the truth. The vast majority of students, however, have said that they would prefer being lied to in such a situation.

Suppose that health is rated on a ten-point scale, and a doctor knows that the best possible outcome after a certain procedure is a six—but that will occur only if the patient expects a ten. If the patient expects less than ten, the most likely outcome is four or less. Should the doctor lie so that the patient expects a ten? Note: A patient who expects ten and ends up with six is likely to be angry and think the doctor incompetent. He may sue.

TIPS ESPECIALLY FOR PATIENTS

Patients should recognize that factors such as how doctors greet patients, diplomas they have hanging on the wall, and general office décor can profoundly affect patients' expectations and, therefore, treatment outcomes. So patients need to make sure that they and their doctor are a good fit. If the doctor gives instructions without asking questions about the patient's condition or values or pays little attention to the patient's answers, the patient might do better with another doctor.

If a doctor indicates that there are alternative treatments for a patient's condition and the patient believes strongly in one of them, she or he should choose that even if the doctor prefers a different alternative. The patient's expectations about the treatments may override any other factors. (Of course, patients should keep in mind that the doctor is the expert and make sure they understand the reasons for the doctor's preference.)

Patients may want to meet with or read about patients who have been treated and had successful outcomes. The more positive cases a patient can be made aware of, the more favorable his or her expectations are likely to be.

LOOKING AHEAD

In this chapter we've shown that expectation effects often play a huge role in medical outcomes. In the next chapter, we evaluate various complementary and alternative practices; we show that expectation effects account for many, although not all, of the benefits.

COMPLEMENTARY
AND ALTERNATIVE MEDICINE

A BRIEF REVIEW

In previous chapters we addressed psychological aspects of medical care as they play out in the doctor-patient relationship and in the context of expectation effects. We saw that interpersonal relationships between doctors and patients impact patient health *separate and apart* from any biomedical treatment the doctor recommends. We discussed how this is partly a result of satisfaction with care and adherence to recommended treatments, and partly a result of the placebo effect benefits of these doctor-patient encounters.

In the chapter on expectation effects, we also looked in detail at what doctors can do to enhance the placebo effect of the medical visit. We made some recommendations:

- Inspire confidence and trust (through appearance, visible credentials, positive prognoses, clear expectations, and directions for self-care).
- Be enthusiastic about the recommended treatment, and provide a reason for patient optimism.

- Consider patients' preferences and beliefs about what will work.
- Provide a diagnosis.
- Make sure patients know they're getting a treatment.

With that review as a backdrop, we're now going to watch those and other issues play out by following a hypothetical patient, Mary Brown, as she makes her way through decisions about her medical care. The text in italics is Mary's story; the plain text following the italics is discussion on points raised by the portion of the story just presented.

As part of her attempt to address her medical problem, Mary pursues acupuncture, a form of what is referred to as complementary and alternative medicine (CAM). Of particular relevance to this book, we end this chapter with a discussion of the category of CAM referred to as mind-body therapies.

CONVENTIONAL MEDICINE DOESN'T CURE EVERYTHING

Our hypothetical patient, Mary Brown, just got a new job as an attorney with the Natural Resources Defense Fund and will be changing her health-care plan as a result. She's had a painful health condition for years and wants to get it dealt with once and for all now because it has caused her to miss work in the past and she's worried about doing that at a new job.

Mary's health concern is chronic lower back pain. To date, she's received no definitive diagnosis as to the cause of her pain. She has been treating it with over-the-counter pain relief medication, specifically ibuprofen. She's read up on problems with ibuprofen, however, and is concerned about potential side effects such as developing ulcers or gastrointestinal bleeding if she continues to use it regularly.

Conventional medicine often fails to find cause of an illness or to completely cure or even relieve it. Lower back pain is a common example. More than 70 percent of people in developed countries will experience lower back pain.[1] Of this group, pain is not specific (meaning not attributable to a recognizable pathology) for about 85 percent of patients.[2] Chronic lower back pain, like many forms of chronic pain, is often treated conventionally by medications that control the pain—but that bring their own medical problems and risks.

THE CONVENTIONAL CARE DOCTOR VISIT

Mary makes an appointment with a new doctor, Dr. Jones. The day before the appointment, Mary goes for a hike in the woods and brushes her arm against some poison oak. It itches a lot, so when Dr. Jones comes in and says, "What can I do for you today?" Mary starts her response with, "Well I think I have poison oak. . . ." At that point, Dr. Jones asks her to roll up her sleeve so he can take a look.

Finishing the poison oak conversation takes a few minutes. When it's done, Dr. Jones opens Mary's file and reads through the new patient questionnaire she filled out in the waiting room. When he feels he needs to, he asks her for more information about her answers to family health history questions and her answers to questions about her lifestyle.

When they finish going through Mary's file it's been about fifteen minutes since Dr. Jones came into the room. He closes the file and looks at her, saying, "Is there anything else?"

Mary feels a little awkward about bringing up her back pain at this point since Dr. Jones appears to think the visit is coming to a close, but she wants to make sure to address it since that was her primary concern. She describes her problem to Dr. Jones. He asks about its onset and severity, where the pain is located and how long it's lasted. He orders some diagnostic tests to rule out potential, unlikely, possibilities, refers to it as "nonspecific low back pain," and writes Mary a prescription for a muscle relaxant. This part of the visit takes about five minutes. After he writes the prescription, he asks again, "Anything else?" When she says no, he says good-bye.

Our hypothetical Dr. Jones[3] is probably a fine doctor, and he's certainly not shockingly bad at the interpersonal aspect of care: he asks what Mary came to see him for, he thoroughly reviews her medical history, he questions her in some detail about her back pain, and he twice gives her an opportunity to raise additional concerns. He's not perfect, though. He didn't effectively set the agenda at the beginning of the interaction, meaning that Mary's main concern was left until the end and might have felt rushed. (At around twenty minutes long, the interaction was about the average length of a U.S. primary care visit.)[4] He didn't engage in real collaborative treatment planning with Mary in terms of making sure the treatment approach he chose was a good fit with her values and preferences. He asked whether there was "anything" else rather than if there was "something" else, which we now know to be the less effective version of that question (see chapter 1). Finally, he didn't give her dosing instructions or tell her about potential side effects for the medication he prescribed, an omission we also now know to be common in conventional care.

Patient Dissatisfaction

Mary fills her prescription and goes home. The pharmacy had been busy, so she didn't ask questions about her medication there but decided to do her own research. She looks online and finds information there that the drug she was prescribed has some concerning potential side effects. She also sees that there is consensus on the online sites that it shouldn't be taken for more than a couple of weeks at a time. She realizes that she doesn't know for how long Dr. Jones intended her to take the medication. She is worried about the side effects and her confusion about how to take the medication, and she feels unhappy that her interaction with Dr. Jones has left her so bewildered. In addition, a lot of the online information Mary finds suggests that lifestyle changes are very important for treating lower back pain; she wishes Dr. Jones had talked to her about these types of changes she could make that could help her condition. She feels unconvinced that her prescribed treatment is right in general, let alone right for her specifically.

Many patients get information online. Although some online information is trustworthy, much of it is not—and even the trustworthy information can be hard to interpret. For example, it can be hard to figure out how to weigh the risk of very rare but serious side effects. This problem is exacerbated when patients don't understand or feel confident about why their doctors made the choices they did.

As noted in chapter 1, doctors often give incomplete drug prescribing information. Dr. Jones's failure to adequately share the prescription information with Mary meant that not only did she not have the information necessary to comply with his recommended treatment, she also began to question the quality of his decision making about her care. And because he didn't engage her in collaborative decision making, she didn't get to express her preference for implementing lifestyle changes rather than taking medication.

ANOTHER OPTION: COMPLEMENTARY AND ALTERNATIVE MEDICINE

Mary talks to a friend about her visit with the doctor and her concerns. The friend is sympathetic and tells Mary that a colleague of hers tried an alternative treatment for her back pain—that person had been similarly unhappy about taking prescription medication and decided to try acupuncture, with great success. The friend puts Mary in touch with her colleague, and the woman raves about how well acupuncture worked for her. She gives Mary the name of the acupuncturist who treats her.

In the medical world, acupuncture belongs to a category of treatments called complementary and alternative medicine (CAM). CAM is defined by the National Center for Complementary and Alternative Medicine (NCCAM) as "a group of diverse medical and health care systems, practices, and products that are not generally considered part of conventional medicine."[5] Complementary medicine is used together with conventional medicine, whereas alternative medicine is used in place of conventional medicine. According to a 2007 National Institute of Health survey, approximately 38 percent of adults and 12 percent of children use some form of CAM.[6] CAM use is greater by women than men, people with higher educational levels,[7] people who have been hospitalized in the past year, and former smokers.

CAM encompasses a wide range of treatment modalities. These are often separated into five categories: alternative medical systems (e.g., acupuncture), biologically based therapies (e.g., megavitamin therapy), manipulative and body-based therapies (e.g., chiropractic care), energy healing therapy (e.g., reiki), and mind-body therapies (e.g., meditation).[8]

Researchers posit a variety of reasons that people choose to use CAM. Some have dubbed them the push factors (those things that drive people from conventional care) and the pull factors (those things that attract people to CAM).[9] In our hypothetical scenario, we have so far seen some of the push factors at work. People, including our Mary, are often "pushed" from conventional care because of

- **A general dissatisfaction with conventional care.** CAM users are more likely than non-CAM users to be dissatisfied with, and lack confidence in, conventional care.[10]
- **A perception of conventional care as too aggressive and dangerous.** The tools of conventional care, surgery and pharmaceuticals, are scary—with good reason. Even when things go well, recovery from surgery can be difficult, and drug side effects can be unpleasant. When things go wrong, the tools are so powerful that consequences can be very serious. A statistic that can be shocking, especially when not viewed in the context of how many people conventional medicine *helps*, is that death caused by conventional medical care is the third leading cause of death in the United States.[11]
- **Having a condition not responsive to conventional care.** As noted above, conventional medicine does not always offer clear-cut diagnoses or effective treatment for chronic pains and discomfort. Similarly, with some serious diseases, conventional care may offer symptom control but no possible treatment option for recovery.
- **A sense that conventional care ignores the individuality of the patient.** Conventional care can have a one-size-fits-all approach that focuses on formulaic responses to symptoms and disease rather than on the totality and uniqueness of the person being treated.
- **Conventional care expense.** CAM is often less expensive than conventional care. People who, because of cost, delay needed conventional medical care are more likely to use CAM than people for whom cost is not a concern.[12]
- **An unsatisfying doctor-patient relationship.** As addressed in chapter 1, doctor-patient relationships are a powerful and important part of the provision of medical care. If their needs for interpersonal aspects of care aren't met by their conventional doctors, patients may be "pushed" to try to get those needs met elsewhere.

DOES CAM WORK? PART 1: THE SCIENTIFIC RESEARCH

Intrigued, Mary looks up acupuncture for back pain online and finds many studies that indicate its effectiveness. She likes that it's been around for thousands of years and has been used by literally countless people. Its potential side effects appear negligible when done by a skilled practitioner, and it feels natural to her in a way that strong pharmaceuticals don't. After reading many testimonials and numerous studies on the use of acupuncture to treat back pain, the fact that Dr. Jones didn't even mention it to her as an option makes her question his knowledge and approach even more.

Much of the research into CAM is not methodologically strong and therefore of questionable probative value. Problems, for example, may take the form of lack of randomization, no or inadequate controls, failure to double-blind, or inadequate sample size. Observational studies may be subject to bias in terms of representativeness of participants. Therapy definitions may be vague and vary from study to study.

Regarding acupuncture for back pain, however, reliable research has indicated some benefits. A 2005 Cochrane review of the effectiveness of acupuncture for lower back pain concludes,

> For chronic low-back pain, acupuncture is more effective for pain relief and functional improvement than no treatment or sham treatment immediately after treatment and in the short-term only. Acupuncture is not more effective than other conventional and "alternative" treatments. The data suggest that acupuncture and dry-needling may be useful adjuncts to other therapies for chronic low-back pain. Because most of the studies were of lower methodological quality, there certainly is a further need for higher quality trials in this area.[13]

It is worth noting that at least one randomized trial conducted since the Cochrane review was published found that sham acupuncture is as effective as real acupuncture, highlighting the continued uncertainty as to whether acupuncture's benefits derive from physiologically important stimulation or from placebo effects.[14]

THE CAM PRACTITIONER VISIT

Mary makes an appointment to see the acupuncturist. In the attractive and comfortable waiting room, she fills out an extensive form asking about her diet, exercise, lifestyle, health history and experience, and goals for treatment. The receptionist brings Mary to the office of the acupuncturist, Lila, who greets Mary warmly. Lila goes through the form with Mary, making sure she understands each answer. She notes that Mary has two sons and tells Mary that she does as well. They talk briefly about their kids and joke about the challenges of raising two boys. Lila clarifies that she understands Mary's treatment goals—specifically, the relief of lower back pain. She does a thorough physical exam.

Lila then creates Mary's treatment plan. In addition to acupuncture, the plan includes specific diet, exercise, and other lifestyle changes. Lila carefully explains the plan and the rationale behind it. She also explains how the acupuncture will work, what it will entail, and what kind of results Mary can expect and when. Lila is enthusiastic about acupuncture's ability to treat lower back pain and tells Mary how well it's worked for other patients. After making sure Mary has no remaining questions or concerns, they move to the treatment room, and Lila gives Mary a first acupuncture treatment.

When the treatment is over, Mary feels positive. She has a complete treatment plan, including lifestyle changes, whose rationale she understands. She feels enormously encouraged by Lila's confidence and the fact that Lila has helped other patients who decided not to use conventional medicine. Two hours have elapsed since her arrival.

We talked above about factors that can push people from conventional medicine. At play in this portion of our hypothetical scenario are factors that can *pull* people to CAM. These include

Trusting the source that recommends the CAM treatment.
Some CAM treatments are licensed and regulated by state governments; this legitimizes them for many potential patients. Some people use CAM because they hear or read positive reports about it in the media. Some try a CAM therapy because someone they know recommends it.

Having a desire to feel in control. People use CAM in part to gain a sense of control over their life and illness experience.[15] Choosing which CAM modality to use gives people a sense of control. Also, if the relationship between the practitioner and patient is good, they can collaborate on treatment goals within that CAM modality.

Having a preference for a holistic approach. Some people believe that CAM treatments offer an approach to care that emphasizes all aspects of health, whereas conventional practitioners treat only specific, localized problems.[16]

Inadequacy of conventional care to address illness or condition. As noted above, conventional medicine often doesn't adequately cope with chronic conditions such as arthritis, cancer, and low back pain, and people may therefore seek out alternatives that promise the possibility of relief.[17] Additionally, some people try CAM to deal with symptoms or side effects from conventional treatments.

Alignment with patient's belief and values. Astin found that CAM users were more likely than nonusers to be committed to causes such as environmentalism or feminism and more interested in spirituality and personal-growth psychology.[18]

Belief that CAM treatments are more natural. Some CAM users may be drawn to it because the remedies and methods feel more "natural" than conventional medicine. This may mean to them that it's safer or more healthful.[19]

DOES CAM WORK? PART 2—THE PATIENT EXPERIENCE

Mary follows Lila's treatment plan to the letter, including suggested exercise and weight loss strategies. She looks forward to her appointments with Lila and doesn't miss a single one. Her back typically feels better immediately after her appointments. Within a month, as Lila predicted, her back feels consistently better than it has for years.

The most compelling reason for people to continue to use CAM is that it works for them. And users perceive that this is the case. In Astin's survey on reasons for CAM use, relief of symptoms was the main reported benefit; the perceived efficacy of CAM was cited almost twice as often as other reported benefits.[20]

Whether they work because of the reasons their advocates claim, because of the placebo effect, or because of benefits of successful provider-patient communication, users perceive real relief from CAM treatments.

PATIENTS AND CONVENTIONAL CARE PRACTITIONERS: TALKING ABOUT CAM

Two months later, Mary needed to see a conventional care doctor for an unrelated health question. She decided not to return to Dr. Jones and found a new doctor, Dr. Andrews, recommended by a colleague. She liked Dr. Andrews and told her the story about her back pain and her approach to treating it. Dr. Andrews was interested in CAM and how patients used CAM to resolve their health issues. She knew the literature about acupuncture and back pain very well. Mary told her that she was getting acupuncture once a week and that her back pain had lessened. Conventional doctors such as Dr. Andrews are likely to respond to such news with anything from approval and encouragement to abject horror.

Whereas hypothetical Mary told her doctor about visiting an acupuncturist, many patients believe that their doctors are not open to alternative approaches; so they don't acknowledge CAM use. Some doctors believe that patients do not think that disclosing CAM use is important.[21] Doctors also often feel uncomfortable discussing CAM with their patients and so don't ask about it.[22] Their discomfort might be based on a doctor's lack of knowledge about CAM modalities.[23] But some CAM treatments are dangerous in conjunction with conventional care, so doctors should encourage their patients to discuss CAM treatments they are exploring; then the doctors can communicate the risks. Also, doctors who learn the care options their patients are pursuing can better understand the patient's concerns, needs, and health-care preferences. Candid communication can also help reduce the risk that patients will abandon conventional care in their pursuit of unproven alternatives.[24]

What doctors should say to patients about CAM is both important and complicated. A few different scenarios may arise. First, as in the acupuncture example, a patient may be exploring a relatively risk-free modality whose efficacy is supported by scientific studies. In this situation a doctor, even if skeptical about the claimed benefits, might feel comfortable supporting the patient's choice to use it. Second, a patient may be using a therapy that has risks associated with its use either alone or in conjunction with conventional care. In this case a doctor will likely feel that it is important to discuss her or his concerns with the patient.

Finally, a patient may be interested in a therapy that the doctor believes has no clear risks but also no benefits beyond placebo effects. There are different perspectives on the best way for doctors to handle such situations. Some authors point out that doctors regularly use placebos in conventional care and that these typically take the form of active agents such as painkillers, sedatives, and antibiotics—which bring dangers such as antibiotic-resistant organisms and painkiller abuse.[25] Given this backdrop, support of innocuous treatments that provide effective results via the placebo effect seems reasonable. Additionally, at times, the placebo effect offered by CAM is the only available treatment option. As Kaptchuk asks, "Should a patient with chronic neck pain who cannot take diazepam because of unacceptable side effects be denied acupuncture . . . because such an effect is 'bogus'?"[26]

But others argue that honesty is critical in the doctor-patient relationship. As articulated by Singh and Ernst, "[t]he question is simple—do we want our healthcare to consist of honest, evidence-based treatments or do we want it built upon a foundation of lies and deceit."[27]

MIND-BODY THERAPIES

The types of CAM referred to as mind-body therapies (MBTs) "focus on the interactions among the brain, mind, body, and behavior, with the intent to use the mind to affect physical functioning and promote health."[28] They are thus particularly relevant to the discussion of psychological aspects of medical care.

The different therapies typically included in the category of MBT are meditation (including mantra meditation, mindfulness meditation, yoga, tai chi, and qi gong), guided imagery, progressive relaxation, deep breathing exercises, and hypnosis.[29] Researchers vary in what they include as part of MBT. For example, NCCAM includes acupuncture as a mind-body therapy, and other researchers include biofeedback.

A 2002 national survey revealed that 16.6 percent of U.S. adults had used at least one mind-body therapy in the prior year.[30] In descending order of use, the percentage of U.S. adults using each therapy was as follows:[31]

deep breathing	11.4 percent
meditation (excluding yoga, tai chi and qi gong)	7.5 percent
yoga	5.0 percent
progressive muscle relaxation	3.0 percent
guided imagery	2.0 percent
tai chi	1.2 percent
qi gong	0.7 percent
hypnosis	0.2 percent
biofeedback	0.1 percent

The survey found that 30 percent of users chose MBT to treat specific medical conditions. Back pain was the most common condition for which an MBT was used, followed by joint pain and hypertension. Among adults who used MBT to treat a specific condition, significant percentages believed it effective—belief that the therapy helped "a great deal" or "to some degree" ranged from a low of 68 percent (for those whose medical concern was anxiety and depression) to a high of 90 percent (for those whose concern was asthma).

Despite users' high levels of belief in the efficacy of these treatments, as with CAM in general, rigorous positive scientific studies are often lacking—and many researchers have reported lack of effectiveness for many of the treatments. For example, such studies have found

- There is inadequate evidence to determine the effectiveness of hypnosis in treating schizophrenia,[32] reducing anxiety and behavioral problems in pediatric dentistry,[33] treating irritable bowel syndrome,[34] or smoking cessation.[35]
- There is inadequate evidence to determine the effectiveness of yoga for treating epilepsy[36] or of meditation in treating attention deficit/hyperactivity disorder[37] or anxiety disorders.[38]
- In an analysis of the effectiveness of meditation on substance abuse, the three highest-quality studies were inconclusive on the effectiveness of mindfulness meditation, relaxation response, and yoga.[39]

- Transcendental meditation was not significantly better than health education at improving blood pressure, heart rate, cholesterol levels, body weight, dietary intake, physical activity stress, or measures of stress, anger, and self-efficacy.[40]
- Relaxation response training did not produce significantly greater benefits on blood pressure than did biofeedback.[41]
- Yoga did not produce clinically or statistically significant effects on blood pressure when compared to no treatment.[42]
- There were no significant differences between yoga and mindfulness-based stress reduction in controlling anxiety in cardiovascular patients.[43]
- Yoga was no better than exercise at producing changes in body weight.[44]

However, some reliable studies support the use of mind-body therapies. For example:

- Some evidence supports the benefits of hypnosis in relieving labor pain[45] and treating nighttime bed-wetting in children.[46]
- Tai chi improved the range of motion in people with rheumatoid arthritis (though it did not approve ability to do chores, joint tenderness, or grip strength).[47]
- In a study of fibromyalgia sufferers, a group using tai chi, compared to the control group, reported less severe symptoms and had improved sleep quality, mood, and quality of life.[48]
- Progressive muscle relaxation may help to reduce blood pressure. (The authors note that "some of the reduction in blood pressure was almost certainly due to aspects of treatment that were not related to relaxation, such as frequent contact with professionals who were trying to help.")[49]
- Qi gong was significantly more effective than a waiting list in reducing systolic blood pressure.[50]
- Relaxation techniques were more effective at reducing self-rated depressive symptoms than no or minimal treatment (although not as effective as psychological treatment).[51]
- Transcendental meditation produced significantly greater benefits in blood pressure than did progressive muscle relaxation.[52]

- Zen Buddhism produced significantly greater reduction in systolic blood pressure, though not in diastolic blood pressure when compared to blood pressure checks.[53]
- When compared to health education, yoga had significant benefits in controlling stress and reducing diastolic, though not systolic, blood pressure.[54]

Many researchers have concluded that more high-quality research is needed in order to assess the effectiveness of mind-body therapies.

TIPS ESPECIALLY FOR PATIENTS

This chapter seeks to remind us of the importance of a good provider-patient relationship. Because of the importance of this relationship, patients should try to select doctors (or other providers) who they believe to be good listeners and effective communicators. In addition, patients using CAM should

- tell their conventional care doctors about all CAM treatments they are using: some treatments may have direct adverse effects or adverse interactions with conventional treatments.
- be informed consumers of CAM care. Some treatments are dangerous, and some patients delay or reject necessary conventional treatment altogether because of their reliance on CAM.

LOOKING AHEAD

This chapter looked at the experience of a hypothetical patient seeking resolution for a specific condition. We saw that individual differences make some people more likely than others to seek out CAM modalities. In the following chapter, we delve further into the impact of psychosocial factors on health—specifically, the relationship of a person's outlook and social connectedness with physical health outcomes. Positive affect, anger/hostility, depression, optimism, sense of control, and social connectedness all vary among individuals and are all related to physical health.

⑩

PATIENT OUTLOOK
AND SOCIAL CONNECTEDNESS

The mind has great influence over the body, and maladies often
have their origin there.

—Molière

People differ in the ways they experience and interpret the world and
the things that happen to them. People also vary in their expectations
about what will happen to them in the future. There is also a wide range
in the ways people connect with the world in terms of their social bonds
and participation. In this chapter we address relationships between
health outcomes and positive/negative outlook, optimism/pessimism,
and perceived control. We end by discussing the correlation between
health outcomes and patient social connectedness.

HAPPY VERSUS HOSTILE/ANGRY AND DEPRESSED

Patient affect is widely studied in relation to health outcomes. Positive
affect has been defined as "feelings that reflect a level of pleasurable
engagement with the environment such as happiness, joy, excitement,
enthusiasm, and contentment."[1] Negative affect includes a range of

attitudes, most significantly hostility, anger, and depression. In general, positive affect is correlated with better health outcomes and negative affect with worse health outcomes.

Happy (Positive Affect)

Self-help books have been saying it for years, and there's some evidence that it's true: happy people tend to be healthier. People with high positive affect are less likely to get the common cold[2] or experience adverse events such as stroke.[3] Long-term studies have found an inverse link between positive affect and mortality; the evidence is strong for community-residing older adults.[4] For example, a 2004 study looked at the impact of positive life orientation (defined by answering yes to being satisfied with life, having zest for life, having plans for the future, feeling needed, and seldom feeling lonely or depressed) in an aged population.[5] Five years after baseline assessments, 2.9 percent of the participants with positive life orientation were in permanent institutional care as compared with 17.5 percent of the remaining participants. At ten years, 54.5 percent of those with positive life orientation were alive as compared with 39.5 percent of the remaining participants.

Though less consistent, a correlation between positive affect and reduced risk of mortality has also been revealed in studies on younger healthy populations. For example, one study scored the emotional content of autobiographies of 180 nuns (mean age twenty-two years old).[6] A strong inverse association was found between positive emotional content in an autobiography and the nun's risk of mortality in late (age seventy-five to ninety-five) life.

Positive affect is also linked to better outcomes among sick people. It has been associated with lower risk of all-cause mortality in people with diabetes[7] and with lower risk of AIDS mortality in HIV-positive men.[8] A 2008 meta-analysis found that psychological well-being was associated with reduced cardiovascular mortality in healthy populations and improved survival in patients with renal failure and HIV infection.[9]

Patients with higher positive affect typically report less pain and fewer symptoms. For example, Zautra and colleagues conducted weekly interviews with women with osteoarthritis and/or fibromyalgia. Higher levels of positive affect predicted lower levels of pain in subsequent weeks.[10] A complicating factor is that people with negative affect may overreport symptoms and people high in positive affect may underreport symptoms.[11]

Quantifying the impact of positive affect is challenging for other reasons. Positive affect may be related to improved health outcomes partly because it often exists alongside other protective psychosocial characteristics. In a sample of 716 people aged fifty-eight to seventy-two, Steptoe and colleagues found that positive affect was associated with greater social connectedness and support, optimism and coping responses, and lower depression, all of which have been independently linked to better health outcomes.[12]

Angry and Depressed (Negative Affect)

As positive affect correlates with better health outcomes, negative affect correlates with worse. The following sections discuss components of negative affect, namely anger/hostility and depression, that have been strongly linked with health outcomes.

Hostile and Angry   Hostility and anger have been researched most extensively for their connection with coronary heart disease (CHD). The constellation of behaviors and attitudes referred to as "type A" was at one time believed linked to the development of CHD. When additional research didn't support such a connection, researchers looked more narrowly at the relationship of anger/hostility, a component of the type A personality, and CHD.[13]

While noting that "hostility" and "anger" are often used interchangeably, Chida and Steptoe define the former as "a negative attitude or cognitive trait directed toward others" and anger as "an emotional state that consists of feelings that vary in intensity from mild irritation or annoyance to intense fury or rage."[14] Their 2009 review concluded that both anger and hostility were associated with increased CHD events in both healthy and high-risk groups.

Chida and Steptoe note that the studies they reviewed were observational and, as such, cannot conclusively establish causation. And other variables may come into play in the relationship. Some studies have found that hostility predicts CHD independent of sociodemographic characteristics and behavioral factors such as alcohol and cigarette use.[15] Other research, however, supports the possibility that anger and hostility impact CHD by influencing high-risk health behaviors such as poor diet, less physical activity, and smoking, or that hostility and anger may be associated with sociodemographic characteristics linked with increased CHD risk.[16] In fact, Chida and Steptoe found that the impact of anger and hostility on CHD was no longer significant after fully controlling for potential confounders such as smoking or socioeconomic status.

There is less research on the relationship of hostility and anger with health outcomes other than those associated with CHD. However, some studies have found that these affective states are associated with greater sensitivity to pain stimuli. The repression of angry feelings is a strong predictor of pain intensity.[17] Likewise, high levels of "anger-out" (management of anger via direct expression) are associated with greater responsiveness to pain stimuli.[18] High anger intensity also correlates with high perceived pain.[19] One study found that anger toward oneself was significantly associated with pain and depression, and overall anger was related to perceived disability.[20]

Depressed   As with hostility/ anger, the relationship of depression with health outcomes has been extensively studied in the context of CHD. Depression in healthy persons almost doubles the risk of developing CHD.[21] Depression is also more prevalent in patients already suffering from CHD: it is also about three times more common in patients after acute myocardial infarctions (MI) than in the general community.[22] After adjusting for disease severity and other potential confounders, depression remains linked with at least double the risk of cardiac events in the one to two years following an MI.[23]

Because depression is so strongly correlated with worsened health outcomes in patients with cardiovascular disease, screening and treatment for depression in those patients is often recommended.[24] A recent review assessed the benefits of screening and treatment, however, and found no evidence that depression treatment improved cardiac outcomes.[25]

In addition to links with cardiovascular disease, depression has also been correlated with an increased risk of developing cancer[26] and with worse outcomes in people with diabetes.[27] Depression during pregnancy has been linked to worsened infant health status.[28] Depression in patients with pain is also associated with more pain complaints.[29] Benefits of depression reduction have been shown to include decreased pain in patients suffering from arthritis.[30]

Biological mechanisms and behaviors such as lessened adherence to treatment and modification of risk factors have been proposed to explain the impact of depression on physical health outcomes. Patients are less compliant with treatment plans when they are depressed. A meta-analysis of studies correlating compliance with depression found that depressed patients are three times more likely to be noncompliant with treatment recommendations than nondepressed patients.[31] In one study, patients assessed as mildly to severely depressed within five days of suffering an MI reported lower adherence to a low-fat diet, regular exercise, reducing stress, and increasing social support four months later.[32] In the same study, patients with major depression also reported taking medications as prescribed less often than those without major depression, and diabetic patients with major depression were less likely to follow a diet for patients with diabetes than those not suffering from depression.

OPTIMISTIC VERSUS PESSIMISTIC

Optimism, the general belief that good things will happen, is firmly tied to better health. Authors of a 2009 meta-analysis of eighty-four studies investigating the link between optimism and physical health concluded that "in the aggregate, these studies strongly suggest that optimism is a significant predictor of physical health."[33]

Objective measures of optimism's link with better health have been found related to a diverse array of health conditions. Such measures include correlations between optimism and better postoperative cognitive performance[34] and levels of pulmonary function in older men.[35] Optimism predicts a lower rate of rehospitalization after coronary artery bypass graft surgery.[36] It has also been linked to reduced risk of postoperative delirium,[37] coronary heart disease,[38] cardiovascular death,[39] and death from cancer.[40]

Not all studies on objective measures find correlations between optimism and negative outcomes, and an important cautionary note is sounded by the authors of one study that found no link between optimism and reduced cancer mortality. The authors warn of the potential pressure patients face from heavy emphasis on the impact of psychosocial factors on health. They note, "Encouraging patients to 'be positive' only may add to the burden of having cancer while providing little benefit, at least in patients with NSCLC [nonsmall cell lung carcinoma]."[41]

Optimism is also correlated with better subjective health outcomes. Optimists report lesser pain severity.[42] They also report fewer symptoms.[43] Rasmussen and colleagues point out, however, the complicated relationship between these subjective (i.e., self-reported or physician-reported) outcomes and results. Self-reports may be biased by the psychosocial attributes of the persons reporting. In their meta-analysis of eighty-four studies, the mean effect size for studies with subjective outcomes was almost twice as high as for objective outcomes (although the effect size for objective outcomes was still statistically significant).[44]

Optimism and pessimism have been treated conceptually both as distinct constructs and as opposite extremes on the same scale.[45] This complicates interpretation of research findings. If optimism and pessimism are extreme ends of the same construct, it is unclear which is most important to physical health—and the apparent benefits of optimism, or costs of pessimism, may simply reflect the absence of the other. If they are mutually independent, both constructs may contribute separately to outcomes. Most researchers construe optimism and pessimism as a single bipolar trait.[46]

Not surprisingly, then, as studies focusing specifically on optimism have uncovered links to improved health outcomes, studies focusing on pessimism have identified correlations with worse health outcomes. One study on the long-term effects of pessimism found that pessimistic explanatory style at age twenty-five predicted poor health at ages forty-five to sixty, even after controlling for physical and mental health at twenty-five.[47] Other health outcomes in studies looking at the impact of pessimism have found correlations in numerous areas. For example, a prospective cohort study of more than 23,000 Finnish people revealed that participants with low pessimism had a 48 percent lower risk for stroke over the seven-year follow-up period.[48] Pessimists also report more pain experience. For example, a 2010 study of 702 patients who had undergone knee replacements found that pessimists reported significantly more moderate to severe pain at two years post-op.[49]

As with all of the psychosocial constructs addressed in this chapter, optimism and pessimism intertwine in various ways with other aspects of outlook and with health behaviors. For example, optimism is associated with taking proactive steps to protect one's health, while pessimism is associated with health-damaging behaviors.[50]

PERCEIVED CONTROL

Perceived control has been defined as "the belief that one can determine one's own internal states and behavior, influence one's environment, and/or bring about desired outcomes."[51] The belief that one has control over one's life provides significant benefits. In an early study, Langer and Rodin assessed the effects of an intervention designed to encourage elderly nursing home residents to feel more control over day-to-day events.[52] Staff gave a talk to the experimental group emphasizing their responsibility for themselves; the residents in this group were also given plants to care for. Staff gave a talk to the control group emphasizing staff's responsibility for them as patients; the residents in this group were given plants to be watered by staff. The authors found that residents belonging to the group in which control was emphasized became more active, reported feeling happier, and showed significant improvements in alertness and involvement in social activities. In addition, when assessed eighteen months later, this group showed higher health and lower mortality rates.

Later research has supported the finding that high levels of perceived control are associated with lower mortality rates.[53] Perceived control has also been well studied in patients with asthma and consistently associated with better outcomes.[54] Perceived control has also been shown to be correlated with less postsurgery physical disability in older women[55] and less disability in patients with Parkinson's disease.[56]

Perceived control has also been studied in the context of social class and appears to play a moderating role in the impact of low socioeconomic status on health. People with lower income tend to have lower perceived control as well as worse health.[57] People in the lowest income group with high perceived control, however, have levels of health and well-being comparable to higher-income groups.[58]

Some beneficial outcomes of perceived control may lie in adherence and lifestyle choices. People with high levels of perceived control tend to take more responsibility for their health, including adherence to treatment recommendations and healthful lifestyle modifications.[59]

A challenging feature of research in this area is that many of these psychosocial attitudes and perceptions have complicated relationships with other aspects of personality and can be hard to tease apart. For example, a 2007 study examined the perceptions of older adults about their risk of suffering a hip fracture compared to the risk for similar individuals.[60] The researchers found that for participants with high perceived control, optimism (perceiving a comparatively low risk) was associated with better psychological and physical well-being relative to pessimism (perceiving a comparatively high risk). Among participants with low perceived control, there were no differences in well-being between optimists and pessimists. The authors suggest that this indicates that "the protective effect of comparative optimism on well-being is limited to older adults who have a strong sense of control."

SOCIAL SUPPORT

Level of social support can be evaluated by the quantity or quality of relationships or by the type of support provided: emotional (including encouragement of health-promoting behaviors and discouragement of health-damaging behaviors) and/or practical (e.g., instrumental support, assistance, reminders).

In an influential early study on the impact of social support on health, Berkman and Syme reported on the results of a nine-year follow-up of nearly seven thousand adults who had been measured for social and community ties at baseline.[61] They found that significantly more people who lacked such ties had died in the follow-up period than those with more extensive contacts. Compared to men with the most social contacts, 2.3 times as many of the most isolated men had died. Compared to women with the most social contacts, 2.8 times as many of the most isolated women had died. These differences were independent of physical health status at the time of the initial survey, socioeconomic status, and health practices.

Many subsequent studies have found correlations between social support and all-cause mortality. For example, Croezen and colleagues followed participants for nineteen years; low positive experience of support at baseline was associated with a significant increased mortality risk after adjusting for socioeconomic factors, lifestyle factors, and indicators of health status.[62] Another study found that perceptions by young adults of having warm relationships with their parents predicted later health status; thirty-five years after an initial assessment, 45 percent of participants who perceived themselves to have had a warm relationship with their mother, and 91 percent of those who had not, had a diagnosed disease. A similar association held for relationships with fathers.[63]

Many studies have investigated the link between social support and specific diseases, especially cardiovascular disease.[64] For example, Brummett and colleagues investigated social isolation as a predictor of mortality in 430 patients with significant CAD.[65] Patients with small social networks had a higher risk of mortality that was not attributable to confounding with disease severity, demographics, or psychological distress.

Social support plays a role in cancer outcomes. A 2010 meta-analysis found that high levels of perceived support, larger social network, and being married were associated with decreased relative risk for mortality of, respectively, 25 percent, 20 percent, and 12 percent.[66] Coping with the challenges of a cancer diagnosis through reliance on social support correlates with improved outcomes. Lutgendorf and colleagues found that patients who sought instrumental support at diagnosis had lower interleukin-6 (elevated IL-6 is associated with a poorer prognosis in ovarian and cervical cancers), better clinical status, and less disability at one year.[67]

Social support has been linked with better outcomes in patients with infectious diseases. In particular, higher satisfaction with social support has been correlated with a slower progression to AIDS in men with HIV type-1 infection.[68]

Social support may impact health outcomes through its relationship with other risk factors. Brummett and colleagues concluded that the relation between social support and longevity is partly accounted for by the inverse association between support and sedentary behavior. (They found no support for the idea that smoking or depression play into the association.)[69]

Similarly, social support may interact with depression in ways that reduce risks of mortality. Frasure-Smith and colleagues assessed depression and social support of 887 patients one week after a myocardial infarction (MI) and followed the patients for one year.[70] They found that post-MI depression predicted cardiac mortality but that social support was not directly related. High social support did, however, appear to buffer the impacts of depression on mortality.

DiMatteo posits that the link between social support and health may lie with patient adherence to treatment recommendations.[71] Her meta-analysis revealed that risks of nonadherence were

- almost twice as high for patients without practical support (e.g., assistance, reminders, organizational support).
- 1.35 times higher for patients without emotional support.
- 1.74 times higher for patients with low family cohesion.
- 1.53 times greater for patients with high conflict in their families
- 1.13 times higher for unmarried patients
- 1.35 times higher for children of unmarried parents
- 1.17 times higher for patients living alone

An interesting final note is that providing support to others is also beneficial. One study found that support given was more important to the well-being of older adults than support received except when received from a spouse or a sibling.[72]

TIPS ESPECIALLY FOR PATIENTS

Although there is a strong link between positive patient outlook and better health, this does not imply that a patient is *responsible* for bringing on an illness or failing to cure it because of his or her outlook. Pressuring patients to control and potentially change well-established parts of their personality could add significantly to an already substantial illness burden. With that said, there are some steps that patients could take in this area that may improve health outcomes:

- Depression is tightly linked to worsened health outcomes. The connection may be through biological mechanisms or because depressed people are less likely to adhere to treatment or modify their risk factors. In either case, treating depression may lead to improved health outcomes.

- Patients who feel in control of their internal states, the environment, and ultimate outcomes stand the best chance of responding favorably to treatment. One way for patients to have a stronger sense of control is to choose doctors who engage them in shared decision making.
- Good social support is correlated with improved health outcomes. Strengthening social ties is a valuable goal for many reasons, including, potentially, staying and getting healthy.

LOOKING AHEAD

In this chapter we looked at how psychosocial factors are related to health outcomes in both healthy and patient populations. In the following chapter, we address another variable with strong correlations to health outcomes: the environment in which patients heal.

HEALING ENVIRONMENTS

Health care cannot be separated from the setting in which it is done.

—Jain Malkin[1]

Windows, sounds of nature, a room with a foldout couch for family, clear signage. This chapter addresses health facility features such as these that help patients heal. We discuss specifically the research on the impact of light, nature, sound, room and facility layout, and way finding in helping patients achieve positive health outcomes and maintain well-being.

HEALING ENVIRONMENT OVERVIEW

The concept of a healing environment suggests that the physical space in which health care happens can play a significant role in the effectiveness of treatment. In some cases this is due directly to physical effects—cleanliness lessens the spread of infections, for example, and loudness can impact patient sleep. As discussed in this chapter, there are also psychological responses to aspects of the environment that can impact healing.

The ideal inpatient medical experience includes a quiet, well-lit, private room with a window looking out onto a natural scene, an easily accessible bathroom, space for family and friends to visit comfortably, and a highly navigable facility outside the room. These may seem like fairly obvious preferences. What is perhaps more surprising is the myriad positive health outcomes that come from experiencing this type of environment. Positive outcomes that derive from physical aspects of the environment include

- Improved medical history taking
- Reduced medication errors
- Reduced patient stress, anxiety, and depression
- Reduced pain experience and reduced pain medication usage
- Increased patient satisfaction
- Improved sleep
- Increased supportive social interaction
- Shortened hospital stay
- Reduced cost of care

LIGHT

The quality and amount of lighting in health-care settings can affect patient health and well-being. We first address how lighting impacts patients directly and then look at how lighting may impact health-care staff in ways that, positively or negatively, affect the patients they treat.

Impact of Lighting on Patients

Numerous studies have shown that variations in lighting have a significant impact on a wide range of patient outcomes. Effective lighting is associated with decreased patient pain and pain medication use, decreased length of hospital stay, better patient orientation, improved emotional well-being, and even lessened mortality rates.

Pain   The amount of sunlight in hospital rooms may influence patients' pain and need for pain medication. Walch and colleagues investigated the pain medication use of postsurgery patients who were randomly assigned to either bright or dim hospital rooms. Patients in the bright rooms (which averaged 46 percent higher intensity sunlight than dim rooms) required 22 percent less pain medication than those in the dim rooms. The patients also reported less stress and less pain. The reduction in pain medication led to a 21 percent decrease in medication costs.[2]

Length of Hospital Stay   Better light exposure is associated with shortened patient hospital stays. Beauchemin and Hays compared durations of stays of depressed patients in sunny rooms with those in dim rooms. The patients in the sunny rooms had an average length of stay 2.6 days shorter than those in dull rooms.[3]

The same authors looked at the impact of natural light on length of hospital stay in patients who had experienced myocardial infarctions. All patients in the sunny room stayed a shorter time, although the difference was significant for the females only.[4]

Benedetti and colleagues compared bipolar inpatients randomly assigned to rooms exposed to direct sunlight in the morning to patients in rooms without direct morning sunlight. Those in the sunny rooms had a mean 3.67-day shorter hospital stay than patients in the dimmer rooms.[5]

Finally, a study at Veterans Health Administration hospitals found that centers in locations with more light have shortest patient length of stay, and centers in cold climates have the longest patient stays in winter and fall.[6]

Orientation   Windows may help patients feel connected to the outside world and remain oriented during hospital stays. Keep and colleagues surveyed two groups of patients who had spent at least forty-eight hours in an intensive therapy unit: one group in a unit without windows and the other in a unit with translucent windows. The patients from the windowless unit had less accurate memories of their stay and were less oriented in time during their stay. They also had more sleep disturbance and twice the incidence of hallucinations and delusions as the patients in windowed rooms.[7]

Depression   Bright light reduces depression among patients with seasonal affective disorder as well as with nonseasonal depressions. A 2005 meta-analysis of randomized, controlled trials on the efficaciousness of light therapy for mood disorders concluded that "bright light treatment and dawn simulation for seasonal affective disorder and bright light for nonseasonal depression are efficacious, with effect sizes equivalent to those in most antidepressant pharmacotherapy trials."[8]

Exposure to light is also correlated with positive mood effects in healthy individuals. Partonen and Lonnqvist repeatedly exposed office employees to bright light during the winter and found reduced depressive symptoms in employees both with and without season-dependent symptoms.[9] In another study, the impact of exercise on mood was compared in two conditions: bright light and normal light.[10] Exercise reduced depression in both conditions, but significantly more so when combined with bright light exposure.

Mortality   Beauchemin and Hays assessed the relationship between natural light exposure and mortality in myocardial infarction patients. In dull rooms, 39 of 335 patients (11.6 percent) died; in sunny rooms, 21 of 293 (7.2 percent) died.[11]

Impact of Lighting on Staff

In addition to impacting patients directly, lighting affects the staff who care for them. For example, bright lighting reduces medication errors. Furthermore, staff whose lighting and other environmental preferences are accommodated are likely to be happier. Happy staff generally leads to reduced turnover, fewer sick days taken, and greater continuity of care for patients.[12]

Effective lighting has been correlated with reduced employee stress and improved job satisfaction, reduced medication dispensing errors, and better employee reports of well-being.

Stress and Job Satisfaction   Access to daylight decreases stress and increases job satisfaction of medical staff. In a study of 141 nurses in Turkey, exposure to daylight for at least three hours a day was associated with less stress and higher satisfaction.[13] The study authors concluded that daylight exposure may be effective at reducing job burnout. Similarly, an employee satisfaction survey at a newly constructed medical center examined sources of staff satisfaction; of all items surveyed, light had the most positive effect.[14] Seventy percent of respondents rated the increased natural light as having a very positive or a positive impact on their work life.

Reduced Errors   The intensity and quantity of light impacts health-care worker error rates. During one study, five pharmacists dispensed a total of 10,888 prescriptions; during days when the workplace was brightly lit, there was a 30 percent reduction in medication dispensing errors.[15] A study of hospital worker medication errors in Alaska, where the daily length of darkness ranges from 4.5 hours in June to 18.6 hours in December, found that 58 percent of all errors happened in the first quarter of the year.[16]

Well-being   Verderber and Reuman assessed the impact of poorly windowed rooms on patients and staff. Patients in rooms with few or no windows experienced negative consequences such as worse health status or lower feeling of well-being. And staff who worked more than forty hours a week or commuted to work experienced feelings of lessened well-being in the poorly windowed environment.[17]

NATURE

Windows provide more than just light. They also offer a way for people to visually connect to the outside world through what they see beyond the glass. Thus, the content of the view may have a large impact.

In this section we look at the healing benefits of windows that look onto natural views. Since windows looking onto nature are not always available, the impact of nature views in other forms has also been researched. It is addressed below, first in the form of representational images in art and second in the form of gardens. Exposure to nature, in a variety of forms, has a beneficial impact on patient health.

View from a Window

A nature view from a window can positively affect patient outcomes. Such views have been associated with reduced health-care needs. For example, prisoners whose cells faced outward toward an exterior natural landscape made use of health services considerably less than those whose cells faced the interior courtyard.[18]

Nature views have been associated with shorter hospital stays and decreased pain. Ulrich found that, compared with surgery recovery patients whose windows looked out onto a brick wall, surgery recovery patients whose windows offered a natural view had shorter postoperative hospital stays, took less pain medication, and had fewer negative nursing notes in their hospital charts.[19]

Given the correlation between pain and window views, Ulrich and colleagues suggest that in addition to hospital rooms, other areas in medical facilities where pain may be experienced (such as procedure spaces, treatment rooms, and waiting areas) should also be provided with window views.[20]

Images of Nature

Images of nature can provide many of the same healing benefits as windows looking onto natural settings. Interestingly, people may intuitively compensate for lacking windows by finding other ways to view nature: one 1986 study found that people in windowless offices used twice as many images to decorate their offices as people in offices with windows, and that the images in the windowless offices tended to be nature scenes.[21] Art (including two-dimensional, video, and sounds) representing nature can decrease stress and anxiety and reduce pain and pain medication usage.

Ulrich and colleagues examined the impact of images of nature on the health of patients recovering from heart surgery.[22] They randomly assigned patients to rooms with images of nature, abstract art, or no art. Patients in the rooms with nature images needed less strong pain medication and reported less anxiety than the patients in the other rooms.

Tse and colleagues used video to assess the impact of natural imagery on pain. The researchers induced pain in healthy subjects, divided into two groups. One group watched a soundless video of natural scenery, and the other group watched a blank screen. Participants who viewed the nature video had significantly higher pain thresholds and pain tolerance.[23]

One study had patients undergoing flexible bronchoscopy (looking inside the air passages leading to the lungs) either view a nature mural while listening to nature sounds or receive normal treatment (no images or sounds).[24] The patients exposed to the nature scenes and sounds reported significantly less pain.

Gardens

Many hospitals offer gardens for the use of patients, visitors, and staff. The gardens reduce stress and improve mood.[25] Ulrich posits that the stress-reducing benefit of gardens derives from their ability to provide a sense of control and access to privacy (by allowing patients to choose to escape, even briefly, negative situations); social support (gardens provide opportunities for social interaction); opportunities for physical movement and exercise; and access to nature and other positive distractions. Gardens can also increase patient and visitor satisfaction with the quality of care.[26]

SOUND

Loud noise can have detrimental impacts on those subjected to it. In recognition of this concern, the World Health Organization (WHO) set guidelines for background noise and peak levels in hospitals. The WHO suggests limiting noise to 30dB(A) for background noise in patient rooms, 35dB(A) for background noise in other rooms in which patients are being treated or observed, and 40dB(A) or less for peak noise levels.[27]

Substantial research indicates that those levels are regularly far exceeded.[28] One recent study of five surgical wards revealed a highest peak noise level of 95.6dB, a level comparable to the noise from a heavy truck, and frequent noise levels exceeding 80dB.[29] The study authors sound the alarm, writing, "It is likely that these findings will translate to other hospitals. Urgent measures are needed to rectify this."

As discussed below, excessive noise is detrimental to both patients and health-care providers in many ways. Among other negative outcomes, excess noise can lead to increased anxiety and pain perception, loss of sleep, and prolonged convalescence.[30]

Impact on Patients

Noisy surroundings can increase patient stress, compromise their sleep, weaken rehabilitation, and adversely affect physiologic and behavioral outcomes.

Stress Noise in hospital settings can increase patient stress levels. Topf asked 105 female volunteers to try to sleep overnight in either a quiet condition or a condition simulating the sounds in a critical care unit (CCU). The group in the CCU sound simulation experienced greater subjective stress.[31]

Jordanian patients in CCUs who heard buzzers and alarms from machinery named the noises as one of the main stressors they experienced.[32] Ulrich noted that stress experienced by patients is both negative on its own and directly affects other health outcomes "related to psychological, physiological, neuroendocrine, and behavioral changes associated with stress responses."[33]

Sleep Excessive noise is a major source of sleep disruption in health care settings. Freedman and colleagues reported that noise in the intensive care unit (ICU) contributes to more than 25 percent of patient awakenings per subject during the night.[34] Topf and colleagues compared self-reports of sleep of female subjects exposed to either recorded critical care unit noise or quiet. Patients in the noise condition reported taking longer to fall asleep, more awakenings, and poorer sleep than at home. They used more negative adjectives when describing their sleep.[35] Disturbed sleep is associated with adverse health impacts such as increase in heart rate and medicine use and subsequent insomnia.[36]

Physiologic and Behavioral Effects Excessive noise negatively affects physiologic and behavior outcomes. Hagerman and colleagues compared patients admitted to an intensive coronary heart unit that had good or poor acoustic conditions. Patients in the good acoustics group had a lower rate of rehospitalization.[37] They also considered the staff attitude much better than those in the poor acoustics group. Noise reduction (via use of earmuffs) in neonatal intensive care units led to significantly higher oxygen saturation levels, less frequent behavioral state changes, and better and longer sleep.[38]

Impact on Staff

Researchers have looked at two main impacts of noise on health-care providers. First, noise may increase stress, which in turn can lead to burnout. Second, noise may impact errors committed by medical staff.

Stress Noise can increase stress for health-care providers. Morrison and colleagues monitored ambient sound levels and nurses' heart rates continuously over three-hour periods while nurses provided patient care. The researchers also collected nurse stress/annoyance reports every half hour. Higher sound levels significantly predicted higher heart rates and increased stress and annoyance.[39] In another study, Blomkvist and colleagues compared the impact of sound reflecting or sound absorbing tiles placed in a CCU. The sound absorbing tiles positively affected the work environment; staff experienced significantly lower work demands and reported less stress.[40]

Increased stress can lead to dissatisfaction with work. In a study of one hundred critical care nurses, Topf and Dillon found that noise-induced occupational stress was positively related to burnout.[41]

Errors and Work Performance Noise in all arenas may lead to worsened task performance.[42] Hospital workers perceive facility noise to interfere with their work performance and to negatively affect patients' comfort and recovery.[43] Noisy distractions such as pagers and overhead announcements are associated with pharmacy dispensing errors.[44]

Strategies for Reducing Noise

Many sources of excessive noise are unnecessary. Cropp and colleagues, for example, recorded thirty-three sounds commonly heard in an ICU and found that only ten were critical alarms.[45] Moreover, staff in the unit could correctly identify only 50 percent of the critical alarms and only 40 percent of the noncritical alarms. The authors concluded that "the myriad of alarms that regularly occur in the ICU are too much for even experienced ICU staff to quickly discern. Patient and caregiver alike could benefit by a graded system in which only urgent problems have audible alarms."

In addition to eliminating unnecessary sources of noise, Ulrich and colleagues recommend the use of single rooms and installation of sound-absorbing materials on ceilings, floors, and walls as important strategies in combating the problem of noise in health-care environments.[46]

Music and White Noise

Pleasant sounds such as music and white noise may positively impact patient well-being. A 2009 Cochrane review found that music listening may beneficially affect blood pressure, heart rate, respiratory rate, anxiety, and pain.[47] It may also improve patient and family satisfaction with care.[48]

White noise may also improve patient outcomes. Williams studied night sleep patterns of patients posttransfer from the ICU.[49] Patients who received ocean sounds reported better sleep experiences than controls (no white noise). The groups were significantly different in sleep depth, awakening, return to sleep, and quality of sleep.

LAYOUT AND DÉCOR

Layout and décor impact patient outcomes, most notably in differences between single and multibed rooms. Esthetically pleasing environments and well-positioned furniture in common areas have positive effects.

Single Rooms

The most studied aspect of layout is the comparison of single to multibed rooms. Single rooms offer a host of significant patient benefits such as increased privacy, better accommodation of visitors, and fewer medical transfers and errors.

Privacy Patients in health-care settings usually must disclose highly personal information and submit themselves to often emotionally uncomfortable physical scrutiny. Patients who perceive their privacy in these settings as inadequate may have decreased satisfaction with their care. Even more troubling, patients who do not feel their privacy is well protected may withhold relevant information out of fear of being overheard or refuse to be examined out of fear of being seen.[50]

Single rooms are significantly better at satisfying patients' privacy concerns.[51] Nurses also prefer single rooms for privacy-related reasons. In one survey, nurses reported that single rooms are most appropriate for patient examinations and patient history taking.[52] One respondent commented that confidentiality can't be assured if another patient is in the same room.

Fewer Transfers and Errors Patient transfers between rooms may lead to communication breakdowns among attending practitioners, loss of information, and changes in computers used. Medical errors increase.[53] Single-patient rooms are associated with fewer patient transfers and fewer medication errors.

Visitor Accommodation   Social support by way of visits by family and friends improves patient psychological and physical well-being. Support has been linked with reduced patient stress, fear and anxiety, and improved patient adherence to treatment plans and physiological outcomes.[54]

Single rooms are better than multibed rooms at facilitating social support. Single rooms offer privacy for visits and, unlike multibed rooms, don't give rise to concerns about bothering other patients. They are also more often able to physically accommodate guests, with greater space capacity and furniture types (e.g., daybeds or pull-out sofas) that allow visitors to stay comfortable during extended visits.

Waiting Areas

Another source of support for beneficial patient social interactions is the availability of comfortable waiting areas with movable furniture.[55] Seating arrangements have a large impact on patients' social interactions.[56] The common pattern of arranging seating in a line against walls lessens social interaction. Furniture should be comfortable and support expected behaviors. For instance, if a television is placed in the waiting room, furniture should be oriented to allow for watching it.

Esthetically Pleasing Environment

Attractive environments are associated with increased patient satisfaction, higher patient ratings for attending doctors and hospitals, increased intentions to use the hospital again and recommend it to others, and lessened patient anxiety.

Leather and colleagues compared patient response to an outpatient waiting area prior to and after renovations. The renovations included changes to layout, furniture, curtains, and information provision. The new waiting area was associated with more positive environmental appraisals, better mood, altered physiological state, and greater reported satisfaction.[57] In another study, patients placed in attractive rather than unattractive rooms evaluated their doctors and nurses more positively and had more positive opinions about the quality of the hospital service.[58]

WAY FINDING

Health-care facilities should provide easy cues to help patients and visitors find their destinations, yet way finding can be difficult, especially in large hospitals.[59] Carpman asserts that health facilities are among the most complex facilities people encounter, in part because of their large size and often confusing nomenclature. In addition, many facilities have grown incrementally, sometimes leading to unrelated destinations being close to each other and related destinations far apart.[60]

Way-finding systems are how hospitals and other health-care delivery sites help patients and visitors navigate these complex physical health-care environments. Ineffective systems have a number of costs. Patients and visitors may get frustrated by difficult way-finding experiences, and this can hurt their perception of the institution they are navigating. Poor way-finding experiences may also impact patients' health. The spatial disorientation that results can lead to stress, raised blood pressure, headaches, and fatigue.[61]

Another cost attributable to poor way finding is the resulting direction giving required of staff members who are not employed for that purpose. Zimring found the actual monetary cost of this activity in a 604-bed hospital to be more than $220,000 per year, the cost equivalent of 4,500 staff hours (two full-time positions).[62] In addition to the financial cost, productivity and patient care are also reduced when the time of staff members is used giving directions instead of providing health care to patients.

Effective way-finding systems are comprehensive and not implemented piecemeal. This can be a challenge for existing facilities. Good systems include clear signage, both outside and inside a facility, but signage alone is typically inadequate to compensate for a complex and confusing structure. In addition to signage, high-quality way-finding systems should include: accessible and clear information provision and orientation aids (such as information desks, maps, and directories) available both previsit and within the facility, understandable nomenclature for departments, architectural and design differentiation for different areas, landmarks to help visitors orient themselves, and a comprehensible overall floor plan.

TIPS ESPECIALLY FOR PATIENTS

Patients will ideally spend any hospital time in quiet and attractive single rooms with good light and nature views. This ideal is not always possible. Still, appreciate that aspects of the environment impact health and healing. So seek ways to make it as supportive of healing as possible. If there's no window in their room, for example, patients can see whether they can get nature artwork for the walls.

LOOKING AHEAD

As discussed in this final chapter, once patients have communicated with their doctors and been diagnosed with conditions for which they are treated, the place in which they are treated and heal now takes its turn to impact health outcomes. As final topics of interest, we close this book with three appendices. The first examines psychiatric diagnosis. The second presents a discussion of the field of Darwinian medicine. The third addresses general wellness strategies to employ to help avoid the need for medical interventions as long as possible.

APPENDIX I

PSYCHIATRIC DIAGNOSIS

The *Diagnostic and Statistical Manual* (*DSM*) was first published in 1952 as an official manual of approved psychiatric diagnostic terms. *DSM-II* followed in 1968, with the goal of improving the quality of the statements that described proper usage of the terms. Although both versions were widely used, critics claimed that their diagnostic descriptions were insufficiently detailed, raising serious questions about reliability.

Then, in 1973, psychologist David Rosenhan published an article that shook the psychiatric community.[1] Rosenhan had arranged for himself and seven other normal people to show up at psychiatric hospitals and say they were hearing a voice. That was their only symptom—no delusions or thought disorder. All were admitted, at which point they stopped feigning their symptom. One pseudopatient was diagnosed as manic depressive, the rest as schizophrenic.

Rosenhan arranged a follow-up study with the staff of a well-known research and teaching hospital. They knew of his prior results and claimed that similar errors were inconceivable at their institution. So he told them that during a three-month period, one or more pseudopatients would attempt to gain admission. The staff agreed to rate the likelihood that each incoming patient was an impostor. They rated 41 of 193 patients as impostors and 42 more as suspect. But Rosenhan had sent no pseudopatients—all the patients were genuine. Rosenhan concluded that "any diagnostic process that lends itself too readily to massive errors of this sort cannot be a very reliable one."

In 1974, Spitzer and Fleiss published an influential paper indicating that psychiatric diagnosis remained a serious problem.[2] Over the next few years, studies indicated that the likelihood of two psychiatrists agreeing on a diagnosis often hovered around 50 percent. Recognition of the problem provided impetus for revision of the *DSM*. *DSM-III* was published in 1980 to improve reliability. It added explicit diagnostic criteria and structured interviews. *DSM-III-R* in 1987 deleted some categories and added others, and its introductory section claims far greater reliability than previously obtained with *DSM-II*. For example, Riskind and colleagues had sixteen psychologists use *DSM-III* to diagnose seventy-five psychiatric patients suffering from either depression, generalized anxiety, or some other disorder. There was 83 percent agreement.[3]

DSM-IV, published in 1994, was the culmination of the work of several groups of approximately twenty expert advisers. Each group reviewed the literature of the diagnoses for which they were responsible and then sought data from researchers to determine which criteria required change. Whereas *DSM-I* identified sixty categories of disorders, *DSM-IV* lists 410. *DSM-IV* is even more reliable than its immediate predecessor and is the official manual for psychiatric diagnosis in the United States. Most health insurance companies require a *DSM-IV* diagnosis as a condition for approving therapy. Thirteen different work groups are currently developing *DSM-V*. A release of the final, approved version is expected in May 2013.

An unreliable diagnostic procedure is useless. After all, what value could a procedure have if, after viewing the results, some doctors concluded that the patient was diabetic and others that she had hepatitis C? However, although *DSM*'s reliability problems may have been solved, there are deeper concerns. Suppose this book's authors were invited to help with the writing of *DSM-V* and we introduced a new diagnostic category: Leavitt Absent Book Syndrome (LABS). Patients would be asked to provide verifiable proof of having bought a copy of this book. Failing that, they would receive a LABS diagnosis. The prognosis for such people would be grim, with years of aimless toil followed by slow descent into madness. The reliability of the LABS tests would be higher than that of any diagnostic category in the *DSM*.

Despite the silliness of the example, it underscores an important point: the process of determining whether a certain constellation of symptoms is worthy of inclusion in the *DSM* is much less objective than proponents claim. Social values play an important role. For example, after gay activists protested at the American Psychiatric Association annual conference in 1974, the *DSM* stopped listing homosexuality as a category of disorder.

Money plays a huge role. Cosgrove and colleagues reported that 95 of 170 psychiatrists who developed the *DSM-IV* had financial ties to drug companies. In six out of eighteen panels, more than 80 percent of members had financial ties. And the percentage was 100 percent for those who worked on sections devoted to severe mental illnesses such as schizophrenia.[4] For those diagnostic areas, drugs are typically the first line of treatment. Critics claim that diagnoses such as social phobia are invented to create a market for antidepressants or other drugs.

Psychiatrists are unique in the medical field in that they often make a diagnosis even though the patient has no discernible physical abnormality and makes no complaints. A diagnosis may have devastating effects, including loss of self-confidence and permanent stigma. In addition, patients diagnosed with certain conditions may lose the right to make decisions about their legal and medical affairs, may lose health insurance or be forced to pay exorbitant premiums, and may lose child custody. The website http://www.psychdiagnosis.net gives many personal stories.

The *DSM* developers made the disease descriptions gender-neutral. But, as noted by Westly, gender influences every aspect of depression and other mental illnesses—from the symptoms experienced to response, to treatment, to the course of the disorder throughout the person's entire life.[5] For example, women most typically express depression as sadness. For men, the most typical expression is anger or irritability, often coupled with recklessness. Depressed women respond better than depressed men to SSRIs, probably because the SSRIs work best in the presence of estrogen.

APPENDIX 2

DARWINIAN MEDICINE

Nothing in biology makes sense except in the light of evolution.

—Theodosius Dobzhansky, evolutionary biologist

Randolph Nesse and George Williams are cofounders of the field they called Darwinian medicine. Their seminal article on the subject, which appeared in the March 1991 *Quarterly Review of Biology* and was followed by the 1994 book *Why We Get Sick*, describes how an understanding of evolutionary principles can help doctors and patients make better choices.[1] Unfortunately, however, Darwinian medicine has not yet had a significant impact in U.S. medical schools. Nesse and Stearns wrote, "We know of no medical school that teaches a course in evolutionary biology as a basic medical science, and none that requires evolution as a prerequisite."[2]

Nesse and Williams wrote that the great mystery of medicine is why, in a machine of exquisite design, "there are a thousand flaws and frailties that make us vulnerable to disease." They ask why natural selection hasn't shaped ways to prevent nearsightedness, heart attacks, and Alzheimer's disease. "Why hasn't it selected for genes that would perfect our ability to resist damage and enhance repairs so as to eliminate aging? The common answer—that natural selection just isn't powerful enough—is usually wrong."

The real answer, they say, is that the body is a bundle of compromises. Like any machine, it has design trade-offs. By understanding how evolution has shaped that design, medicine can become more effective. Patients would benefit if doctors took an evolutionary approach. Some illnesses would be redefined and others explained.

Nesse[3] gave six main reasons why selection has left us vulnerable to disease:

- Pathogens evolve faster than humans do. The generation times of *E. coli* are one million times faster than ours, and every time we get better at treating a disease, the disease gets better. The co-evolutionary arms race is never ending. Vaccinating large populations changes the pathogen's environment, and imperfect vaccines can create selection pressures for increased virulence. Not only can pathogens evolve ways to avoid our defenses, but our defenses and counterdefenses are costly. One consequence is that we become vulnerable to autoimmune diseases. (See below.)

- We do not evolve fast enough to keep up with changing environments, which explains much chronic disease in modern populations. Our Paleolithic ancestors had strong appetites for sugars and fats, which are valuable energy sources.[4] This proclivity persists— we are programmed to store fat reserves when possible, against lean times. But sugars and fats are no longer rare commodities. As a result, too many people indulge themselves endlessly in rich, tasty, fatty foods. The price is obesity and heart disease.

- Natural selection has limitations. It cannot maintain uncorrupted DNA information, and it is constrained by dependence on evolutionary history. The vertebrate eye is an example. Nerves and vessels run between the light and the visual receptors, and the resulting blind spot at their exit causes further problems. But that's because the eye was not designed from scratch; it evolved from preexisting parts, and there is no way to go back and set things right.

- Every feature of the body involves trade-offs and is less than perfect. The bones in the wrist could be larger and less prone to breakage, but only at the cost of wrist mobility. Increased investment in immune response would require more calories and risk damaging tissues. Decreased anxiety would result in more individuals dying young because they would take insufficient precautions against serious threats. People who inherit a single copy of a certain gene are protected from malaria and do not develop sickle-cell anemia; but people who inherit a copy of the gene from both parents do develop the deadly disease. There's a trade-off: relatively few people get two copies of the gene, and those who inherit a single copy have a huge advantage in areas rife with malaria.

- Some traits increase reproduction even though they decrease health. Males of most species have shorter average life spans than females, because investments in competitive ability give greater reproductive payoffs for males. So males invest more in body size, armor, and weaponry, less in safety and tissue repair.

- Symptoms such as pain, fever, vomiting, coughing, inflammation, depression, and anxiety are often positive bodily defenses shaped by natural selection. They are useful, although in many cases they are expressed too readily. This can be explained by the smoke-detector principle: failure to respond to a real threat can be catastrophic, so the normal system is set to a threshold that yields many false alarms.

Medical symptoms represent a deviation from normality, and doctors generally assume that deviations are bad. (See also p. 73.) Most doctors treat symptoms to try to restore normality. Proponents of Darwinian medicine behave differently. Because they view health and disease from an evolutionary perspective, they recognize that symptoms may reflect any of three possible causes. Some symptoms, such as jaundice or seizures, arise from defects in the body's machinery. They have no utility and should be corrected. But many symptoms are defensive strategies—adaptations shaped through eons of natural selection. In fact, according to Nesse and Stearns, most symptoms of infectious disease are not caused directly by the pathogens; they result from useful defenses. Some symptoms are parts of the inflammation and immune systems that attack pathogens. Others, such as cough, diarrhea, and vomiting, extrude pathogens. Proponents of Darwinian medicine urge physicians to recognize the implications of treating such symptoms. Doing so is likely to prolong and exacerbate illness. A third cause of symptoms is adaptations that have gone awry, such as chronic pain or dehydration from diarrhea.

Following are several examples that show the importance of considering symptoms from an evolutionary perspective. Then we discuss why it is important to search for novel factors in the modern environment in trying to understand the cause of certain diseases. We conclude by considering policy implications for dealing with infectious diseases.

Although an understanding of evolutionary principles may eventually change the way doctors treat certain medical conditions, we must raise a cautionary note. Many assertions of the Darwinian medicine proponents are difficult to test and remain largely speculative. Supportive evidence is sparse—but see below for a sampling. At the least, the ideas are exciting and provocative and have already stimulated lots of research.

SYMPTOMS MAY BE VALUABLE DEFENSES

Fever is a potentially harmful consequence of infection, and high fever should be promptly treated. But Darwinian practitioners ask why the body responds as it does to injury or illness, so they ask whether fever might promote healing. It often does, by making the body's environment less hospitable to pathogens and enabling the immune system to work faster. Kluger and colleagues, while acknowledging that fever has metabolic costs, argued for the benefits of fever in controlling infection.[5] They cited the work of Julius Wagner-Jauregg, who injected patients in the late stage of syphilis with organisms that cause malaria. This caused them to undergo several cycles of extreme fevers. When medicine was finally administered to treat the malaria, 30–40 percent of patients showed marked improvement of their syphilis symptoms. For his work, Wagner-Jauregg in 1927 became the first psychiatrist to win the Nobel Prize for Medicine.

Kluger and colleagues noted that both fish and lizards, if inoculated with harmful bacteria, seek to raise their body temperature; fish swim toward warmer waters, and lizards move to sunny spots. Styrt and Sugarman inhibited the fever response in rabbits infected with pneumococci; their death rate increased.[6] Doran and colleagues administered acetaminophen or placebo for four days to children with chicken pox.[7]

The placebo group recovered faster. Graham and colleagues infected volunteers with rhinovirus (the cause of the common cold).[8] Aspirin and acetaminophen suppressed immune responses, and aspirin increased nasal symptoms such as nasal obstruction.

Barlow and colleagues examined more than four hundred records of patients with pneumonia.[9] One third of those whose temperature was below 36°C died within thirty days of admission, whereas only 8 percent of patients with higher-than-normal temperatures died within the same period, and not one of those admitted with fevers of 40°C or higher. The team also tracked patients with bloodstream infections and found that those with higher temperatures did better. If additional research supports the view that fever is often a useful bodily defense, doctors might offer a choice to patients with bad colds: Take aspirin to lower the fever and feel better sooner but remain sick and infectious longer, or let the fever run and recover more quickly.

A cold or flu sufferer who sneezes and coughs around others is spreading the pathogenic microorganisms. In such instances, the symptoms should be suppressed. But sneezing and coughing are often beneficial, by helping people rid their bodies of irritating substances. Diarrhea is also a defense that helps hosts rid themselves of parasites. DuPont and Hornick found that patients infected with *Shigella* who did not take antidiarrheal medication recovered faster, developed fewer complications, and were less likely to become carriers than those who did take medication.[10]

Sprains and broken bones cause the affected regions to become hot to the touch, swell up, and hurt. Those symptoms are typically treated with ice, anti-inflammatory drugs, and pain medication. Darwinian practitioners consider the possibility that the standard treatments are counterproductive. After all, heat makes cells divide faster; swelling pushes cells apart, enabling fluid to go between them to carry in necessary nutrients and remove dead cells; and pain restricts movement when movement could cause further damage.

Iron deficiency sometimes represents a defense rather than a defect. Murray and colleagues gave Somali nomads with low serum iron levels either a placebo or an iron supplement.[11] After one month, 50.7 percent of the individuals in the supplement group and only 10.6 percent of the placebo recipients had episodes of infection. Microbes require iron to multiply, and a temporary reduction in the body's iron stores can serve as a defense against them. The Somalis' "deficiency" was actually an evolved defense that protected them from pathogens. When it was removed, latent infections resurfaced.

Margie Profet asked why women get morning sickness. Why do women's bodies reject food at a time when their fetuses need nourishment the most? Is it an evolutionary mistake, or does it have a purpose? Profet, taking the Darwinian perspective, speculated that such a common condition is unlikely to be pathological. She and other researchers found that women who experience moderate morning sickness are less likely to miscarry.[12] Their nausea typically occurs after they smell or taste foods containing chemicals or pathogens potentially harmful to the developing fetus, even though harmless to the mother. These include meat, eggs, strong-tasting vegetables like broccoli, and caffeinated beverages. By rejecting those foods through nausea or vomiting, the mother's body is protecting the baby. So women with a genetic tendency toward morning sickness are more likely to reproduce and pass on the trait to the next generation. If morning sickness is a bodily defense rather than a defect, then working to develop a treatment for it is probably unwise.

Mervyn Singer, an intensive care specialist, takes the Darwinian view that our bodies evolved to deal with various threats to health faced by our ancestors.[13] So our immune system fights off infections, our blood clots to prevent excessive bleeding, tissues regenerate, bone fractures heal, and we respond adaptively to temperature extremes and shortage of food. Singer's perspective recognizes the possibility that many changes seen in severe illness are coping strategies rather than pathologies. For example, critically ill patients may suffer multiple organ failure which, according to the generally accepted view, is the leading cause of death in intensive care units. But Singer cites evidence suggesting that organs do not fail so much as adaptively shut down in response to the extreme physiological stress of critical illness. By slowing metabolism, organs have a better chance of resuming their normal function if the critical illness passes. Similarly, a strong local inflammatory immune response at the site of injury or infection helps fend off microorganisms that might enter the body and also rallies immune cells to break down damaged tissue. The responses cause local tissue damage prior to healing, but they protect the body as a whole.

Singer's view has important practical implications. He noted, "We haven't evolved to cope with being sedated, put on a ventilator, and pumped full of drugs." In fact, many drugs and interventions have been linked to a worse outcome for critically ill patients. He added, "Virtually all the advances in intensive care in the past ten years have involved doing less to the patient."

Nesse and Williams argue that evolutionary principles should be applied to psychiatric disorders. Negative emotions such as anxiety and depression were shaped by natural selection along with the mechanisms that regulate them, and disorders are due to dysregulation of often normal and useful responses. They write that "psychiatrists now divide anxiety disorders into nine subtypes, and many researchers treat each as a separate disease, investigating its epidemiology, genetics, brain chemistry, and response to treatments." But anxiety is not a disease—it is a defense.

Suppose doctors studied cough the way psychiatrists study anxiety.

> First, internists would define cough disorder and create objective criteria for diagnosis. Perhaps the criteria would say you have cough disorder if you cough more than twice per hour over a two-day period or have a coughing bout that lasts more than two minutes. Then researchers would look for subtypes of cough disorder based on factor-analytic studies of clinical characteristics, genetics, epidemiology, and response to treatment. They might discover specific subtypes of cough disorders such as mild cough associated with runny nose and fever, cough associated with allergies and pollen exposure, cough associated with smoking, and cough that usually leads to death. Next, they would investigate the causes of these subtypes of cough disorder by studying abnormalities of neural mechanisms in people with cough disorders. The discovery that cough is associated with increased activity in the nerves that cause the chest muscles to contract would stimulate much speculation about what neurophysiological mechanisms could make these nerves overly active. The discovery of a cough control center in the brain would give rise to another set of ideas as to how abnormalities in this center might cause cough. The knowledge that codeine stops cough would lead other scientists to investigate the possibility that cough results from deficiencies in the body's codeine like substances.

Of course, cough is not treated as above. The reason, say Nesse and Williams, is that doctors recognize that the cough reflex is normally protective. So, given a coughing patient, they try to find a provoking cause. Rarely, a cough may be caused by an abnormality of the cough regulation mechanisms. An anxiety response may also in some cases be due to an abnormal brain mechanism, but it more frequently serves a useful function. Nesse and Williams note that doctors treat normal defensive reactions such as cough and pain, and they should do the same with psychological reactions such as anxiety and depression. Nesse's website makes available many of his writings on evolutionary approaches to treating psychological disorders.[14]

SEARCH FOR NOVEL FACTORS
IN THE MODERN ENVIRONMENT

Nesse and Stearns suggest that, when looking for risk factors for common diseases, ask whether the condition is equally common in hunter–gatherer populations. If not, then novel factors in the modern environment should top the list of suspects. Some already do, such as too much fat and too little exercise.

The invention of the light bulb introduced a major change in people's lives. We no longer go to sleep as soon as darkness falls, which may increase our susceptibility to certain diseases. Melatonin levels increase in the dark. Visually impaired women tend to have higher than normal melatonin levels and a lower rate of breast cancer than other women.[15] Shift workers and others exposed to light at night have higher than normal cancer rates.[16] These findings suggest simple public health advice—sleep with the lights off.

Improved hygiene in developed countries has vastly changed our internal environments from the environment in which we evolved. Until relatively recently, most humans lived with parasitic worms in the gut. Modern societies have eliminated that problem, but at a cost. The absence of parasitic worms may account for the vastly increased rates of autoimmune diseases (diseases caused by the reaction of antibodies to substances occurring naturally in the body). The worms may have evolved a capacity to make a protein to reduce the activity of immune cells that would otherwise attack them. Without the worms, the immune cells become hyperactive. In countries where parasites persist, autoimmune diseases are still comparatively rare. The parasite *Schistosoma mansoni* causes the disease schistosomiasis. People infected with *S. mansoni* tend to have milder courses of asthma.[17]

In places where treatment has been initiated to rid people of worms, asthma and Crohn's disease rates have gone up. These observations provided the basis for a novel treatment of patients with ulcerative colitis or Crohn's disease.[18] The patients swallowed the live ova of pig whipworm in a beverage every three weeks for twenty-four weeks. Many reported considerable reduction in symptoms such as abdominal pain, bleeding, and diarrhea. The treatment achieved 50 percent remission in ulcerative colitis and 70 percent remission in Crohn's disease.

Epidemiological studies suggest that hookworm infection protects against asthma. Therefore, Feary and colleagues randomly assigned volunteers with asthma to be injected with either ten hookworm larvae or placebo.[19] During sixteen weeks of follow-up, the hookworm group had a greater (although nonsignificant) improvement in airway responsiveness.

PUBLIC POLICY IMPLICATIONS SHAPED FROM A DARWINIAN APPROACH

Darwinian doctors such as Paul Ewald have gained important insights about infectious disease control.[20] They understand that viruses and bacteria evolve as humans do, although much more rapidly. Some diseases, like colds and flu, are transmitted from person to person. Their transmission depends upon mobile hosts; thus, the pathogens have evolved to be relatively benign. But malaria and yellow fever spread through disease-carrying organisms, and cholera spreads through water. A bedridden malaria patient is easy prey for an infected mosquito. The excretions of a cholera patient are likely to find their way into the water supply. The victims do not have to survive very long, so there is no selection pressure for the diseases to be mild. As a result, malaria and cholera (in places where the water supply is contaminated) remain virulent. Ewald emphasizes that if we understand what the disease pathogens evolved to do, we can take steps to make the disease more benign. He argues that cholera can be tamed by designing water purification systems that prevent infection from bedridden patients. Then the selective advantage would go to mild organisms whose infected but mobile victims can spread them.

Ewald also discussed the HIV virus, which has a fairly long latency period before causing AIDS. If people were largely monogamous, with rare sexual activity outside their primary relationship, the virus would have few chances for transmitting its genes to another host and would benefit from remaining latent. Only the variants that allowed their host to stay healthy and active would eventually be transmitted through sexual intercourse. So natural selection would favor milder forms of the virus. But when people are actively involved with many different sexual partners, an HIV strain that reproduces vigorously has the potential for soon infecting several new hosts; and a strain with a long latency period is at a disadvantage. So HIV virulence is positively correlated with rates of sexual contact. A greater number of sexual partners favors HIV variants that replicate rapidly, that is, are more virulent. The public policy message would be to limit the number of sexual partners and to always use condoms.

APPENDIX 3

WELLNESS STRATEGIES

The strategies for a healthful lifestyle can be summarized in a few lines:

- Exercise on a regular basis, but don't overdo it.
- Get enough sleep.
- Eat the right foods—fresh fruits and vegetables, whole grains, nuts, fish.
- Don't overeat.
- Don't smoke.
- Use alcohol in moderation, if at all.
- Try to reduce the stressors in your life.
- Stay away from hungry polar bears.

We could not be comprehensive about wellness practices in a short chapter—or even in a good-sized book. Instead, we explore some complexities and uncertainties about day-to-day practices. It is important to recognize that almost all the information comes from correlational, not experimental, research. Therefore, while it would be reasonable to conclude, for example, that people who eat a Mediterranean diet tend to live longer than people who don't, it may not be the case that they live longer *because* of the Mediterranean diet. See pp. 31–33 for further discussion.

EAT

Glassner compared the official dietary guidelines issued by the governments of several countries.[1] Following is a sample:

Dietary Guidelines of Several Countries

> *Australia: Enjoy a wide variety of nutritious foods.*
> *Ireland: Enjoy your food!*
> *Japan: Happy eating makes for happy family life; sit down and eat together and talk; treasure family taste and home cooking.*
> *Korea: Enjoy homemade meals to be happy with families.*
> *Canada: Enjoy a variety of foods.*
> *Norway: FOOD + JOY = HEALTH.*
> *United States: Aim for fitness.*
> *Cardiologists' recommendation: If it tastes good, spit it out.*

Glassner inferred that people in the United States do not seem to enjoy food as much as people do in other countries. Ironically, when the focus is on eating for health, a food's health value may be diminished. In a series of studies, Hallberg and colleagues asked Swedish and Thai women to eat various foods.[2] The Thai women absorbed almost 50 percent more iron from a spicy Thai meal than did the Swedish women. When the same ingredients were served as a mushy paste, the Thai women absorbed 70 percent less iron than they had before. Similar differences in iron absorption were obtained when Swedish women ate a meal of hamburger, string beans, and mashed potatoes served either in the usual way or as a mix.

The diets of French and American people differ considerably. The French diet features many foods regarded by Americans as unhealthful—cheese, butter, cream, foie gras, eggs, rich sauces, pastries, and wine—and they eat three times as much saturated animal fat as Americans do. Yet the French live a little longer and have a 30 percent lower rate of heart disease.[3] Part of the explanation of the "French paradox" is that the French derive much more pleasure from their meals. Rozin compared food attitudes in the two countries.[4] Americans, particularly women, think of food—"one of the great pleasures of life"—as an ambivalent thing. Whereas the French are more likely to think of fried eggs in a culinary context, as breakfast, Americans think of them as cholesterol, a supposedly harmful nutrient. Asked to free associate to "heavy cream," the French said "whipped," and the Americans said "unhealthy." Rozin wrote, "We tend to think about what's in the food that's either good or bad for us, and the French think about it as an experience: it's eating. They're thinking about it in the mouth, and we're thinking about it in the bloodstream."

He concluded that because the French appreciate and enjoy food, they eat less and thus weigh less. He wrote, "What Americans love is getting a deal on a big bowl of food. The French, on the other hand, love a small bit of delicious food." Their focus on quality and pleasure allows them to be satisfied with smaller portions. Rozin concluded that small portions of a highly flavored dish will have roughly the same effect in memory as a large portion.

Eat Sweets

In 1988, Lee and Paffenbarger surveyed 7,841 men, free of cardiovascular disease and cancer, who had entered Harvard University between 1916 and 1950.[5] They asked the men about the average number of servings of candy eaten in the past year. Response options ranged from "almost never" to "6+ per day." They also asked about other health habits. Between 1988 and 1993, 514 of the men died. Mortality was lowest among those consuming candy one to three times a month. They lived longer than those indulging three or more times a week and almost a year longer than did abstainers, who had the highest mortality overall. The results are suggestive, but before reaching for your Halloween leftovers, keep in mind that the study was correlational. Consumers and nonconsumers (those who responded "almost never") of candy differed in several ways. The abstainers were older, leaner, and more likely to smoke. They drank more, ate less red meat and vegetables, and were more likely to take vitamin or mineral supplements.

Chocolate lovers, rejoice—chocolate is officially a health food. Cocoa beans, from which chocolate is made, contain large quantities of flavonoids. (The concentration of flavonoids is much higher in dark than milk chocolate.)[6] Flavonoids prevent fatlike substances in the bloodstream from clogging the arteries, and they make blood platelets less likely to clot.[7] They induce coronary vasodilation and improve coronary vascular function.[8] They help the body process nitric oxide, a compound critical for healthy blood flow and blood pressure. So chocolate can help reduce the risk of cardiovascular disease.[9]

Free radicals, formed when oxygen interacts with certain molecules, can react with important cellular components such as DNA or cell membranes and cause the cells to function poorly or die. Antioxidants help protect the body from the harmful effects of free radicals. Cocoa powder, dark chocolate, and milk chocolate are all powerful antioxidants.[10]

Volunteers who rated themselves as highly stressed ate about an ounce and a half of dark chocolate for two weeks. Their levels of stress hormones were substantially reduced.[11]

Eat Whole Foods

Akbaraly and colleagues collected diet data on 3,500 middle-aged people.[12] Those who ate the most processed foods were 58 percent more likely to suffer from depression five years later than those who ate the least. Those who ate the most whole foods were 26 percent less likely to suffer from depression in five years than those who ate the least. Whole foods included fruits and vegetables. Processed foods included high-fat dairy, processed meats, refined grains, fried food, and sweetened desserts. The study was correlational.

DRINK

Drink Water

Adults lose slightly more than six cups of water per day in urine output, and more is lost through breath, perspiration, and bowel movements. It must be replenished. The Mayo Clinic listed three approaches to approximate water needs for the average, healthy adult living in a temperate climate.[13] Their website also notes that a person who rarely feels thirsty and produces 6.3 cups or more of colorless or slightly yellow urine a day is probably consuming enough fluids.

- Consuming eight cups of water or other beverages each day will typically replace the lost fluids. Food intake provides, on average, about 20 percent of total water intake.
- Although no scientific evidence exists to support the claim that people should drink eight 8-ounce glasses of water per day, it's a reasonable guideline.
- The Institute of Medicine advises that men consume roughly thirteen cups of total beverages a day and women consume nine cups.

Sweating, whether exercise induced or caused by living in a hot or humid climate, boosts the need for water intake. During long bouts of intense exercise, sports drinks containing sodium are useful for replacing sodium lost in sweat. Exercisers should continue to replace fluids even after they have stopped exercising.

Women who are expecting or breast-feeding need additional fluids. The Institute of Medicine recommends that pregnant women drink about ten cups of fluids daily and women who breast-feed about thirteen cups.

W. C. Fields had a different perspective. He said, "I never drink water because of the disgusting things that fish do in it."

It is possible to drink too much water. When a person's kidneys are unable to excrete the excess water, the electrolyte content of the blood is diluted, resulting in low sodium levels. Endurance athletes, such as marathon runners, who drink large amounts of water put themselves at risk. Electrolyte imbalance can cause an irregular heartbeat and allow fluid to enter the lungs. Swelling puts pressure on the brain and nerves, which can cause behaviors resembling alcohol intoxication. Swelling of brain tissues can cause seizures, coma, and even death.

Drink Alcohol

Recent studies on the harmful and beneficial effects of alcohol are confusing and contradictory. Four points are worth noting at the outset. First, almost all of the research is correlational—which is important, because heavy drinkers, moderate drinkers, and abstainers differ in many ways that affect health other than their drinking habits. For example, many poor people abstain because they can't afford alcohol. They may also be unable to afford decent health care. Their financial status may cause high levels of stress and, eventually, stress-related diseases.

Holahan and colleagues examined the association between alcohol consumption and mortality over twenty years among 1,824 adults between the ages of fifty-five and sixty-five.[14] Abstainers (people who abstained from alcohol at baseline) had more than double the mortality risk of moderate drinkers (people who had from one to less than three drinks per day at baseline). Compared with moderate drinkers, heavy drinkers had a 70 percent and light drinkers a 23 percent increased risk. But the abstainers were more likely than moderate drinkers to be obese and smoke cigarettes. They had more initial health problems, depressive symptoms, and avoidance coping. They were lower on income and education, physical activity, number of close friends, and quality of friend support. They were less likely to be married. All those factors were associated with increased mortality. So when Holahan and colleagues used a model that controlled for them, the mortality effect for abstainers compared to moderate drinkers was substantially reduced. Nevertheless, abstainers and heavy drinkers showed increased mortality risks of 49 percent and 42 percent, respectively, compared with moderate drinkers.

A second complicating factor, which Holahan and colleagues noted, is that many current abstainers were at one time heavy drinkers who stopped because drinking had caused them health problems. A third consideration is that, as shown in the next paragraph, pattern of drinking may be as important as amount drunk. Fourth, most of the suggested benefits concern the cardiovascular system. But alcohol consumption can cause liver, brain, and pancreatic illnesses. Heavy drinking increases the risk of stroke and is associated with cardiomyopathy, a disease of the heart muscle that can lead to premature death.

Marques-Vidal and colleagues compared patterns of drinking in Northern Ireland and France.[15] In Belfast, 66 percent of alcohol is consumed on weekends. In France it is consumed evenly throughout the week. Blood pressure was higher among Northern Irish drinkers on Mondays and decreased through Thursdays. French drinkers' blood pressure remained constant throughout the week. The researchers concluded that for cardiovascular health, people should drink small amounts daily.

Arriola and colleagues asked 41,500 men and women to document their alcohol drinking habits over a ten-year period.[16] The researchers differentiated between those who had never drunk and those who had quit because of ill health. During the duration of the study, women drinkers had slightly fewer coronary events than women abstainers. Differences were much greater for men. Moderate drinkers (type of alcohol was irrelevant) were 35 percent less likely to develop coronary heart disease; and heavy drinkers (between three and more than eleven shots of hard liquor a day) were 50 percent less likely. At least part of the explanation is that alcohol raises high-density lipoproteins ("good" cholesterol), which prevents bad cholesterol from accumulating in the arteries.

Spaak and colleagues had volunteers drink wine, ethanol, and water on three occasions two weeks apart.[17] One drink of either red wine or ethanol (no difference between them) dilated blood vessels. After two drinks, heart rate, amount of blood pumped out of the heart, and sympathetic nervous system activity all increased; and the ability of blood vessels to expand in response to an increase in blood flow diminished. These effects counteracted the beneficial effect of one drink.

Streppel and colleagues monitored the health of 1,373 fifty-year-old men between the years 1960 and 2000.[18] Over the forty years, 1,130 of the men died, about half from cardiovascular disease. The men who drank only wine, and less than half a glass a day, lived approximately 2.5 years longer than those who drank beer and spirits. Life expectancy was slightly less for the men who drank more than half a glass a day—and about five years less for total abstainers. The results held no matter the socioeconomic status, diet, and other lifestyle habits of the men.

Brown and colleagues reviewed recent findings and concluded that too much drinking causes multiple organ damage.[19] But low to moderate drinking, especially of red wine, reduces mortality. "The breadth of benefits is remarkable—cancer prevention, protection of the heart and brain from damage, reducing age-related diseases such as inflammation, reversing diabetes and obesity, and many more." The authors attributed many of the benefits of red wine to one of its constituents, resveratrol, and they made an important observation: Resveratrol is largely inactivated by the gut or liver before it reaches the blood stream. So, when red wine is drunk, most of the resveratrol does not reach the circulation.

If absorbed through the mucous membranes in the mouth, however, resveratrol can reach blood levels around a hundred times higher. For this to happen, the wine must be drunk slowly rather than gulped down.

The cancer prevention effect of alcohol is questionable, at least in women. Allen and colleagues followed more than one million middle-aged British women for an average of 7.2 years.[20] They found that even moderate alcohol drinking was associated with increased incidence of cancers of the rectum, mouth, throat, and esophagus—and especially breast and liver cancers. They estimated that alcohol, whether in the form of wine, beer, spirits, or a combination of beverages, was responsible for 13 percent of the cancers. Each additional drink increased risk. Women who smoked and drank alcohol had an increased risk of oral, throat, and esophageal cancer that was greater than the risk associated with smoking alone.

ENJOY CAFFEINE

Coffee is the second-most-traded commodity in the world, after oil.[21] According to the U.S. Department of Agriculture database, the average American drinks 1.64 cups of coffee per day. Moderate amounts of caffeine (250–500 milligrams per day) offer several benefits. Most people report increased alertness and arousal and lower levels of fatigue after as little as 25 to 50 milligrams.[22] Trained runners and cyclists showed greater endurance after a dosage of 9 milligrams of caffeine per kilogram of body weight.[23] Table A.1 lists the amount of caffeine in various products.

Many people who drink coffee because of its effects on alertness start their days by having a cup or two with breakfast, another cup or two at lunchtime, and a final cup in early afternoon. That is not a good strategy. When drunk, caffeine reaches peak blood levels within about forty-five minutes and has a half-life of about four hours. So caffeine levels soar after the morning coffee, often to such an extent that they cause some of the problems listed below. Then, because no coffee is drunk for a period of about sixteen hours (say, 3 p.m. to 7 a.m.), blood levels are depleted by morning. People who drink caffeine to stay alert would be better off taking frequent low doses (about a quarter of a cup) throughout the day

Table A.1. Amount of Caffeine in Various Products

Product	Serving Size	Milligrams of Caffeine
Brewed coffee	8 oz.	100–200
Instant coffee	8 oz.	25–175
Decaffeinated coffee	8 oz.	3–12
Brewed tea	8 oz.	40–120
Mountain Dew	12 oz.	71
Diet Coke, Coca-Cola Classic	12 oz.	47, 35
TAB	12 oz.	46
Dr. Pepper	12 oz.	42
Pepsi, Diet Pepsi, Pepsi One	12 oz.	38, 36, 54
Red Bull	8.3 oz.	80
Rockstar Energy Drink	8 oz.	80
SoBe Adrenaline Rush	8.3 oz.	79
Häagen-Dazs coffee ice cream	8 fl. oz.	58
Starbucks coffee ice cream	8 fl. oz.	50–60
Hershey's chocolate bar	1.55 oz.	9
Hershey's Kisses	41g (nine pieces)	9
Hot cocoa	8 oz.	3–13
NoDoz (Maximum Strength)	one tablet	200
Extra Strength Excedrin	two tablets	130

until midafternoon. Wyatt and colleagues found that that was the best way to overcome performance decrements due to sleep deprivation.[24]

However, a recent study questions coffee's effects on alertness.[25] Rogers and colleagues tested 379 volunteers who abstained from caffeine for sixteen hours before being given either caffeine or placebo. Then they performed several computer tasks that tested memory, attentiveness, and vigilance. The volunteers who normally drank medium to high levels of coffee and received a placebo reported both more headaches and reduced levels of alertness than those who received caffeine. However, alertness levels of the caffeine recipients were comparable to those of normally non- or light drinkers who received placebo—and caffeine did not increase the alertness of the latter. The authors inferred that the heavy users had been experiencing the fatiguing effects of acute caffeine withdrawal and that caffeine pills merely returned them to normal.

Caffeine may protect against certain diseases. A correlational study found that men and women who consumed coffee on a daily or almost daily basis had a lower risk of liver cancer than those who almost never drank coffee; cancer incidence decreased with the amount of coffee consumed.[26] According to the *Johns Hopkins News-Letter*,[27] an antioxidant found only in coffee reduces risk of colon cancer, and coffee consumption is linked to decreases in Parkinson's disease and type 2 diabetes. Among postmenopausal women, a clear relationship was shown between coffee drinking and both total mortality and mortality attributed to cardiovascular disease, cancer, and other diseases with a major inflammatory component. Andersen and colleagues concluded that "consumption of coffee . . . may inhibit inflammation and thereby reduce the risk of cardiovascular disease and other inflammatory diseases in postmenopausal women."[28]

Ritchie and colleagues studied more than seven thousand men and women over the age of sixty-five.[29] Participants took several tests to determine their memory skills and took them again two and then four years later. Women who initially reported that they drank three or more cups of tea or coffee each day had smaller subsequent test score reductions than women who consumed a maximum of one cup daily. The important factor was the amount of caffeine consumed on a daily basis. There was no relationship between caffeine intake and test scores in men.

Eskelinen and colleagues studied middle-aged people for an average of twenty-one years. Those who drank three to five cups of coffee a day in their midlife years were less likely to develop dementia or Alzheimer's disease in old age compared with those who drank either no coffee at all or very little.[30]

Unfortunately, caffeine has a bad side. Tolerance develops, and discontinuation results in a withdrawal syndrome. Caffeine increases blood pressure even in habitual users, although some tolerance develops. Caffeinism, a syndrome that includes restlessness, nervousness, excitement, insomnia, a flushed face, ringing in the ears, muscle tenseness and tremor, and diarrhea, has been reported following ingestion of as little as 250 milligrams of caffeine per day and is common in people with an intake above 600 milligrams per day. Drinking more than 1,000 milligrams per day is well into the toxic range.

Coffee, whether regular or decaffeinated, relaxes the muscle that keeps stomach acids from rising into the throat, so people with heartburn or reflux disease should avoid or strictly limit coffee. Cafestol, a compound found in coffee, is the most potent dietary cholesterol-elevating agent known.[31] French press coffee, boiled Scandinavian brew, and espresso contain the highest levels of cafestol, which is removed by paper filters used in most other brewing processes. Removing caffeine does not remove cafestol. Consuming five cups of French press coffee per day (30 milligrams of cafestol) for four weeks raises cholesterol in the blood 6 to 8 percent.

The next paragraph is included for people who are *very* particular about their coffee.

For Coffee Snobs

Britain's newspaper The Telegraph *reported on a very special coffee sold by the British department store Peter Jones.*[32] *The coffee is harvested from the dung of Indonesian jungle cats and sold for £50 (about $100) a cup. "The cats select the best beans to chew. It's rather like a natural filtering process," said Carie Barkhuzen, a spokeswoman for the upmarket store. The blend is made by Italian company De Longhi. A De Longhi spokesman said, "It is in high demand from coffee aficionados. They will relish the chance to buy such a rare coffee. After all, only 200 kg of Kupi Luwak coffee is produced each year."*

EXERCISE

Regular exercise helps lower blood pressure and levels of bad cholesterol. It boosts high-density lipoprotein (HDL, good) cholesterol and, by reducing body fat, helps prevent and control type 2 diabetes. Men who were physically active during leisure time had a lower risk of death from coronary heart disease, cancer, and all causes.[33] Regular weight-bearing exercise promotes bone formation and thus reduces the risk of osteoporosis. It is an important adjunct to any weight-loss program. Exercise helps the entire cardiovascular system, which leads to increased energy. Regular physical activity improves mood and, when done no later than midafternoon, improves nighttime sleep.

Exercise decreases acute pain perception to a variety of stimuli. People with chronic low back pain reduced their pain perception for up to thirty minutes after a moderate workout on an exercise bike. Regular exercisers had higher pain thresholds to a painful pressure stimulus and a higher threshold for noxious cold than did normally active controls.[34]

Boecker and colleagues compared runners' brains before and after a two-hour run. Endorphins produced during running attached themselves largely to the limbic and prefrontal areas, and ratings of happiness correlated directly with the production of the endorphins.[35]

Exercise stimulates the formation of new brain cells that are responsible for memory and learning. Older adults who engage in regular physical activity have better performances in tests measuring decision making, memory, and problem solving.[36]

Can People Overexercise?

Scientists disagree about whether people can exercise too much.

Too Much Exercise Is Bad   Some of the risks of overexercising are as follows:

- Immune dysfunction: Excessive exercise without adequate recovery stresses the body, decreasing immune function and increasing the chance of respiratory infection.
- Reproductive health problems: Women whose body-fat level falls below 13 to 17 percent may stop menstruating.
- Mood and cognition problems: People who have lengthy daily workouts may experience disturbed sleep, depression, anxiety, confusion, and difficulty concentrating if they miss a day of exercise.
- Bone health: People who exercise too much increase their risk of developing osteoporosis and stress fractures.
- Too much exercise can destroy muscle mass, especially if the body is not getting enough nutrition.
- Vigorous exercise regimens can lead to injury.

Murphy and colleagues assigned mice to one of two groups: exercise or control. The exercise group was forced to run on a treadmill for approximately 120 minutes on three consecutive days. The controls rested in their cages. Fifteen minutes after the last bout of exercise or rest, the mice were inoculated with influenza virus. Exercise stress was associated with an increase in susceptibility to upper respiratory tract infection (morbidity, mortality, and symptom severity).[37]

On the Other Hand   The federally recommended exercise guidelines call for half an hour a day, including a portion at moderate to high levels of intensity. Except for Olympic hopefuls, few runners who merely follow the guidelines would reach twenty miles per week. Yet Paul Williams, who studied more than 100,000 runners over nearly twenty years and published more than forty articles in peer-reviewed journals, found progressively greater health benefits for runners topping as many as forty-nine miles a week. Runners who exceeded the guidelines were much less likely to experience stroke, heart attack, glaucoma, cataracts, macular degeneration, diabetes, gout, gall stones, diverticulitis, or prostate enlargement.[38] Williams assumes that similar effects would be gained from increased workloads among swimmers, cyclists, and other aerobic athletes.

Although intriguing, Williams's research suffers from two serious limitations. First, the runners, rather than examining physicians, provided his information. Second, his work is correlational. Not all people are capable of running marathons. Those who are, or who engage in other extreme exercise, are almost surely more fit than the rest of the population at the outset. They are also probably more concerned about their fitness and make sure to eat right, get enough sleep, and so forth.

SIT UP STRAIGHT

McGonigal cited several studies showing the value of adopting proper habits of posture, facial expression, muscle tension, and breathing.[39] For example, Briñol and colleagues had volunteers write down their best and worse qualities while sitting with back erect and chest pushed out (confident posture) or slouched forward with back curved.[40] The confident posture led participants to rate themselves as better candidates for the job market, better interviewees for a new position, better on-the-job performers, and more satisfied as future employees.

SLEEP

Although the need for sleep is unquestionable, no current theory about its function is convincing.[41] The National Sleep Foundation (http://www .sleepfoundation.org), which offers a great deal of information on sleep and strategies for dealing with sleep problems, recommends that adults get at least seven hours each night. Anything less and our immune systems function poorly, making us more vulnerable to various diseases. Insufficient or irregular sleep slows reaction times, causes memory impairment, and increases the risk for colon cancer, breast cancer, heart disease, and diabetes. Much obesity may be due to sleep deprivation, as deprivation disrupts the hormones ghrelin (stimulates hunger) and leptin (induces satiation). Being awake more than twenty-four hours impairs performance as much as having a blood-alcohol level of 0.1 percent—which is legally drunk.

Yet whereas adults in 1910 averaged nine hours of sleep a night, today's average is less than seven hours. More than one-third of U.S. adults report daytime sleepiness that interferes with their work and social functioning at least a few days each month, and an estimated 70 million Americans have chronic sleep loss or sleep disorders.[42]

Below are quotations from three sleep experts, the first two from *Harvard Magazine* online, the third from *The Utne Reader* online:[43]

- David White, professor of sleep medicine: "You can make up for *acute* sleep deprivation, but we don't know what happens when people are chronically sleep-deprived over years."
- Robert Stickgold, a cognitive neuroscientist specializing in sleep research: "We are living in the middle of history's greatest experiment in sleep deprivation and we are all a part of that experiment. It's not inconceivable to me that we will discover that there are major social, economic, and health consequences to that experiment. Sleep deprivation doesn't have any good side effects."
- Thomas Roth of the Henry Ford Sleep Disorders Center in Detroit: "The percentage of the population who need less than five hours of sleep per night, rounded to a whole number, is zero."

Nap

Even people who get enough nighttime sleep can benefit from daytime naps. Milner and Cote reviewed the literature and summarized many of the important recent findings.[44] Naps of ten, twenty, and thirty minutes, but not five minutes, improve mood and increase vigor while decreasing fatigue. Napping benefits performance on tasks such as addition, logical reasoning, reaction time, and symbol recognition. The benefits following ten-minute naps are seen immediately but are delayed following longer naps. Horne and colleagues reported that a twenty-minute nap approximately eight hours after awakening does more for stamina than sleeping another twenty minutes in the morning.[45]

Napping at least three times a week for a half-hour was associated with a significantly decreased risk of death from heart disease.[46] People who regularly took a siesta had a 37 percent lower coronary death rate than those who never napped. Many people in Mediterranean and certain Central American countries take regular siestas, and those countries have low rates of heart disease. However, the habit of taking frequent long naps has been associated with higher morbidity and mortality, especially among the elderly.[47] All the studies are correlational—taking regular naps may reflect a leisurely, stress-free lifestyle that is the real reason for reduced risk of heart disease; elderly people who are particularly feeble may require long naps.

Walker and colleagues divided thirty-nine healthy adults into nap and no-nap groups.[48] At noon, all the participants were subjected to a rigorous learning task, and the two groups performed at comparable levels. At 2 p.m., one group took a ninety-minute nap while the other group stayed awake. At 6 p.m., they were all exposed to new learning exercises. Those who had remained awake became worse at learning, whereas the nappers did markedly better.

The best time to nap depends on factors such as individual sleep need, stability and timing of sleep/wake schedule, morningness-eveningness tendencies, quality of sleep during the preceding night, quality of sleep during the nap, and amount of prior wakefulness. People other than night-shift workers typically have a dip in alertness between 3 and 5 in the afternoon, so sleep efficiency may be better with naps taken between those hours. Trying to take a nap too early in the day is inefficient, because the body is not ready for more sleep. Taking a nap too late in the day can impair nighttime sleep.

Reyner and Horne recommended drinking coffee just before taking a fifteen-minute nap as a way to counteract sleepiness upon awakening.[49] They tested their strategy with sleepy volunteers who, upon awakening, drove a car simulator continuously for two hours. Compared with subjects who received placebos, the number of negative incidents was reduced substantially. Caffeine takes about thirty minutes to have an alerting effect, so people can get in a short sleep without interference by the caffeine and then experience its stimulating effects just as they are waking up.

WHEN ANXIOUS OR IN PAIN, PUT IN A CD

In his 1697 play *The Mourning Bride*, William Congreve had one of the characters say, "Musick has Charms to sooth a savage Breast." His observation was correct. Several studies have shown that music reduces patients' anxiety and pain right before, during, and after surgery. They need smaller amounts of sedative drugs to achieve a comparable degree of sedation. Music helps people lower their blood pressure and heart rate.[50] Cochrane reviewers concluded that patients who listen to music after surgery report less pain and less need for morphine-like drugs than patients who don't listen.[51] Although the effects are small, the reviewers recommend trying music.

CHOOSE THE RIGHT ENVIRONMENTS

Enjoy the Sun

Exposure to too much sunlight is harmful, but solar radiation is the primary source of vitamin D for most Americans and Europeans. Dietary sources are inadequate, and supplements have to be used carefully. Midday summer sun is the best source, as minimal exposure time is needed. Grant suggested that people go into the sun for ten to fifteen minutes without sunscreen to generate a day's worth of vitamin D. He claimed that more than twenty thousand Americans die prematurely annually from insufficient vitamin D.[52]

Avoid Hospitals

Hospitals are no places for sick people. According to the World Health Organization guidelines, health-care–associated infections affect hundreds of millions of patients worldwide every year.[53] The infections lead to serious illness, prolong hospital stays, and cause long-term disability. In the United States, one in 136 hospital patients becomes seriously ill as a result of acquiring an infection in the hospital. This is equivalent to about two million cases and eighty thousand deaths annually.

Lipsky reported that 27 percent of skin or muscle infections that required hospitalization originated from microbes acquired in a clinic, hospital, or other medical care setting.[54] The infections typically followed trauma, surgery, or an invasive medical procedure such as kidney dialysis. People with such infections were more likely to die in the hospital because the microbe involved was more likely to be resistant to some drugs.

According to the WHO guidelines, hand hygiene is the primary measure to reduce health-care–associated infection. Yet compliance with hand hygiene is very low throughout the world. Meengs and colleagues reported that an unacceptably high proportion of physicians fail to take hand-washing breaks between patient contacts.[55] Widmer and colleagues observed health-care workers as they washed.[56] A fluorescent dye was added to the disinfectant to assess the number of areas missed. At baseline, only 31 percent used proper technique. Training improved compliance and increased the reduction of bacteria by almost 50 percent. (Note, however, on p. 84, that French physicians have a much different view of hygiene.)

Jones and colleagues surveyed emergency care providers working in a university-affiliated community hospital about their stethoscope-cleaning measures.[57] Only 48 percent of 150 health-care providers cleaned their stethoscopes daily or weekly. Another 37 percent did so monthly, 7 percent yearly, and 7 percent never. Culturing of each stethoscope indicated that 133 grew staphylococci and twenty-five yielded *Staphylococcus* aureus, a bacterium that can cause a range of illnesses, including several that are life threatening. Cleaning the stethoscope diaphragm resulted in immediate reduction in the bacterial count: alcohol swabs were the most effective cleaner. The authors concluded that stethoscopes used in emergency practice are often contaminated and are a potential vector of infection. This contamination is greatly reduced by frequent cleaning with alcohol.

Even scissors can be a problem. Embil and colleagues sampled the scissors of 232 health-care workers and found that 182 were colonized with bacteria.[58] The scissors of nurses and those for communal use were most frequently contaminated. The medical personnel cleaned their scissors infrequently, even though wiping with an alcohol swab was sufficient to disinfect them.

Especially Avoid Teaching Hospitals in July

Each year around July 1, U.S. teaching hospitals receive an influx of interns, residents, nurses, and other health-care workers. Fresh from college and receiving little direct supervision, they immediately begin writing medication orders. As a result, more errors occur in July than in other months. Phillips and Barker analyzed more than 62 million death certificates from 1979 to 2006 and found that fatal medication errors consistently spiked in July by about 10 percent—but only in counties with many teaching hospitals.[59] There was no measurable increase in counties with facilities that don't employ residents, such as community hospitals, and no increase in deaths from surgical errors, hospital-acquired infection, or other causes.

Avoid Everything

Tucson Weekly magazine published an article about respected microbiologist Charles Gerba, whose nickname is "Dr. Germ."[60] Gerba said, "We import half of our food now, a lot of which comes from developing countries with Third World sanitation. We import 23 percent of our fresh fruit, 16 percent of vegetables and 40 percent of tomatoes. Fifty percent of food-borne outbreaks since 1974 involved produce. The explosion in worldwide travel exposes us to organisms we've never seen before. And new diseases keep emerging, such as bird flu, SARS and others that make our aging population more vulnerable." He added, "Good hygiene has prevented more disease than every vaccine and antibiotic ever invented. But we've forgotten that lesson. We need to reinvent hygiene in the 21st century."

Gerba talked about dangerous microbes on common objects. Reading the list makes it seem amazing that any of us are still alive.

- Office water-cooler handles: "Where does everybody go when they have a cold or diarrhea? The water cooler. Go there for conversation, not to drink."

- Office coffee cups: "Sixty percent have fecal bacteria on them."
- Airplanes: "All those people sharing toilets in a short period. By the time the plane lands, a thin layer of E. coli covers those little bathroom sinks."
- Cell phones: "Talk about a germ-collection device. The germs on your hand go onto the phone, and a lot of respiratory viruses are put out when you talk, sneeze or cough. People are talking dirty and don't realize it." Gerba recommended that cell phone users wipe cell phones down with a disinfectant wipe or spray a towel with disinfectant and wipe the phones off at least once a day.

  The reason most people don't get sick from exposure to cell phones is that the phones are coated with only their own germs, to which they have built immunity. We get sick when exposed to new germs. So phones should not be shared with others except in emergencies. People should carry wipes with them and clean phones before sharing.

- Women's purses: "Never touch the bottom of a woman's purse. One-third have coliform bacteria in them."
- Grocery carts: "Let's see. Baby's wearing a diaper, and mom puts the baby in the seat facing her, and the next person comes along and puts broccoli there. Fifty percent of grocery carts have fecal bacteria on them."
- Kitchen sponges: "Great places for microbes to live: nice and moist, bacteria cafeterias, soaking up food all the time. The bacteria multiply overnight. In the billions. Ten percent of households' sponges have salmonella."
- Kitchen sinks: "If you're cutting carrots, and one falls into the sink, and you use it again, it has more fecal bacteria on it than if it fell into the toilet."
- Public swimming pools: "I don't go to public pools anymore, especially if there are children in them. They're basically large toilets."

  The Centers for Disease Control and Prevention analyzed data from more than 121,000 routine public pool inspections in fifteen states in 2008.[61] They reported in their *Morbidity and Mortality Weekly Report* that more than 12 percent violated safety standards designed to reduce the risk of infection. The most frequently reported type of recreational water illness is gastroenteritis (inflammation of the stomach and the intestines, with vomiting and diarrhea). The violations involved either insufficient levels of chlorine or improper pH levels, both of which increase the risk that pathogens will multiply in the water. The pH should fall between 7.2 and 7.8. Pools in child-care settings had the highest percentage of serious violations.

Swimmers should ask pool operators what the pH of the water is or test it themselves with free strips available from the Health Pools website. Swimmers should shower with soap before entering a pool, avoid swallowing pool water, and wash their hands upon exiting. Children or adults suffering from diarrhea should not use public pools. Parents should check children's diapers both before and after children swim, and diapers should never be changed near the water.

- Office phones and desks have four hundred times more germs than toilets; toilets are frequently cleaned. Also worse than toilets: restroom faucets, kitchen sinks, sponges, and dishcloths.
- Ninety-three percent of shoes worn for at least ninety days have *E. coli* on them.

Gerba tested five Tucson Fire Department firehouses for MRSA—methicillin-resistant staphylococcus aureus—an antibiotic-resistant staph infection that, in 2005, killed more people than AIDS. MRSA was commonplace—on keyboards, pens, couches, remote controls, kitchen counters, classrooms, and tools. It was also found on 47 percent of household hairbrushes and 20 percent of home desks.

Rhinovirus causes at least half of common colds. Hendley and colleagues obtained mucus samples from adults with active rhinovirus infections and asked them to spend at least seven hours awake in a hotel room.[62] Afterward, the researchers tested several surfaces in the rooms, such as television remote controls, doorknobs, telephones, and light switches. Fifty-two of 150 tested surfaces had detectable rhinovirus traceable to the volunteer who had stayed there.

The researchers stored the rhinovirus-laden mucus and several weeks later brought back some of the volunteers. Before each person's arrival, they placed drops of his or her mucus on light switches, telephone handsets, and the phones' keypads in two hotel rooms. In one room, the samples were placed the night before, and in the other room, a half-hour before arrival. The volunteers, now rhinovirus-free, touched each object and were then tested for the virus. (They were immune to reinfection.) The virus was present in ten of thirty instances in which they touched surfaces infected the night before and in eighteen of thirty instances of freshly infected surfaces.

In subsequent studies, Hendley and colleagues found that 21 percent of toys sampled in a pediatric waiting room and 41 percent of surfaces in the homes of adults with rhinovirus colds were positive for viral RNA.[63]

LAUGH?

> A clown is like an aspirin, only he works twice as fast.
>
> —Groucho Marx

After reading the preceding paragraphs it might be hard to laugh, but there may be some (although overstated) benefits. Norman Cousins's 1979 book *Anatomy of an Illness* described how he reversed the painful disease ankylosing spondylitis, which causes degeneration of the connective tissue. Cousins's therapy program involved taking high doses of vitamin C and frequently watching movies and reading books that made him laugh. He reported that ten minutes of hearty laughter produced two hours of pain-free sleep. His symptoms gradually lessened, and eventually he regained most of his lost freedom of movement. Several researchers since then have claimed that laughter has a wide range of health benefits.

But Martin, in a lengthy review, concluded that the majority of humor research either negates or is insufficient to support the stated claims.[64] The studies provide little evidence for unique positive effects of laughter on health-related variables. Many of the positive studies did not control for the effects of normal variations, distraction, and emotional arousal apart from humor. Most authors failed to check to see whether their participants found the material funny. They rarely measured frequency of laughter. They measured many different health outcomes without introducing appropriate statistical corrections, so many of the positive findings are probably due solely to chance.[65]

Although exposure to comedy temporarily increases pain threshold and tolerance, similar changes occur in negative emotion control conditions. There is no convincing evidence that exposure to comedy significantly affects endorphin concentration or lowers levels of heart rate or blood pressure. Laughter may reduce minor postsurgical pain but not severe pain that requires major analgesics. Although correlations between sense of humor and S-IgA[66] have been reported, the findings have generally not been replicated in studies with larger sample sizes.

MAKE FRIENDS

Berkman and Syme surveyed a random sample of 6,928 adults in Alameda County, California, in 1965 and then did a nine-year mortality follow-up.[67] Both men and women who lacked social and community ties were more likely to die in the follow-up period than those with more extensive contacts. The association between social ties and mortality was independent of self-reported physical health status at the time of the 1965 survey and also independent of socioeconomic status and health practices such as smoking, alcohol consumption, obesity, and physical activity.

BE GRATEFUL

Emmons and McCullough randomly assigned both healthy college students and adults with various neuromuscular disorders to one of three groups.[68] One group's members were asked to keep journals in which they recorded things for which they were grateful; another recorded things they found annoying and/or irritating; and a third recorded things that had a major impact on them. After two, three, or ten weeks, the grateful group reported the highest levels of overall well-being. The group that recorded annoyances and/or irritations was least happy. Several other studies show that the expression of gratitude plays a significant role in a person's sense of well-being.[69] The benefits may last for months.[70]

Practicing gratitude also has physical health benefits. These include higher levels of alertness, vitality, enthusiasm, determination, attentiveness, and energy; better quality of sleep; fewer headaches, coughing, nausea, or pain; and heightened immunity in both healthy and sick persons.[71] Alspach described a procedure for practicing gratitude. The suggestions below are adapted from her discussion.

A Procedure for Practicing Gratitude

Compile a mental list of three to five things for which you are grateful; they need not be complex or lengthy and may sound trivial to someone else. The only person they need to be meaningful to is you. Following are some examples:

- *It did not rain today, when I once again forgot my umbrella.*
- *I found a parking space right away.*
- *My husband is my best friend.*
- *My Pap smear was negative again this year.*
- *We got eight inches of snow today instead of the predicted ice storm.*
- *I made a difference in this patient's life today from something I learned at last week's conference.*
- *The sound of rain helped me fall asleep last night.*
- *Work on the committee was enormously frustrating for nearly eighteen months, but since Jen volunteered to help us, we've made huge progress.*
- *I lost five pounds last month.*
- *Our daughter has only one more year of college bills that we'll need to pay.*
- *Those same maple trees that drop branches and cut off our power during summer thunderstorms give us breathtaking beauty with spectacular foliage every autumn.*
- *I don't have to see the dentist for another six months.*

If benefactors are identifiable, share what you are grateful for and why it means so much to you. Some strategies for expressing gratitude:

- *Send thank-you notes that detail the basis for your gratitude.*
- *Meet with special people to explain what their thoughtfulness means to you.*

- *At a staff meeting, laud the accomplishments of a colleague or point out some kindness that a colleague extended to you that others were not aware of.*
- *Ask a colleague how you can reciprocate when he or she needs some assistance.*
- *Let your coworkers know how much you enjoy working with them.*
- *Spend a few moments in thankful repose at your place of worship or at any naturally quiet or beautiful setting.*

DIRECT YOURSELF TO ACTION

This appendix lists several scientifically based suggestions for improving health. Readers may be pleased with some of the recommendations, such as eating for enjoyment and taking daily naps. Other recommendations may not be eagerly welcomed, and for those, a strategy called directed thinking may be helpful. Directed thinking involves asking people to think about information that directs them to action. Over an eight-week period, Ten Eyck and colleagues had sedentary college students think about ideas for exercising regularly.[72] Some students were asked to list the reasons why they should increase the performance of a target cardiovascular exercise they had previously selected, such as to be healthier or lose weight. Others were asked to list actions they could take to increase exercise performance, such as joining a gym or working out with a friend.

The students who listed actions they could take to increase exercise performance began exercising more and improved their cardiovascular fitness. The students who repeatedly brought to mind the reasons for exercising did not increase time spent exercising.

NOTES

CHAPTER 1: DOCTOR-PATIENT COMMUNICATION

1. Starfield, B., et al. (1981). The influence of patient-practitioner agreement on outcome of care. *Am J Public Health* 71:127–31; Stewart, M., et al. (1979). The doctor/patient relationship and its effect upon outcome. *Journal of the Royal College of General Practitioners* 29:77–82; Freeling, P., et al. (1985). Unrecognised depression in general practice. *Br Med J (Clin Res Ed)* 290:1880–83; Tarn, D., et al. (2006). Physician communication when prescribing new medications. *Arch Intern Med* 166:1855–62; Kessels, R. (2003). Patients' memory for medical information. *J R Soc Med* 96:219–22; Martin, L., et al. (2005). The challenge of patient adherence. *Therapeutics and Clinical Risk Management* 1:189–99; White, J., et al. (1994). "Oh, by the way . . .": The closing moments of the medical visit. *J Gen Intern Med* 9:24–28.

2. Ulrich, R., et al. (2004). The role of the physical environment in the hospital of the 21st century: A once-in-a-lifetime opportunity, report to the Center for Health Design, Concord, Calif.

3. Roter and colleagues define nonverbal behavior as the "variety of communicative behaviors that do not carry linguistic content . . . these include (among others) facial expressivity, smiling, eye contact, head nodding; hand gestures, postural positions (open or closed body posture and forward to backward body lean); paralinguistic speech characteristics such as speech rate, loudness, pitch, pauses, and speech dysfluencies; and dialogic behaviors such as interruptions." Roter, D., et al. (2006). The expression of emotion through nonverbal behavior in medical visits: Mechanisms and outcomes. *J Gen Intern Med* 21:28–34.

4. DiMatteo, M., et al. (1986). Relationship of physicians' nonverbal communication skill to patient satisfaction, appointment noncompliance, and physician workload. *Health Psychol* 5:581–94.

5. Hall, J., et al. (1995). Nonverbal behavior in clinician-patient interaction. *Applied and Preventive Psychology* 4:21–37.

6. See O'Callaghan, T. (2010). Patients more content, confident when doctors sit to talk. *Time Healthland*, http://www.healthland.time.com, discussing a recent University of Kansas study.

7. Buller, M., & Buller, D. (1987). Physicians' communication style and patient satisfaction. *Journal of Health and Social Behavior* 28:375–88.

8. Griffith, C., et al. (2003). House staff nonverbal communication skills and standardized patient satisfaction. *J Gen Intern Med* 18:170–74.

9. Roter, D., & Hall, J. (2006). *Doctors talking with patients/patients talking with doctors: Improving communication in medical visits* (p. 150) (2nd ed.). Westport, Conn.: Praeger.

10. Buller & Buller, Physicians' communication style.

11. Husson, O., et al. (2010). The relation between information provision and health-related quality of life, anxiety and depression among cancer survivors: A systematic review. *Ann Oncol*, first published online September 24, 2010, DOI:10.1093/annonc/mdq413.

12. Edwards, A., & Elwyn, G. (2006). Inside the black box of shared decision making: Distinguishing between the process of involvement and who makes the decision. *Health Expect* 9:307–20.

13. Golin, C., et al. (2002). Impoverished diabetic patients whose doctors facilitate their participation in medical decision making are more satisfied with their care. *J Gen Intern Med* 17:866–75.

14. Beach, M., et al. (2006). Are physicians' attitudes of respect accurately perceived by patients and associated with more positive communication behaviors? *Patient Educ Couns* 62:347–54.

15. Ibid.

16. Hall, J., et al. (2002). Liking in the physician-patient relationship. *Patient Educ Couns* 48:69–77.

17. Martin et al., The challenge of patient adherence.

18. Ibid.

19. Osterberg, L., & Blaschke, T. (2005). Drug therapy: Adherence to medication. *N Engl J Med* 353:487–97.

20. Martin et al., The challenge of patient adherence. An important caveat to this point is that not all patients want to be fully involved in decision making about their care. As always, patient preferences should be taken into account and supported where possible. Doctor-patient agreement about how involved in their care patients should be also improves adherence.

21. Wright, K., et al. (2008). *Health communication in the 21st century* (p. 39). Oxford: Blackwell.

22. Williams, S., et al. (2007). The therapeutic effects of the physician-older patient relationship: Effective communication with vulnerable older patients. *Clinical Interventions in Aging* 2:453–67.

23. Heisler, M., et al. (2003). When do patients and their physicians agree on diabetes treatment goals and strategies, and what difference does it make? *J Gen Intern Med* 18:893–902.

24. Sudore, R., & Schillinger, D. (2009). Interventions to improve care for patients with limited health literacy. *J Clin Outcomes Manag* 16:20–29.

25. In addition to being less likely to comply with treatment plans, limited health literacy impacts patients in numerous other ways. Patients with limited health literacy often have worse health, fail to seek preventive care, are at higher risk for hospitalization and longer hospital stays, and obtain more emergency room care. Ibid.

26. Williams, M., et al. (1995). Inadequate functional health literacy among patients at two public hospitals. *JAMA* 274:1677–82.

27. Katz, M., et al. (2007). Patient literacy and question-asking behavior during the medical encounter. *J Gen Intern Med* 22:782–86; Koo, M., et al. (2006). Enhancing patient education about medicines: Factors influencing reading and seeking of written medicine information. *Health Expect* 9:174–87; Schillinger, D., et al. (2003). Closing the loop: Physician communication with diabetic patients who have low health literacy. *Arch Intern Med* 163:1745–46.

28. Martin et al., The challenge of patient adherence.

29. Note that doctors often cannot identify which patients have limited health literacy. It cannot be assumed based on educational levels or intelligence, so doctors should use strategies for ensuring comprehension with all their patients. See Nelson, W., et al. (2008). Clinical implications of numeracy: Theory and practice. *Annals of Behavioral Medicine* 35:261–74.

30. Tarn, Physician communication.

31. Kessels, Patients' memory.

32. Wright et al., *Health Communication*, 38.

33. Roter, D., & Hall, J. (2006) *Doctors Talking with Patients*, 15.

34. Ibid., 157.

35. See, for example, Stewart, M. (1995). Effective physician-patient communication and health outcomes: A review. *Can Med Assoc J* 152:1423–33; Kaplan, S., et al. (1989). Assessing the effects of physician-patient interactions on the outcomes of chronic disease. *Med Care* 27:S110–S127; Headache Study Group of the University of Western Ontario. (1986). Predictors of outcome in headache patients presenting to family physicians—A one year prospective study. *Headache* 26:285–94; Schillinger, D., et al. (2003). Closing the loop: Physician communication with diabetic patients who have low health literacy. *Arch Intern Med* 163:83–90; Mumford, E., et al. (1982). The effect of psychological intervention on recovery from surgery and heart attacks: An analysis of the literature. *Am J Public Health* 72:141–51; Greenfield, S., et al. (1985). Expanding patient involvement in care: Effects on patient outcomes. *Ann Intern Med* 102:520–28.

36. Street, R., et al. (2009). How does communication heal? Pathways linking clinician patient communication to health outcomes. *Patient Educ Couns* 74:295–301.

37. Roter & Hall, *Doctors Talking with Patients* (pp. 158–59).

38. Street et al., How does communication heal?

39. Hall, J. (2003). Some observations on provider-patient communication research. *Patient Educ Couns* 50:9–12.

40. Franks, P., et al. (2005). Are patients' ratings of their physicians related to health outcomes? *Ann Fam Med* 3:229–34.

41. Ramirez, A., & Graham, J. (1996). Mental health of hospital consultants: The effect of stress and satisfaction at work. *Lancet* 347:724–28.

42. Mello, M., et al. (2004). Caring for patients in a malpractice crisis: Physician satisfaction and quality of care. *Health Affairs* 23:42–53.

43. Ramirez & Graham, Mental health of hospital consultants.

44. Suchman, A., et al. (1993). Physician satisfaction with primary care office visits. *Med Care* 31:1083–92.

45. Roter, D., et al. (1997). Communication patterns of primary care physicians. *JAMA* 270:350–55.

46. Dauphiness, D., et al. (2007). Physician scores on a national clinical skills examination as predictors of complaints to medical regulatory authorities. *JAMA* 298:993–1001; Shapiro, R., et al. (1989). A survey of sued and nonsued physicians and suing patients. *Arch Intern Med* 149:2190–96.

47. Beckman, H., et al. (1994). The doctor-patient relationship and malpractice: Lessons from plaintiff depositions. *Arch Intern Med* 154:1365–70.

48. Levinson, W., et al. (1997). The relationship with malpractice claims among primary care physicians and surgeons. *JAMA* 277:553–59.

49. Ambady, N., et al. (2002). Surgeons' tone of voice: A clue to malpractice history. *Surgery* 132:5–9.

50. Hickson, G., et al. (1994). Obstetricians' prior malpractice experience and patients' satisfaction with care. *JAMA* 272:1583–87.

51. Shapiro et al. (1989), A survey of sued and nonsued physicians.

52. Beach, M., et al. (2006). Is the quality of the patient-provider relationship associated with better adherence and health outcomes for patients with HIV? *J Gen Intern Med* 21:661–65.

53. Stewart, M. (2005). Reflections on the doctor-patient relationship: from evidence and experience. *British Journal of General Practice* 55:793–801. Stewart's other four components of the patient-centered clinical method are: finding common ground, incorporating prevention and health promotion, enhancing the patient-doctor relationship, and being realistic.

54. Ibid.

55. Ibid.

56. Saha, S., et al. (2008). Patient centeredness, cultural competence and healthcare quality. *J Natl Med Assoc* 100:1275–85.

57. Wright, *Health Communication* (p. 101).

58. Little, P., et al. (2001). Observational study of effect of patient centredness and positive approach on outcomes of general practice consultations. *BMJ* 323:908–11.

59. Little, P., et al. (2001). Preferences of patients for patient centered approach to consultation in primary care: Observational study. *BMJ* 322:1–7. Little et al. identified three distinct domains of patient centeredness: communication, partnership, and health promotion.

60. Stewart, M., et al. (2000). The impact of patient-centered care on outcomes. *Journal of Family Practice* 49:796–804.

61. Beach et al., Is the quality of the patient-provider relationship . . . ?

62. Waitzkin, H. (1985). Information-giving in medical care. *Journal of Health and Social Behavior* 26:81–101.

63. Roter, D., et al. (2002). Physician gender effects in medical communication: A meta-analytic review. *JAMA* 288:756–64.

64. Hall, J., & Roter, D. (2002). Do patients talk differently to male and female physicians? A meta-analytic review. *Patient Educ Couns* 48:217–24.

65. Hall et al., Liking in the physician-patient relationship.

66. Sandhu, H., et al. (2009). The impact of gender dyads on doctor-patient communication: A systematic review. *Patient Educ Couns* 76:348–55.

67. Hooper, E., et al. (1982). Patient characteristics that influence physician behavior. *Med Care* 20:630–38.

68. Cooper-Patrick, L., et al. (1999). Race, gender and partnership in the patient-physician relationship. *JAMA* 282:583–89.

69. Street, R., et al. (2007). Physicians' communication and perception of patients: Is it how they look, how they talk, or is it just the doctor? *Soc Sci Med* 65:586–98.

70. Collins, K., et al. (2002). Diverse communities, common concerns: Assessing health care quality for minority Americans, findings from the Commonwealth Fund 2001 health care quality survey. The Commonwealth Fund.

71. Johnson, R., et al. (2004). Patient race/ethnicity and quality of patient-physician communication during medical visits. *Am J Public Health* 94:2084–90.

72. Cooper, L., et al. (2003). Patient-centered communication, ratings of care, and concordance of patient and physician race. *Ann Intern Med* 139:907–15.

73. Ibid.; Saha, S., et al. (1999). Patient-physician racial concordance and the perceived quality and use of health care. *Arch Intern Med* 159:997–1004.

74. Robert Wood Johnson Foundation. (2002). New survey shows language barriers causing many Spanish-speaking Latinos to skip care. Cited in Williams et al. (2007), The therapeutic effects.

75. Hall, J., et al. (1993). Physicians' liking for their patients: Further evidence for the role of affect in medical care. *Health Psychol* 12:140–46.

76. Hall, J., et al. (1996). Patients' health as a predictor of physician and patient behavior in medical visits. A synthesis of four studies. *Med Care* 34:1205–18.

77. Hall, J., et al. (1990). Older patients' health status and satisfaction in an HMO population. *Med Care* 28:261–70.

78. Willems, S., et al. (2005). Socio-economic status of the patient and doctor patient communication: Does it make a difference? *Patient Educ Couns* 56:139–146.

79. Waitzkin, Information-giving in medical care.

80. Hooper et al., Patient characteristics.

81. Ibid.

82. Mauksch, L., et al. (2008). Relationship, communication, and efficiency in the medical encounter. *Arch Intern Med* 168:1387–95.

83. Marvel, M., et al. (1999). Soliciting the patient's agenda: Have we improved? *JAMA* 281:283–87.

84. Ibid.

85. Ibid.

86. Heritage, J., et al. (2007). Reducing patients' unmet concerns in primary care: The difference one word can make. *J Gen Intern Med* 22:1429–33.

87. Beach, M., et al. (2005). Do patients treated with dignity report higher satisfaction, adherence, and receipt of preventive care? *Ann Fam Med* 3:331–38.

88. Johnson, A., et al. (2003). Written and verbal information versus verbal information only for patients being discharged from acute hospital settings to home. Cochrane Database of Systematic Reviews 2003, Issue 4. Art. No.: CD003716.

89. Sudore & Schillinger, Interventions to improve care.

90. Martin, L., et al. (2003). Physician facilitation of patient involvement in care: Correspondence between patient and observer reports. *Behavioral Medicine* 28:159–164.

91. Schillinger et al., Closing the loop.

92. O'Connor, A., & Stacey, D. (2005). Should patient decision aids (PtDAs) be introduced in the health care system? Copenhagen, WHO Regional Office for Europe (Health Evidence Network report, http://www.euro.who.int/Document/E87791.pdf, accessed August 12, 2010).

93. O'Connor, A., et al. (2007). Do patient decision aids meet effectiveness criteria of the international patient decision aid standards collaboration? A systematic review and meta-analysis. *Med Decis Making* 27:554–74.

94. O'Connor & Stacey, Should patient decision aids . . . ?

95. Shaffer, V., & Hulsey, L. (2009). Are patient decision aids effective? Insights from revisiting the debate between correspondence and coherence theories of judgment. *Judgment and Decision Making* 4:141–46.

96. O'Donnell, S., et al. (2006). Understanding and overcoming the barriers of implementing patient decision aids in clinical practice. *Journal of Evaluation in Clinical Practice* 12:174–81.

97. Mauksch et al., Relationship, communication, and efficiency; Chen, J., et al. (2008). Impact of physician-patient discussions on patient satisfaction. *Med Care* 46:1157–62; Krupat, E., et al. (2001). When physicians and patients think alike: Patient centered beliefs and their impact on satisfaction and trust. *Journal of Family Practice* 50; Heisler et al., When do patients and their physicians agree . . . ?; Kenny, D., et al. (2009). Interpersonal perception in the context of doctor-patient relationships: A dyadic analysis of doctor-patient communication. *Soc Sci Med* 70:763–68.

98. Schattner, A., et al. (2006). Information and shared decision-making are top patients' priorities. *BMC Health Services Research* 6. The six options were: increased information and autonomy; continuity of care; time spent with doctor; easier access to sophisticated medical services; shorter queue for tests; cost of medications.

99. Swenson, S. L., et al. (2004). Patient-centered communication: Do patients really prefer it? *J Gen Intern Med* 19:1069–79.

100. Flynn, K., & Smith, M. (2007). Personality and health care decision-making style. *J Gerontol B Psychol Sci Soc Sci* 62:261–67.

101. Ibid.

102. Golin et al., Impoverished diabetic patients.

103. Jahng, K., et al. (2005). Preferences for medical collaboration: Patient-physician congruence and patient outcomes. *Patient Educ Couns* 57:308–14.

104. Egbert, L., et al. (1964). Reduction of postoperative pain by encouragement and instruction of patients: A study of doctor-patient rapport, *N Eng J Med* 270:825–27; see Roter & Hall, *Doctors talking with patients* (p. 167), for a discussion of the body of later studies that support this finding.

105. Fallowfield, L., & Jenkins, V. (2004). Communicating sad, bad, and difficult news in medicine. *Lancet* 363:312–19.

106. Parker, P., et al. (2001). Breaking bad news about cancer: Patients' preferences for communication. *J Clinical Oncology* 19:2049–56.

107. Lamont, E., & Christakis, N. (2001). Prognostic disclosure to patients with cancer near the end of life. *Ann Intern Med* 134:1096–1105.

108. Ibid.

109. Fallowfield & Jenkins, Communicating sad, bad, and difficult news.

110. Jurkovich, G., et al. (2000). Giving bad news: The family perspective. *J Trauma* 48:865–70.

111. Back, A., & Curtis, J. (2002). Evidence-based case reviews: Communicating bad news. *West J Med* 176:177–80.

112. Jurkovich et al., Giving bad news.

113. Back & Curtis, Evidence-based case reviews.

114. Sharp, M., et al. (1992). Communicating medical bad news: Parents' experiences and preferences. *J Pediatr* 121:539–46.

CHAPTER 2: INTERPRETING MEDICAL INFORMATION

1. Ramnarayan, P., & Britto, J. (2002). Paediatric clinical decision support systems. *Archives of Disease in Childhood* 87:361–62.

2. Burnside, E. (2005). Bayesian networks: Computer-assisted diagnosis support in radiology. *Academic Radiology* 12:422–30.

3. Drug companies cannot legally promote a drug before the FDA approves it and cannot legally promote a drug for off-label use. But journal articles are considered as protected speech, so the FDA doesn't regulate their content.

4. Scott, T. (2006). *America fooled: The truth about antidepressants, antipsychotics and how we've been deceived*. Victoria, Tex.: Argo Publishing.

5. Wilson, D. (2008, December 12). Wyeth's use of medical ghostwriters questioned. *New York Times*, http://www.nytimes.com/2008/12/13/business/13wyeth.html?_r=2&ref=business (accessed on May 2, 2010).

6. Chan, A., & Altman, D. (2005). Identifying outcome reporting bias in randomised trials on PubMed: Review of publications and survey of authors. *BMJ* 330:753–56; Kirsch, I., et al. (2002). The emperor's new drugs: An analysis of antidepressant medication data submitted to the U.S. Food and Drug Administration. *Prevention & Treatment* 5, Article 23, posted July 15, 2002; Lee, K., et al. (2008). Publication of clinical trials supporting successful new drug applications: A literature analysis. *PLoS Med* 5:e191. DOI:10.1371/journal.pmed.0050191.

7. Scott, *America Fooled*.

8. Turner, E., et al. (2008). Selective publication of antidepressant trials and its influence on apparent efficacy. *N Engl J Med* 358:252–60.

9. Rising, K., et al. (2008). Reporting bias in drug trials submitted to the Food and Drug Administration: Review of publication and presentation. *PLoS Med* 5(11):e217. DOI:10.1371/journal.pmed.0050217.

10. Spiro, H. (1997). Clinical reflections on the placebo phenomenon. In A. Harrington (ed.), *The placebo effect: An interdisciplinary exploration* (pp. 37–55). Cambridge, Mass.: Harvard University Press.

11. Bodenheimer, T. (2000). Uneasy alliance: Clinical investigators and the pharmaceutical industry. *Health Policy Report* 342:1539–44.

12. Bero, L., et al. (2007). Factors associated with findings of published trials of drug-drug comparisons: Why some statins appear more efficacious than others. *PLoS Med* 4(6):e184. DOI:10.1371/journal.pmed.0040184.

13. Huss, A., et al. (2007). Source of funding and results of studies of health effects of mobile phone use: Systematic review of experimental studies. *Environmental Health Perspectives* 115:1–4.

14. Lesser, L., et al. (2007). Relationship between funding source and conclusion among nutrition-related scientific articles. *PLoS Med* 4:e5.

15. The Cochrane Collaboration is a group of more than 11,500 volunteers in more than ninety countries who apply a rigorous, systematic process to review the effects of biomedical interventions. The results of these systematic reviews are published in the Cochrane Library.

16. Davidson, R. (1986). Source of funding and outcome of clinical trials. *J Gen Intern Med* 3:155–58.

17. Cho, M., & Bero, L. (1996). The quality of drug studies published in symposium proceedings. *Ann Intern Med* 124:485–89.

18. Walton, R. (1994). Survey of aspartame studies: Correlation of outcome and funding sources. Unpublished study, compiled for the television show *60 Minutes*.

19. Dyer, O. (2004). Journal rejects article after objections from marketing department. *BMJ* 328:244.

20. Yank, V., et al. (2005). Are authors' financial ties with pharmaceutical companies associated with positive results or conclusions in meta-analyses on antihypertensive medications [abstract]? *Proceedings of the 5th International Congress on Peer Review and Biomedical Publication*, Chicago, September.

21. Lurie, P., et al. (2006). Financial conflict of interest disclosure and voting patterns at Food and Drug Administration drug advisory committee meetings. *JAMA* 295:1921–28.

22. Tuller, D. (2004, July 20). Seeking a fuller picture of statins. *New York Times*.

23. Union of Concerned Scientists. Brochure, http://www.ucsusa.org/assets/documents/scientific_integrity/fda-survey-brochure.pdf.

24. Roseman, M., et al. (2011). Reporting of conflicts of interest in meta-analyses of trials of pharmacological treatments. *JAMA* 305:1008–17.

25. Ioannidis, J. (2005). Contradicted and initially stronger effects in highly cited clinical research. *JAMA* 294:218–28.

26. Ioannidis, J. (2005). Why most published research findings are false. *PLoS Med* 2(8):e124. DOI:10.1371/journal.pmed.0020124.

27. Freedman, D. Lies, damned lies, and medical science, http://www.theatlantic.com/magazine/archive/2010/11/lies-damned-lies-and-medical-science/8269/ (accessed on October 26, 2010).

28. Puccio, E., et al. (1990). Clustering of atherogenic behaviors in coffee drinkers. *Am J Public Health* 80:1310–13.

29. Smith, G., & Ebrahim, S. (2002). Data dredging, bias or confounding. They can all get into the *BMJ* and the Friday papers. *BMJ* 325:1435–38.

30. Basoglu, M., et al. (1997). Double-blindness procedures, rater blindness, and ratings of outcome observations from a controlled trial. *Arch Gen Psychiatry* 54:744–48; Moscucci, M., et al. (1987). Blinding, unblinding, and the placebo effect: An analysis of patients' guesses of treatment assignment in a double-blind clinical trial. *Clinical Pharmacology and Therapeutics* 41:259–65; Rickels, K., et al. (1970). Is a double-blind clinical trial really double-blind? *Psychopharmacology* 16:1432–2072.

31. Schulz, K. (1995). Empirical evidence of bias: Dimensions of methodological quality associated with estimates of treatment effects in controlled trials. *JAMA* 273:408–12.

32. Fergusson, D., et al. (2004). Turning a blind eye: The success of blinding reported in a random sample of randomised, placebo controlled trials. *BMJ* 328:432–34.

33. Golomb, B. (2010). What's in placebos: Who knows? Analysis of randomized, controlled trials. *Ann Intern Med* 153:532–35.

34. Kirsch, I., et al. (2008). Initial severity and antidepressant benefits: A meta-analysis of data submitted to the Food and Drug Administration. *PLoS Med* 5(2):e45.

Kirsch also observed that most of the clinical trials sponsored by drug companies showed no significant difference between drug and placebo. The drugs were approved because the FDA requires only that two trials show a statistical difference between drug and placebo—even if the difference has little clinical significance and even if several other trials have failed to show a difference. He further noted that, compared with placebos, the antidepressants produced more side effects such as nausea and sexual dysfunction.

35. Hopewell, S., et al. (2009). Publication bias in clinical trials due to statistical significance or direction of trial results. *Cochrane Database of Systematic Reviews*, Issue 1. Art. No.: MR000006.

36. Sutton, A., et al. (2000). Empirical assessment of effect of publication bias on meta-analyses. *BMJ* 320:1574–77.

37. Simes, R. (1986). Publication bias: The case for an international registry of clinical trials. *J Clinical Oncology* 4:1529–41.

38. Ioannidis, J. P. (2005). Contradicted and initially stronger effects in highly cited clinical research. *JAMA* 294:218–28.

39. Mack, J. (2008). The statin lottery: Number needed to treat statistic. http://phar mamkting.blogspot.com/2008/01/statin-lottery-number-needed-to-treat.html (accessed August 21, 2009).

40. Bridge, J., et al. (2009) Placebo response in randomized controlled trials of antidepressants for pediatric major depressive disorder. *Am J Psychiatry* 166:42–49.

41. Gigerenzer, G. (2007). Helping physicians understand screening tests will improve health care. *Association for Psychological Science* 20:37–38.

42. Naylor, C., et al. (1992). Measured enthusiasm: Does the method of reporting trial results alter perceptions of therapeutic effectiveness? *Ann Intern Med* 117:916–21.

43. Gigerenzer, G., et al. (2007). Helping doctors and patients make sense of health statistics. *Psychological Science in the Public Interest* 8:53–96.

44. Forrow, L., et al. (1992). Absolutely relative: How research results are summarized can affect treatment decisions. *Am J Med* 92:121–24.

45. Carling, C., et al. (2009). The effect of alternative summary statistics for communicating risk reduction on decisions about taking statins: A randomized trial. *PLoS Med* 6(8):e1000134.

CHAPTER 3: DECISIONS: OVERVIEW

1. Croskerry, P. (2005). The theory and practice of clinical decision-making. *Canadian Journal of Anesthesia* 52:R1.

2. De Bono, E. (1992). *Serious Creativity*. New York: HarperCollins.

3. Hamilton, W. (2000). *New Yorker*, January 10.

4. Soelberg, P. (1967). Unprogrammed decision making. *Industrial Management Review* 8:19–29.

5. Wilson, T., & Schooler, J. (1991). Thinking too much: Introspection can reduce the quality of preferences and decisions. *J Pers Soc Psychol* 60:181–92.

6. Halberstadt, J., & Levine, G. (1999). Effects of reasons analysis on the accuracy of predicting basketball games. *J Applied Social Psychology* 29:517–30.

7. Crandall, B., & Getchell-Reiter, K. (1993). Critical decision method: A technique for eliciting concrete assessment indicators from the "intuition" of NICU nurses. *Advances in Nursing Sciences* 16:42–51.

8. Damasio, A. (1994). *Descartes' error: Emotion, reason, and the human brain.* New York: Avon.

9. Hsee, C., & Kunreuther, H. (2000). The affection effect in insurance decisions. *J Risk and Uncertainty* 20:141–59.

10. Isen, A. (2001). An influence of positive affect on decision making in complex situations: Theoretical issues with practical implications. *J Consumer Psychology* 11:75–85; Isen, A. (2004). Some perspectives on positive feelings and emotions: Positive affect facilitates thinking and problem solving. In A. Manstead et al. (eds.), *Feelings and emotions: The Amsterdam Symposium* (pp. 263–81). New York: Cambridge University Press.

11. Isen, A., et al. (1991). The influence of positive affect on clinical problem solving. *Med Decis Making* 11:221–27.

12. Estrada, C., et al. (1994). Positive affect improves creative problem solving and influences reported source of practice satisfaction in physicians. *Motivation and Emotion* 18:285–99.

13. Alexander, J., & Beversdorf, D. (2004). Cognitive consequences of examination stress. Society for Neuroscience Annual Meeting, San Diego, Calif., October 23–27.

14. Cleland, V. (1967). Effects of stress on thinking. *American Journal of Nursing* 67:108–111.

15. Liston, C., et al. (2009). Psychosocial stress reversibly disrupts prefrontal processing and attentional control. *Proceedings of the National Academy of Sciences* 106:912–17.

16. Kontogiannis, T., & Kossiavelou, Z. (1999). Stress and team performance: Principles and challenges for intelligent decision aids. *Safety Science* 33:103–28.

17. Beversdorf, D., et al. (2005). *Annual meeting of the Society for Neuroscience,* Washington, November 12–19. News release, Ohio State University.

18. North, A., et al. (1999). The influence of in-store music on wine selections. *J Applied Psychology* 84:271–76.

19. Nisbett, R., & Wilson, T. (1977). Telling more than we can know: Verbal reports on mental processes. *Psychological Review* 84:231–59.

20. McKinlay, J., et al. (1996). Non-medical influences on medical decision-making. *Soc Sci Med* 42:769–76.

21. Redelmeier, D., & Shafir, E. (1995). Medical decision making in decisions that offer multiple alternatives. *JAMA* 273:302–5.

22. Ganiats, T. (1999). Screening options for colorectal cancer. *American Family Physician* 59:3083–92.

23. Schwartz, J., & Chapman, G. (1999). Are more options always better? The attraction effect in physicians' decisions about medications. *Med Decis Making* 19:315–23; Schwartz, J., et al. (2004). The effects of accountability on bias in physician decision making: Going from bad to worse. *Psychonomic Bulletin & Review* 11:173–78.

24. Adair, R., & Holmgren, L. (2005). Do drug samples influence resident prescribing behavior? A randomized trial. *Am J Med* 118:881–84.

25. Adair, R. (2006). Hidden costs of free samples. *Ethics Journal of the American Medical Association* 8:367–71.

26. Weiner, S., et al. (2010). Contextual errors and failures in individualizing patient care: A multicenter study. *Ann Intern Med* 153:69–75.

CHAPTER 4: DECISIONS: BIASES

1. Galanter, C., & Patel, V. (2005). Medical decision making: A selective review for child psychiatrists and psychologists. *J Child Psychology and Psychiatry* 46:675–89.

2. Poses, R., & Anthony, M. (1991). Availability, wishful thinking, and physicians' diagnostic judgments for patients with suspected bacteremia. *Med Decis Making* 11:159–68.

3. Swinkels, A. (2003). An effective exercise for teaching cognitive heuristics. *Teaching of Psychology* 30:120–22.

4. Berner, E., & Graber, M. (2008). Overconfidence as a cause of diagnostic error in medicine. *Am J Med* 121:(5A), S2–S23.

5. Tversky, A., & Kahneman, D. (1974). Judgment under uncertainty: Heuristics and biases. *Science* 185:1124–31.

6. Strack, F., & Mussweiler, T. (1997). Explaining the enigmatic anchoring effect: Mechanisms of selective accessibility. *J Personality and Social Psychology* 73:437–46.

7. Wilson, T., et al. (1996). A new look at anchoring effects: Basic anchoring and its antecedents. *J Experimental Psychology: General* 125:387–402.

8. Garb, H. (1998). *Studying the Clinician: Judgment Research and Psychological Assessment.* Washington, D.C.: American Psychological Association.

9. Brewer, N., et al. (2007). The influence of irrelevant anchors on the judgments and choices of doctors and patients. *Med Decis Making* 27:203–11.

10. Pothier, D., et al. (2009). Arbitrary coherence in theoretical decision making about surgical training: The effect of irrelevant subliminal anchoring. *J Surgical Education* 66:129–31.

11. Hitinder, S., & Litaker, D. (2000). Is 99% safe the same as a risk of 1 in 100? *Academic Medicine* 75:840–42.

12. Marteau, T. (1989). Framing of information: Its influence upon decisions of doctors and patients. *British J Social Psychology* 28:89–94.

13. McNeil, B., et al. (1982) On the elicitation of preferences for alternative therapies. *N Engl J Med* 306:1259–62.

14. Martin, R., et al. (2006). Method of presenting oncology treatment outcomes influences patient treatment decision-making in metastatic colorectal cancer. *Ann Surg Oncol* 13:86–95.

15. Slovic, P., et al. (2000). Violence risk assessment and risk communication: The effects of using actual cases, providing instruction, and employing probability versus frequency formats. *Law and Human Behavior* 24:271–96.

16. Detweiler, J., et al. (1999). Message framing and sunscreen use: Gain-framed messages motivate beach-goers. *Health Psychol* 18:189–96.

17. Gerend, M., & Shepherd, J. (2007). Using message framing to promote acceptance of the human papillomavirus vaccine. *Health Psychol* 26:745–52.

18. Tversky, A., & Kahneman, D. (1981). The framing of decisions and the rationality of choice. *Science* 221:453–8.

19. See, e.g., Krishnamurthy, P., et al. (2001). Attribute framing and goal framing effects in health decisions. *Organizational Behavior and Human Decision Processes* 85:382–99; Siminoff, L., & Fetting, J. (1989). Effects of outcome framing on treatment decisions in the real world. *Med Decis Making* 9:262–71; O'Connor, A., et al. (1996). Framing effects on expectations, decisions, and side effects experienced: The case of influenza immunization. *J Clinical Epidemiology* 49:1271–76.

20. Ubel, P., et al. (2001). Preference for equity as a framing effect. *Med Decis Making* 21:180–89.

21. Li, M., & Chapman, G. (2009). "100% of anything looks good": The appeal of one hundred percent. *Psychonomic Bulletin & Review* 16:156–62.

22. Asch, D., et al. (1994), Omission bias and pertussis vaccination. *Med Decis Making* 14:118–23.

23. Dawn, A., et al. (2008). Systematic selection bias: A cause of dramatic errors in the inference of treatment effectiveness. *J Dermatological Treatment* 19:68–71.

24. Gehr, B., et al. (2006). The fading of reported effectiveness. A meta-analysis of randomised controlled trials. *BMC Medical Research Methodology* 6:25.

25. Hammers, R., et al. (2010). Neurosurgical mortality rates: What variables affect mortality within a single institution and within a national database? *J Neurosurg* 112:257–64.

26. Bornstein, B., et al. (1999). Rationality in medical treatment decisions: Is there a sunk-cost effect? *Soc Sci Med* 49:215–22.

27. Shafir, E. (1993). Why some options are both better and worse than others. *Memory and Cognition* 21:546–56.

28. Redelmeier, D., & Kahneman, D. (1996). Patients' memories of painful medical treatments: Real-time and retrospective evaluations of two minimally invasive procedures. *Pain* 66:3–8.

29. Weinstein, N. (1989). Optimistic biases about personal risks. *Science* 246:1232–33; Avis, N., et al. (1989). Accuracy of perceptions of heart attack risk: What influences perceptions and can they be changed? *Am J Public Health* 79:1608–12; Niknian, M., et al. (1989). A comparison of perceived and objective risk in a general population. *Am J Public Health* 79:1653–4.

30. Aberegg, S., et al. (2006). Failure to adopt beneficial therapies caused by bias in medical evidence evaluation. *Med Decis Making* 26:575–82.

31. Loewenstein, G. (2005). Projection bias in medical decision-making. *Med Decis Making* 25:96–105.

32. Ubel, P., et al. (2005). Disability and sunshine: Can predictions be improved by drawing attention to focusing illusions or emotional adaptation? *J Experimental Psychology: Applied* 11:111–23; Ubel, P., et al. (2005). Misimagining the unimaginable: The happiness gap and healthcare decision making. *Health Psychol* 24:S57–S62.

33. Wu, A., et al. (1991). Do house officers learn from their mistakes? *JAMA* 265:2089–94.

34. Caplan, R., et al. (1991). Effect of outcome on physician judgments of appropriateness of care. *JAMA* 265:1957–60.

35. Dawson, N., et al. (1988). Hindsight bias: An impediment to accurate probability estimation in clinicopathologic conferences. *Med Decis Making* 8:259–64.

36. Aberegg, S., & O'Brien Jr., J. (2009). The normalization heuristic: An untested hypothesis that may misguide medical decisions. *Medical Hypotheses* 72:745–48.

37. Kahneman, D., & Tversky, A. (1979). Prospect theory: An analysis of decision under risk. *Econometrica* 47:263–91; Tversky, A., & Kahneman, D. (1991). Loss aversion in riskless choice: A reference-dependent model. *Quart J Economics* 106:1039–61.

38. Polak, B., et al. (1972). Blood dyscrasias attributed to chloramphenicol: A review of 576 published and unpublished cases. *Acta Med Scand* 192:409–14.

39. Owens, D., & Nease, R. (1992). Occupational exposure to human immunodeficiency virus and hepatitis B virus: A comparative analysis of risk. *Am J Med* 92:503–12.

40. Wegwarth, O., et al. (2009). Smart strategies for doctors and doctors-in-training: Heuristics in medicine. *Medical Education* 43:721–28.

41. Woolever, D. (2008). The art and science of clinical decision making. *Family Practice Management* 15:31–36.

42. Miller, P., & Fagley, N. (1991). The effects of framing, problem variations, and providing rationale on choice. *Pers Soc Psychol Bull* 17:517–22; Takemura, K. (1994). Influence of elaboration on the framing of decision. *J Psychol* 128:33–39.

43. Almashat, S., et al. (2008). Framing effect debiasing in medical decision making. *Patient Educ Couns* 71:102–7.

44. Bond, W., et al. (2004). Using simulation to instruct emergency medicine residents in cognitive forcing strategies. *Academic Medicine* 79:438–46.

45. Swets, J., et al. (1991). Enhancing and evaluating diagnostic accuracy. *Med Decis Making* 11:9–18.

CHAPTER 5: MEDICAL DIAGNOSIS

1. Sonnenberg, A., & Gogel, H. (2002). Translating vague complaints into precise symptoms: The implications of a poor medical history. *European J Gastroenterology & Hepatology* 14:1–5.

2. National Cancer Institute. Fact sheet. Mammograms. Available at: http://www.cancer.gov/cancertopics/factsheet/Detection/mammograms (accessed August 3, 2010).

3. Payer, L. (1995). *Medicine & culture: Varieties of treatment in the United States, England, West Germany, and France.* New York: Henry Holt.

4. But see p. 267 on calculating life spans.

5. Weisz, G., & Knaapen, L. (2009). Diagnosing and treating premenstrual syndrome in five Western nations. *Social Science & Medicine* 68:1498–1505.

6. Strickland, T., et al. (1988). Diagnostic judgments as a function of client and therapist race. *J Psychopathology and Behavioral Assessment* 10:141–51.

7. Blow, F., et al. (2004). Ethnicity and diagnostic patterns in veterans with psychoses. *Soc Psychiatry Psychiatr Epidemiol* 39:841–51.

8. Bernstein, B., & Kane, R. (1981). Physicians' attitudes toward female patients. *Med Care* 19:600–608.

9. Wells, C., & Feinstein, A. (1988). Detection bias in the diagnostic pursuit of lung cancer. *Am J Epidemiol* 128:1016–26.

10. Khan, S., et al. (1990). Increased mortality of women in coronary artery bypass surgery: Evidence for referral bias. *Ann Intern Med* 112:561–67; Wenger, N. (1985). Coronary disease in women. *Ann Rev Med* 36:285–94; Fiebach, N. (1990). Differences between women and men in survival after myocardial infarction. *JAMA* 263:1092–96; Dittrich, H., et al. (1988). Acute myocardial infarction in women: Influence of gender on mortality and prognosis variables. *Am J Card* 62:1–7.

11. Tobin, J., et al. (1987). Sex bias in considering coronary bypass surgery. *Ann Intern Med* 107:19–25.

12. Katz, J., et al. (1994). Differences between men and women undergoing major orthopedic surgery for degenerative arthritis. *Arthritis Rheum* 37:687–94.

13. Garcia, R. (2004). The misuse of race in medical diagnosis. *Pediatrics* 113:1394–95.

14. Werner, R., et al. (2005). The unintended consequences of coronary artery bypass graft report cards. *Circulation* 111:1257–63.

15. Trokel, M. (2006). Variation in the diagnosis of child abuse in severely injured infants. *Pediatrics* 117:722–28.

16. Boom, R., et al. (1986). Looking for "indicants" in the differential diagnosis of jaundice. *Med Decis Making* 6:36–41.

17. Curran, M., & Jagger, C. (1997). Interobserver variability in the diagnosis of foot and leg disorders using a computer expert system. *The Foot* 7:7–10.

18. Espelid, I., et al. (1994). Variations among dentists in radiographic detection of occlusal caries. *Caries Res* 28:169–75.

19. Lanning, S., et al. (2005). Variation in periodontal diagnosis and treatment planning among clinical instructors. *J Dental Education* 69:325–37.

20. Grady, D. (2007, July 29). Cancer patients lost in a maze of uneven care. *New York Times.*

21. Hashem, A., et al. (2003). Medical errors as a result of specialization. *J Biomedical Informatics* 36:61–69.

22. Kalf, A., & Spruijt-Metz, D. (1996). Variation in diagnoses: Influence of specialists' training on selecting and ranking relevant information in geriatric case vignettes. *Soc Sci Med* 42:705–12.

23. Leape, L., et al. (2002). Counting deaths due to medical errors [letter]. *JAMA* 288:2405.

24. Leape, L., et al. (1991). The nature of adverse events in hospitalized patients: Results of the Harvard Medical Practice Study II. *N Engl J Med* 324:377–84.

25. Elstein, A. (1995). Clinical reasoning in medicine. In J. J. M. Higgs (ed.), *Clinical reasoning in the health professions*. Oxford: Butterworth-Heinemann.

26. Amy, L., et al. (2006). Impact of a web-diagnosis reminder system on errors of diagnosis. In *Proceedings of the American Medical Information Association (AMIA) Annual Conference* (pp. 2–6), 11–15 November, Bethesda, MD,

27. Berner, E., & Graber, M. (2008). Overconfidence as a cause of diagnostic error in medicine. *Amer J Medicine* 121:S2–S23.

28. Berlin, L. (2001). Defending the missed radiographic diagnosis. *Am J Radiol* 176:317–22.

29. Berlin, L., & Hendrix, R. (1998). Perceptual errors and negligence. *Am J Radiol* 170:863–67.

30. Majid, A., et al. (2003). Missed breast carcinoma: Pitfalls and pearls. *Radiographics* 23:881–95.

31. Harvey, J., et al. (1993). Previous mammograms in patients with impalpable breast carcinoma. *Am J Radiol* 161:1167–72.

32. Nuñez, S. (2006). Unscheduled returns to the emergency department: An outcome of medical errors? *Qual Saf Health Care* 15:102–8; O'Dwyer, F., & Bodiwala, G. (1991). Unscheduled return visits by patients to the accident and emergency department. *Arch Emerg Med* 8:196–200; Wilkins, P., & Beckett, M. (1992). Audit of unexpected return visits to an accident and emergency department. *Arch Emerg Med* 9:352–56.

33. Neale, G., et al. (2001). Exploring the causes of adverse events in NHS hospital practice. *J R Soc Med* 94:322–30.

34. Leape, L., et al. (1991). The nature of adverse events in hospitalized patients. Results of the Harvard Medical Practice Study II. *N Engl J Med* 324:377–84.

35. Bartlett, E. (1998). Physicians' cognitive errors and their liability consequences. *J Healthcare Risk Management* (Fall): 62–69.

36. Phillips, R. (2004). Learning from malpractice claims about negligent, adverse events in primary care in the United States. *Qual Saf Health Care* 13:121–6.

37. Thomas, E., et al. (2000). Incidence and types of adverse events and negligent care in Utah and Colorado. *Med Care* 38:261–71.

38. Tai, D., et al. (2001). A study of consecutive autopsies in a medical ICU: A comparison of clinical cause of death and autopsy diagnosis. *Chest* 119:530–36.

39. Wells, C., & Feinstein, A. (1988). Detection bias in the diagnostic pursuit of lung cancer. *Am J Epidemiol* 128:1016–26.

40. Roosen, J., et al. (2000). Comparison of premortem clinical diagnoses in critically ill patients and subsequent autopsy findings. *Mayo Clinic Proceedings* 75:562–67.

41. Scott, I. (2009). Errors in clinical reasoning: Causes and remedial strategies. *BMJ* 339:22–25.

42. Weeks, W., et al. (2001). Tort claims analysis in the Veterans Health Administration for quality improvement. *J Law Med Ethics* 29:335–45.

43. Cited at How common is misdiagnosis? http://www.cureresearch.com/intro/common_printer.htm (accessed March 28, 2010).

44. Gandhi, T., et al. (2006). Missed and delayed diagnoses in the ambulatory setting: A study of closed malpractice claims. *Ann Intern Med* 145:488–96.

45. Schiff, G., et al. (2009). Diagnostic error in medicine: Analysis of 583 physician-reported errors. *Arch Intern Med* 169:1881–87.

46. Scott, I. (2009). Errors in clinical reasoning: Causes and remedial strategies. *BMJ* 339:22–25.

47. McAbee, G., et al. (2008). Medical diagnoses commonly associated with pediatric malpractice lawsuits in the United States. *Pediatrics* 122:e1282–86.

48. Kentsis, A., et al. (2009). Discovery and validation of urine markers of acute pediatric appendicitis using high-accuracy mass spectrometry. *Ann Emerg Med* June 25. [Epub ahead of print.]

49. Over-diagnosed diseases, at http://www.wrongdiagnosis.com/intro/overdiag.htm (accessed November 6, 2009).

50. Ciatto, S., et al. (2000). Prostate cancer screening: The problem of overdiagnosis and lessons to be learned from breast cancer screening. *Eur J Cancer* 36:1347–50.

Zappa, M., et al. (1998). Overdiagnosis of prostate carcinoma by screening: An estimate based on the results of the Florence Screening Pilot Study. *Ann Oncol* 9:1297–1300.

51. Andriole, G. et al. (2009) Mortality results from a randomized prostate-cancer screening trial. *N Engl J Med*, 360:1310–19.

52. Sandblom, G., et al. (2011). Randomised prostate cancer screening trial: 20 year follow-up. *BMJ* 342:d1539.

53. Jørgensen, K., & Gøtzsche, P. (2009). Overdiagnosis in publicly organised mammography screening programmes: Systematic review of incidence trends. *BMJ* 339:206–209.

54. In November 2009, a panel of experts appointed by the Department of Health and Human Services announced revised guidelines for breast cancer screening. The panel recommended that, except for a small group of women with unusual risk factors, women start regular breast cancer screening at age fifty. Just seven years ago, the same group, with different members, urged women to have mammograms starting at age forty. The new panel also recommended that women of age fifty to seventy-four should have mammograms every two years rather than every year and that doctors should stop teaching women to examine their breasts on a regular basis (http://topics.nytimes.com/top/reference/timestopics/organizations/p/preventive_services_task_force/index.html?scp=2&sq=MAMMOGRAM&st=cse (accessed November 10, 2010).

55. Welch, H., & Black, W. (2010). Overdiagnosis in cancer. *J Natl Cancer Inst* 102:605–13.

56. Smith-Bindman, R., et al. (2009). Radiation dose associated with common computed tomography examinations and the associated lifetime attributable risk of cancer. *Arch Intern Med* 169:2078–86.

57. Berrington de González, A., et al. (2009). Projected cancer risks from computed tomographic scans performed in the United States in 2007. *Arch Intern Med* 169:2071–77.

58. Epstein, S., et al. (2001). Dangers and unreliability of mammography: Breast examination is a safe, effective, and practical alternative. *Int J Health Services* 31:605–15.

59. Croskerry, P. (2002). Achieving quality in clinical decision making: Cognitive strategies and detection of bias. *Acad Emerg Med* 9:1184–1204.

60. Under-Diagnosed Diseases, at http://www.wrongdiagnosis.com/intro/underdiag .htm (accessed November 6, 2009).

61. Pope, H., et al. (2000). Missed diagnoses of acute cardiac ischemia in the emergency department. *N Engl J Med* 342:1163–70.

62. Ely, J., et al. (1995). Perceived causes of family physicians' errors. *J Fam Pract* 40:337–44.

63. Vickers, A., et al. (2008). Against diagnosis. *Ann Intern Med* 149:200–203.

64. Patrick, G. (2009). Risk prediction versus diagnosis: Preserving clinical nuance in a binary world. *Ann Intern Med* 150:223.

CHAPTER 6: REDUCING DIAGNOSTIC ERRORS

1. Graber, M. (2008). Taking steps towards a safer future: Measures to promote timely and accurate medical diagnosis. *Am J Med* 121:S43–S46.

2. Berlin, L. (2007). Accuracy of diagnostic procedures: Has it improved over the past five decades? *Am J Roentgenol* 188:1173–78.

Kirch, W., & Schafii, C. (1996) Misdiagnosis at a university hospital in 4 medical eras. *Medicine (Baltimore)* 75:29–40.

3. Shojania, K., et al. (2003). Changes in rates of autopsy-detected diagnostic errors over time: A systematic review. *JAMA* 289:2849–56.

4. Fredrickson, B. (1998). What good are positive emotions? *Review of General Psychology* 2:300–319.

5. Graber, M., et al. (2002). Reducing diagnostic errors in medicine: What's the goal? *Acad Med* 77:981–92; Graber, M., et al. (2005). Diagnostic error in internal medicine. *Arch Intern Med* 165:1493–99.

6. Gandhi, T., et al. (2000). Communication breakdown in the outpatient referral process. *J Gen Intern Med* 15:626–31.

7. Smith-Bindman , R., et al. (2003). Comparison of screening mammography in the United States and the United Kingdom. *JAMA* 290:2129–37.

8. Groopman, J. (2007, March 19). The mistakes doctors make: Errors in thinking too often lead to wrong diagnoses. *Boston Globe*, at http://www.boston.com/news/globe/ health_science/articles/2007/03/19/the_mistakes_doctors_make (accessed December 10, 2009).

9. Berner, E., & Graber, M. (2008). Overconfidence as a cause of diagnostic error in medicine. *Am J Med* 121(5A): S2–S23.

10. Podbregar, M., et al. (2001). Should we confirm our clinical diagnostic certainty by autopsies? *Intensive Care Med* 27:1750–55.

11. Landefeld, C., et al. (1988). Diagnostic yield of the autopsy in a university hospital and a community hospital. *N Engl J Med* 318:1249–54.

12. Potchen, E. (2006). Measuring observer performance in chest radiology: Some experiences. *J Am Coll Radiol* 3:423–32.

13. Hodges, B., et al. (2001). Difficulties in recognizing one's own incompetence: Novice physicians who are unskilled and unaware of it. *Academic Medicine* 76 (suppl): S87–S89.

14. Davis, D., et al. (2006). Accuracy of physician self-assessment compared with observed measures of competence: A systematic review. *JAMA* 296:1094–1102.

15. Friedman, C., et al. (2005). Do physicians know when their diagnoses are correct? Implications for decision support and error reduction. *J Gen Intern Med* 20:334–39.

16. Baumann, A., et al. (1991). Overconfidence among physicians and nurses: The "micro-certainty, macro-uncertainty" phenomenon. *Social Science & Medicine* 32:167–74.

17. Croskerry, P., & Norman, G. (2008). Overconfidence in clinical decision making. *Am J Med* 121 (5A): 524–29.

18. Sanders, L. (2009). *Every patient tells a story*. New York: Broadway Books.

19. Trowbridge, R. (2008). Twelve tips for teaching avoidance of diagnostic errors. *Medical Teacher* 30: 496–500.

20. Chapman, G., et al. (1996). Order of information affects clinical judgment. *J Behavioral Decision Making* 9:201–11.

21. Bergus, G., et al. (1995). Clinical reasoning about new symptoms despite pre-existing disease: Sources of error and order effects. *Fam Med* 27:314–20.

22. Cunnington, J., et al. (1997). The effect of presentation order in clinical decision making. *Academic Medicine* 72 (Suppl. 10): 40–42.

23. Barrows, H., et al. (1982). The clinical reasoning of randomly selected physicians in general medical practice. *Clin Invest Med* 5:49–55; Dawson, N. (1993). Physician judgment in clinical settings: Methodological influences and cognitive performance. *Clin Chem* 39:1468–78.

24. Strohmer, D., et al. (1990). Information processing strategies in counselor hypothesis testing: The role of selective memory and expectancy. *J Counseling Psychology* 37:465–72.

25. Eva, K., & Cunnington, J. (2006). The difficulty with experience: Does practice increase susceptibility to premature closure? *J Continuing Education in the Health Professions* 26:192–98.

26. Poses, R., et al. (1990). What difference do two days make? The inertia of physicians' sequential prognostic judgments for critically ill patients. *Med Decis Making* 10:6–14.

27. Kronz, J., et al. (1999). Mandatory second opinion surgical pathology at a large referral hospital. *Cancer* 86:2426–35.

28. Landrigan, C., et al. (2004). Effect of reducing interns' work hours on serious medical errors in intensive care units. *N Engl J Med* 351:1838–48.

29. Scott, I. (2009). Errors in clinical reasoning: Causes and remedial strategies. *BMJ* 339:22-25.

30. Bordage, G. (1995). Where are the history and the physical? *Can Med Assoc J* 152:1595-98.

31. Ramani, S. (2004). Promoting the art of history taking. *Medical Teacher* 26:374-76.

32. Peterson, M., et al. (1992). Contributions of the history, physical examination, and laboratory investigation in making medical diagnoses. *West J Med* 156:163-65.

33. Ghandi, T., et al. (2006). Missed and delayed diagnoses in the ambulatory setting: A study of closed malpractice claims. *Ann Intern Med* 145:488-96.

34. Sanders, L. (2009). *Every patient tells a story*. New York: Broadway Books.

35. Stillman, P., et al. (1991). Assessment of clinical skills of residents utilizing standardized patients. *Ann Intern Med* 114:393-401.

36. Mangione, S. (2001). Cardiac auscultatory skills of physicians-in-training: A comparison of three English-speaking countries. *Am J Med* 110:210-16; Smith, C. (2006). Teaching cardiac examination skills: A controlled trial of two methods. *J Gen Intern Med* 21:1-6; Criley, J., et al. (2008). Innovative web-based multimedia curriculum improves cardiac examination competency of residents. *J Hospital Medicine* 3:124-33; Favrat, B., et al. (2004). Teaching cardiac auscultation to trainees in internal medicine and family practice: Does it work? *BMC Med* 4:5.

37. Elstein, A., et al. (1978). *Medical problem solving: An analysis of clinical reasoning*. Cambridge, Mass.: Harvard University Press.

38. Yudkowsky, R., et al. (2009). A hypothesis-driven physical examination learning and assessment procedure for medical students: Initial validity evidence. *Medical Education* 43:729-40.

39. Schiff, G. (2008). Minimizing diagnostic error: The importance of follow-up and feedback. *Am J Med* 121 (5A): S38-S42.

40. Arzy, S., et al. (2009). Misleading one detail: A preventable mode of diagnostic error? *Journal of Evaluation in Clinical Practice* 15:804-6.

41. Ramnarayan, P., et al. (2006). Assessment of the potential impact of a reminder system on the reduction of diagnostic error: A quasi-experimental study. *BMC Medical Informatics and Decision Making* 6:6-22.

42. Tang, H., & Ng, J. (2006). Googling for a diagnosis—use of Google as a diagnostic aid: Internet-based study. *BMJ* 333:1143-45.

43. Three free DSS websites that were available as of November 12, 2009, are http://www.wrongdiagnosis.com/checklist.htm; http://symptoms.webmd.com/default.htm; and http://en.diagnosispro.com/.

44. Tsai, T., et al. (2003). Computer decision support as a source of interpretation error: The case of electrocardiograms. *J Am Med Inform Assoc* 10:478-83.

45. Innocent, P., & John, R. (2004). Computer-aided fuzzy medical diagnosis. *Information Sciences* 162:81-104.

46. Croskerry, P. (2005). The theory and practice of clinical decision-making. *Canadian Journal of Anesthesia* 52:R1.

47. Ericsson, K. (2004). Deliberate practice and the acquisition and maintenance of expert performance in medicine and related domains. *Academic Medicine* 10:S1-S12;

Ericsson, K., & Lehmann, A. (1996). Expert and exceptional performance: Evidence on maximal adaptations on task constraints. *Annual Review of Psychology* 47:273–305; Ericsson, K. (2006). The influence of experience and deliberate practice on the development of superior expert performance. In K. Ericsson et al. (eds.), *Cambridge handbook of expertise and expert performance* (pp. 685–706). Cambridge: Cambridge University Press.

48. McDaniel, M., et al. (1988). Job experience correlates of job performance. *J Applied Psychology* 73:327–30.

49. *Sports Illustrated*, October 26, 2009, pp. 72–77.

50. Graber, M. (2007). Perspective, at http://webmm.ahrq.gov/perspective .aspx?perspectiveID=36.

51. Bond, W., et al. (2004). Using simulation to instruct emergency medicine residents in cognitive forcing strategies. *Academic Medicine* 79:438–46.

52. Two simulation sites as of November 10, 2009, are http://www.healthcarefree ware.com/diag_aid.htm and http://www.medicalsimulations.com/.

53. Eddy, D. (1982). Probabilistic reasoning in clinical medicine: Problems and opportunities. In D. Kahneman et al. (eds.), *Judgment under uncertainty: Heuristics and biases* (pp. 249–67). Cambridge: Cambridge University Press.

54. Gigerenzer, G., & Hoffrage, U. (1995). How to improve Bayesian reasoning without instruction: Frequency formats. *Psychological Review* 102:684–704.

55. Sedlmeier, P., & Gigerenzer, G. (2001). Teaching Bayesian reasoning in less than two hours. *J Experimental Psychology: General* 130:380–400.

56. Galesic, M., et al. (2009). Natural frequencies help older adults and people with low numeracy to evaluate medical screening tests. *Med Decis Making* 29:368–71.

57. Andereck, W. (2009, November 15). Docs missing the diagnosis. *San Francisco Chronicle*, p. E8.

58. Richardson, W., et al. (2003). Could our pretest probabilities become evidence based? A prospective survey of hospital practice. *J Gen Intern Med* 18:203–8.

59. Green, L., & Yates, F. (1995). Influence of pseudodiagnostic information on the evaluation of ischemic heart disease. *Annals of Emergency Medicine* 25:451–57.

60. Croswell, J., et al. (2009). Cumulative incidence of false-positive results in repeated, multimodal cancer screening. *Ann Fam Med* 7:212–22.

61. Likelihood ratios, at http://www.mclibrary.duke.edu/subject/ebm/ratios.html.

62. The website http://www.medicine.ox.ac.uk/bandolier/booth/diagnos/Liketab .html lists likelihood ratios for many different tests and medical conditions (accessed October 26, 2009).

CHAPTER 7: PRESCRIPTION FOR PRESCRIBING

1. Cherry, D., et al. (2008). National Ambulatory Medical Care Survey: 2006 summary. *National health statistics reports*, no 3. Hyattsville, Md.: National Center for Health Statistics.

2. Wilson, D. (2009, March 3). Harvard medical school in ethics quandary, at http://www.nytimes.com/2009/03/03/business/03medschool.html?_r=1&emc=etal.

3. AMSA executive summary, updated June 16, 2009, at http://www.amsascorecard.org/executive-summary (accessed on November 10, 2010).

4. Campbell, E., et al. (2007). Institutional academic-industry relationships. *JAMA* 298:1779–86.

5. Cohen, J., & Insel, P. (1996). The Physicians' Desk Reference: Problems and possible improvements. *Arch Intern Med* 156:1375–80.

6. Cohen, J. (2001). Dose discrepancies between the Physicians' Desk Reference and the medical literature, and their possible role in the high incidence of dose-related adverse drug events. *Arch Intern Med* 161:957–64.

7. Mullen, W., et al. (1997). Incorrect overdose management advice in the Physicians' Desk Reference. *Annals of Emergency Medicine* 29:255–61.

8. Harris, G., & Roberts, J. (2007, March 21). Doctors' ties to drug makers are put on close view, at http://www.nytimes.com/2007/03/21/us/21drug.html?_r=4&pagewanted=1&ref=us&oref=slogin (accessed May 5, 2010).

9. Sigworth S., et al. (2001). Pharmaceutical branding of resident physicians. *JAMA* 286:1024–25.

10. Landers, S. Industry support of CME under scrutiny, at http://www.ama-assn.org/amednews/2010/03/08/prsd0310.htm (accessed May 1, 2010).

11. Davis, D. (2004). CME and the pharmaceutical industry: Two worlds, three views, four steps. *Can Med Assoc J* 171:149–50.

12. Fuller Torrey, E. (2002). The going rate on shrinks: Big pharma and the buying of psychiatry, at http://www.schizoaffective.org/torrey.htm (accessed May 3, 2010).

13. Abassi, K., & Smith, R. (2003). No more free lunches. *BMJ* 326:1155–56.

14. Villanueva, P., et al. (2003). Accuracy of pharmaceutical advertisements in medical journals. *Lancet* 361:27–32.

15. Santiago, M., et al. (2008). Accuracy of drug advertisements in medical journals under new law regulating the marketing of pharmaceutical products in Switzerland. *BMC Medical Informatics and Decision Making* 8:61.

16. Othman, N., et al. (2009). Quality of pharmaceutical advertisements in medical journals: A systematic review. *PLoS One* (July 22), 4(7):e6350.

17. Avorn, J., et al. (1982). Scientific versus commercial sources of influence on the prescribing behavior of physicians. *Am J Med* 73:4–8.

18. Matalia, N. (1994). Journal advertising works! Three studies say so! *Medical Marketing and Media* 5:12.

19. Moynihan, R. (2008). Key opinion leaders: Independent experts or drug representatives in disguise? *BMJ* 336:1402–3.

20. Harris, G., & Roberts, J. (2007, March 21). Doctors' ties to drug makers are put on close view, at http://www.nytimes.com/2007/03/21/us/21drug.html?_r=4&pagewanted=1&ref=us&oref=slogin (accessed May 5, 2010).

21. Editorial. Expert or shill? At http://www.nytimes.com/2008/11/30/opinion/30sun2.html (accessed May 4, 2010).

22. Harris, G. (2008, November 22). Radio host has drug company ties, at http://www.nytimes.com/2008/11/22/health/22radio.html (accessed May 4, 2010).

23. UE News. (1999, November). Say it ain't so, Everett! at http://www.ranknfile-ue.org/h&s1199.html (accessed May 4, 2010).

24. Exposing WHO influenza advisers: They're paid by the pharmaceutical industry, at http://preventdisease.com/news/09/111909_WHO_on_big_pharma_payroll.shtml (accessed May 4, 2010).

25. Cited in Millard, W. (2007). Docking the tail that wags the dog: Banning drug reps from academic medical facilities. *Annals News & Perspective* 49:785–91.

26. Wazana, W. (2000). Physicians and the pharmaceutical industry: Is a gift ever just a gift? *JAMA* 283:373–80.

27. Radley, D., et al. (2006). Off-label prescribing among office-based physicians. *Arch Intern Med* 166:1021–26.

28. Walton, S., et al. (2008). Prioritizing future research on off-label prescribing: Results of a quantitative evaluation. *Pharmacotherapy* 28:1443–52.

29. Steinman, M., et al. (2007). Characteristics and impact of drug detailing for gabapentin. *PLoS Med* 4:e134. DOI:10.1371/journal.pmed.0040134.

30. Return on Investment (ROI) of the four major promotional tactics (detailing, DTC advertising, medical journal advertising, and physician meetings & events). The study was first presented to the industry on May 22, 2001, by Scott Neslin, http://rxpromoroi.org/rapp/exec_sum.html (accessed May 5, 2010).

31. Cauchon, D. (2000, September 25). FDA advisers tied to industry. *USA Today*, p. A:1.

32. Lurie, P., et al. (2006). Financial conflict of interest disclosure and voting patterns at Food and Drug Administration drug advisory committee meetings. *JAMA* 295:1921–28.

33. Bekelman, J., et al. (2003). Scope and impact of financial conflicts of interest in biomedical research: A systematic review. *JAMA* 289:454–65.

34. Lurie, P., & Wolfe, S. (1998, December 30). Troubling climate at FDA. *Washington Post*, p. A19.

35. Klein, E. When you can't trust drug companies, who can you trust? at http://www.prospect.org/csnc/blogs/ezraklein_archive?month=01&year=2009&base_name=when_you_cant_trust_drug_compa (accessed May 4, 2010).

36. Harris, G., & Roberts, J. (2007, March 21). Doctors' ties to drug makers are put on close view, at http://www.nytimes.com/2007/03/21/us/21drug.html?_r=4&pagewanted=1&ref=us&oref=slogin (accessed May 5, 2010).

37. Grindrod, K., et al. (2006). What interventions should pharmacists employ to impact health practitioners' prescribing practices? *Annals of Pharmacotherapy* 40:1546–57.

38. Ostini, R., et al. (2009). Systematic review of interventions to improve prescribing. *Annals of Pharmacotherapy* 43:502–13.

39. Jamtvedt, G., et al. *The Cochrane Library*. Oxford: Update Software, 2004. Audit and feedback: Effects on professional practice and health care outcomes.

40. Jamtvedt, G., et al. (2007). Audit and feedback: Effects on professional practice and health care outcomes (Review). The Cochrane Collaboration.

41. The comparisons with placebo are often unfair because people who have been unsuccessful with an earlier drug of the same class are typically dismissed from studies. The reason is that they will probably do no better with the new drug.

42. U.S. Food and Drug Administration Center for Drug Evaluation and Research, Department of Health and Human Services. (2004, January 21). *NDAs approved in calendar years 1990–2003 by therapeutic potentials and chemical types.*

43. Alexander, G., et al. (2009). Does comparative effectiveness have a comparative edge? *JAMA* 301:2488–90.

44. Hochman, M., & McCormick, D. In defense of comparative effectiveness research, at http://www.huffingtonpost.com/michael-hochman/in-defense-of-comparative_b_564678.html (accessed May 7, 2010).

45. Frosch, D., & Grande, D. (2010). Direct-to-consumer advertising of prescription drugs. *Leonard Davis Institute of Health Economics* 15(3) (March/April).

46. Mintzes, B., et al. (2003). How does direct-to-consumer advertising (DTCA) affect prescribing? A survey in primary care environments with and without legal DTCA. *Can Med Assoc J* 169:405–12.

47. Frosch, D., et al. (2007). Creating demand for prescription drugs: A content analysis of television direct-to-consumer advertising. *Ann Fam Med* 5:6–13.

48. Abel, G., et al. (2008). Direct-to-consumer advertising for bleeding disorders: A content analysis and expert evaluation of advertising claims. *J Thromb Haemost* 6:1680–84.

49. Kusuma, S., et al. (2007). DTCA: Improving patient education or simply increasing pharmaceutical profits? American Academy of Orthopaedic Surgeons, at http://www.aaos.org/news/bulletin/dec07/reimbursement1.asp.

CHAPTER 8: EXPECTATION EFFECTS

1. Leavitt, F. (2003). *Evaluating scientific research.* Long Grove, Ill.: Waveland Press.

2. Plassmann, H., et al. (2008). Marketing actions can modulate neural representations of experienced utility. *Proc National Academy of Sciences* 105:1050–54.

3. Rosenthal, R., & Jacobson, L. (1968). *Pygmalion in the classroom.* New York: Holt, Rinehart & Winston.

4. Stone, J., et al. (1997). White men can't jump: Evidence for the perceptual confirmation of racial stereotypes following a basketball game. *Basic and Applied Social Psychology* 19:291–306.

5. Noseworthy, J., et al. (1994). The impact of blinding on the results of a randomized, placebo-controlled multiple sclerosis clinical trial. *Neurology* 44:16–20.

6. Psychologists explain. *ScienceDaily.* Retrieved on April 29, 2008, from http://www.sciencedaily.com/releases/2008/04/080421191418.htm.

7. Steele, C. (1999). Thin ice: Stereotype threat and black college students. Retrieved on July 5, 2009, from http://www.theatlantic.com/doc/199908/student-stereotype.

8. Shih, M., et al. (1999). Stereotype susceptibility: Identity salience and shifts in quantitative performance. *Psychological Science* 10:80–83.

9. Mondloch, M., et al. (2001). Does how you do depend on how you think you'll do? A systematic review of the evidence for a relation between patients' recovery expectations and health outcomes. *Can Med Assoc J* 165:174–79.

10. Southworth, S., & Kirsch, I. (1988). The role of expectancy in exposure-generated fear reduction in agoraphobia. *Behaviour Research and Therapy* 26:113–20; Weinberger, J., & Eig, A. (1999). Expectancies: The ignored common factor in psychotherapy. In I. Kirsch (ed.), *How expectancies shape experience* (pp. 357–382). Washington, D.C.: American Psychological Association; Elkin, I. (1994). The NIMH treatment of depression collaborative research program: Where we began and where we are. In A. Gergin & S. Garfield (eds.), *Handbook of psychotherapy and behavior change* (4th ed.), (pp. 114–49). New York: Wiley; Sotsky, S., et al. (2001). Nonspecific, unintended, and serendipitous effects in psychotherapy. *Professional Psychology: Research and Practice* 32:283–88.

11. Desharnais, R., et al. (1993). Aerobic exercise and the placebo effect: A controlled study. *Psychosom Med* 55:149–54.

12. Levy, B., & Langer, E. (1994). Aging free from negative stereotypes: Successful memory among the American deaf and in mainland China. *J Personality and Social Psychology* 66:935–43.

13. Sievert, L., et al. (2007). Symptom groupings at midlife: Cross-cultural variation and association with job, home, and life change. *Menopause* 14:798–807; Lock, M. (1998). Menopause: Lessons from anthropology. *Psychosom Med* 60:410–19.

14. Talbot, M. (2000, January 9). The placebo prescription. *New York Times Magazine*.

15. Carroll, L., et al. (2009). Recovery in whiplash-associated disorders: Do you get what you expect? *J Rheumatol* 36:1063–70; Ozegovic, D., et al. (2009). Does expecting mean achieving? The association between expecting to return to work and recovery in whiplash associated disorders: A population-based prospective cohort study. *Eur Spine J* 18:893–99.

16. Mahomed, N., et al. (2002). The importance of patient expectations in predicting functional outcomes after total joint arthroplasty. *J Rheumatol* 29:1273–79.

17. Yee, A., et al. (2008). Do patient expectations of spinal surgery relate to functional outcome? *Clin Orthop Relat Res* 466:1154–61.

18. Bausel, R., et al. (2005). Is acupuncture analgesia an expectancy effect? Preliminary evidence based on participants' perceived assignments in two placebo-controlled trials. *Eval Health Prof* 28:9–26.

19. Jones, T. (2000). Mass psychogenic illness: Role of the individual physician. *Am Fam Physician* 62:2649–53, 2655–6.

20. Lorber, W., et al. (2007). Illness by suggestion: Expectancy, modeling, and gender in the production of psychosomatic symptoms. *Annals of Behavioral Medicine* 33:112–16.

21. Voelker, R. (1996). Nocebos contribute to host of ills. *JAMA* 275:345–47.

22. Sternberg, E. (2002). Walter B. Cannon and "voodoo death": A perspective from 60 years on. *Am J Public Health* 92:1564–66.

23. Shapiro, A., & Shapiro, E. (1999). The placebo: Is it much ado about nothing? In A. Harrington (ed.), *The placebo effect*. Cambridge, Mass.: Harvard University Press.

24. Beecher, H. (1955). The powerful placebo. *JAMA* 159:1602–6.

25. Levine, J., et al. (1979). The mechanism of placebo analgesia. *Lancet* 2:654–7.

26. Benedetti, F. (1996). The opposite effects of the opiate antagonist naloxone and the cholecystokinin antagonist proglumide on placebo analgesia. *Pain* 64:535–43.

27. Petrovic, P., et al. (2002). Placebo and opioid analgesia—Imaging a shared neuronal network. *Science* 295:1737–40.

28. Enck, S., & Klosterhalfen, S. (2005). The placebo response in functional bowel disorders: Perspectives and putative mechanisms. *Neurogastroenterol Motil* 17:325–31.

29. Sysko, R., & Walsh, B. (2007). A systematic review of placebo response in studies of bipolar mania. *J Clin Psychiatry* 68:1213–17.

30. Macedo, A., et al. (2008). Placebo response in the prophylaxis of migraine: A meta-analysis. *Eur J Pain* 12:68–75.

31. Shapiro, A., & Shapiro, E. (1997). The placebo: Is it much ado about nothing? In A. Harrington (ed.), *The placebo effect*. Cambridge, Mass.: Harvard University Press.

32. Hoffman, G., et al. (2005). Pain and the placebo: What we have learned. *Perspectives in Biology and Medicine* 48:248–65.

33. Khan, A., et al. (2008). The persistence of the placebo response in antidepressant clinical trials. *J Psychiatric Research* 42:791–96.

34. Shiv, B., et al. (2005). Placebo effects of marketing actions: Consumers may get what they pay for. *J Marketing Research* 42:383–93.

35. Waber, R., et al. (2008). Commercial features of placebo and therapeutic efficacy. *JAMA* 299:1016–17.

36. Marlatt, G., & Rohsenow, D. (1981). The think-drink effect. *Psychology Today* 15:60–93.

37. Colagiuri, B., et al. (2009). Expectancy in double-blind placebo-controlled trials: An example from alcohol dependence. *Psychotherapy and Psychosomatics* 78:167–71.

38. Dar, R., et al. (2005). Assigned versus perceived placebo effects in nicotine replacement therapy for smoking reduction in Swiss smokers. *J Consult Clin Psychol* 73:350–53.

39. Volkow, N., et al. 2003. Expectation enhances the regional brain metabolic and the reinforcing effects of stimulants in cocaine abusers. *J Neurosci* 23:11461–68.

40. Luparello, T., et al. (1968). Influences of suggestion on airway reactivity in asthmatic subjects. *Psychosom Med* 30:819–25.

41. Eccles, R. (2007). The power of the placebo. *Curr Allergy Asthma Rep* 7:100–104.

42. BBC News. (1999, July 5). Placebo effect shocks allergy drugs maker.

43. Broadhurst, P. (1977). Pharmacogenetics. In L. Iverson et al. (eds.), *Handbook of psychopharmacology*, vol. 7. New York: Plenum.

44. Blackwell, B., et al. (1972). Demonstration to medical students of placebo responses and non-drug factors. *Lancet* 1:1279–82.

45. Scott, D., et al. (2007). Individual differences in reward responding explain placebo-induced expectations and effects. *Neuron* 55:325–36.

46. Archer, T., & Leier, C. (1992). Placebo treatment in congestive heart failure. *Cardiology* 81:125–33.

47. McRae, C., et al. (2004). Effects of perceived treatment on quality of life and medical outcomes in a double-blind placebo surgery trial. *Arch Gen Psychiatry* 61:412–20.

48. De la Fuente-Fernandez, R., et al. (2001). Expectation and dopamine release: Mechanism of the placebo effect in Parkinson's disease. *Science* 293:1164–66; Benedetti, F., et al. (2004). Placebo-responsive Parkinson patients show decreased activity in single neurons of subthalamic nucleus. *Nat Neurosci* 7:587–88.

49. Benedetti, F., et al. (2007). Opioid-mediated placebo responses boost pain endurance and physical performance: Is it doping in sport competitions? *J Neurosci* 27:11934–39.

50. Moncrieff, J., et al. (1998). Meta-analysis of trials comparing antidepressants with active placebos. *British J Psychiatry* 172:227–31.

51. Herrnstein, R. (1962). Placebo effect in the rat. *Science* 138:677–78.

52. Hróbjartsson, A., & Gøtzsche, P. (2001). Is the placebo powerless? An analysis of clinical trials comparing placebo with no treatment. *N Engl J Med* 344:1594–1602; Hróbjartsson, A., & Gøtzsche, P. (2004). Is the placebo powerless? Update of a systematic review with 52 new randomized trials comparing placebo with no treatment. *J Internal Medicine* 256:91–100.

53. Spiegel, D., et al. (2001). Is the placebo powerless? *N Engl J Med* 345:1276; Wampold, B., et al. (2007). The story of placebo effects in medicine: Evidence in context. *J Clinical Psychology* 63:379–90.

54. Humphrey, N. (2002). Great expectations: The evolutionary psychology of faith healing and the placebo response. In *The mind made flesh: Essays from the frontiers of psychology and evolution*. Oxford: Oxford University Press.

55. Breznitz, S. (1999). The effect of hope on pain tolerance. *Social Research* 66: 629–52.

56. Meagher, M., et al. (2001). Pain and emotion: Effects of affective picture modulation. *Psychosom Med* 63:79–90.

57. Cummings, N., & Vanden Bos, G. (1981). The twenty years Kaiser-Permanente experience with psychotherapy and medical utilization: Implications for national health policy and national insurance. *Health Policy Q* 1:59–75.

58. Kroenke, K., & Mangelsdorff, D. (1989). Common symptoms in ambulatory care: Incidence, evaluation, therapy, and outcome. *Am J Med* 86:262–66.

59. Shapiro, A., & Shapiro, E. (1999). The placebo: Is it much ado about nothing? In A. Harrington (ed.), *The placebo effect*. Cambridge, Mass.: Harvard University Press.

60. McKenzie, J. (1896). The production of the so-called 'rose-cold' by means of an artificial rose. *Am J Med Sci* 91:45.

61. Siegel, S. (2001). Pavlovian conditioning and drug overdose: When tolerance fails. *Addiction Research & Theory* 9:503–13.

62. Batterman, R., & Lower, W. (1968). Placebo responsiveness: Influence of previous therapy. *Curr Ther Res* 10:136–43.

63. Ader, R., & Cohen, N. (1975). Behaviorally conditioned immunosuppression. *Psychosom Med* 37:333–40.

64. Goebel, M., et al. (2002). Behavioral conditioning of immunosuppression is possible in humans. *FASEB Journal* 16:1869–73.

65. Olness, K., & Ader, R. (1992). Conditioning as an adjunct in the pharmacotherapy of lupus erythematosus: A case report. *J Developmental and Behavioral Pediatrics* 13:124–25.

66. Giang, D., et al. (1996). Conditioning of cyclophosphamide-induced leukopenia in humans. *J Neuropsychiatry Clin Neurosci* 8:194–201.

67. Colloca, L., & Benedetti, F. (2009). Placebo analgesia induced by social observational learning. *Pain* 144:28–34.

68. Walsh, B., et al. (2002). Placebo response in studies of major depression: Variable, substantial, and growing. *JAMA* 287:1840–47.

69. Kemp, A., et al. (2008). What is causing the reduced drug-placebo difference in recent schizophrenia clinical trials and what can be done about it? *Schizophrenia Bulletin*, at http://schizophreniabulletin.oxfordjournals.org/cgi/reprint/sbn110v1 (accessed October 12, 2009).

70. Montgomery, G., & Kirsch, I. (1977). Classical conditioning and the placebo effect. *Pain* 72:107–13.

71. Montgomery, G., & Kirsch, I. (1996). Mechanisms of placebo pain reduction: An empirical investigation. *Psychological Science* 7:174–76.

72. Benedetti, F., et al. (2005). Neurobiological mechanisms of the placebo effect. *J Neurosci* 25:10390–402.

73. Benedetti, F., et al. (2003). Conscious expectation and unconscious conditioning in analgesic, motor, and hormonal placebo/nocebo responses. *J Neurosci* 23:4315–23.

74. Moerman, D., & Jonas, W. (2002). Deconstructing the placebo effect and finding the meaning response. *Ann Intern Med* 136:471–76.

75. Whalley, B., et al. (2008). Consistency of the placebo effect. *J Psychosom Res* 64:537–41.

76. Klosterhalfen, S., & Enck, P. (2008). Neurophysiology and psychobiology of the placebo response. *Curr Opin Psychiatry* 21:189–95.

77. Nierenberg, A. (2003). Predictors of response to antidepressants: General principles and clinical implications. *Psychiat Clin North America* 26:345–52.

78. Schweinhardt, P., et al. (2009). The anatomy of the mesolimbic reward system: A link between personality and the placebo analgesic response. *J Neurosci* 15:4882–87.

79. Cited in Silberman, S. (2009, August 24). Placebos are getting more effective. Drugmakers are desperate to know why. *Wired Magazine*, at http://www.wired.com/medtech/drugs/magazine/17-09/ff_placebo_effect?currentpage=2 (accessed October 12, 2009).

80. Macedo, A., et al. (2008). Placebo response in the prophylaxis of migraine: A meta-analysis. *Eur J Pain* 12:68–75.

81. Moerman, D. (2001). Cultural variation in the placebo effect: Ulcers, anxiety, and blood pressure. *Medical Anthropology Quarterly* 14:51–72.

82. Walach, H., et al. (2005). The therapeutic effect of clinical trials: Understanding placebo response rates in clinical trials—A secondary analysis. *BMC Medical Research Methodology* 5:26.

83. A detailed account of neurobiological mechanisms is beyond the scope of this book. For anyone who wants to supplement this cursory review, the following readings are recommended:

Benedetti, F. (2008). Mechanisms of placebo and placebo-related effects across diseases and treatments. *Annu Rev Pharmacol Toxicol* 48:33–60.

Benedetti, F., et al. (2005). Neurobiological mechanisms of the placebo effect. *J Neurosci* 25:10390–402.

De la Fuente-Fernandez, R., et al. (2001). Expectation and dopamine release: Mechanism of the placebo effect in Parkinson's disease. *Science* 293:1164–66.

Mayberg, H., et al. (2002). The functional neuroanatomy of the placebo effect. *Am J Psychiatry* 159:728–37.

Petrovic, P., et al. (2002). Placebo and opioid analgesia—Imaging a shared neural network. *Science* 295:1737–40.

Price, D., et al. (2008). A comprehensive review of the placebo effect: Recent advances and current thought. *Annual Review of Psychology* 59:565–90.

Price, D., et al. (2007). Placebo analgesia is accompanied by large reductions in pain-related brain activity in irritable bowel syndrome patients. *Pain* 127:63–72.

Scott, D., et al. (2008). Placebo and nocebo effects are defined by opposite opioid and dopaminergic responses. *Arch Gen Psychiatry* 65:220–31.

Scott, D., et al. (2007). Individual differences in reward responding explain placebo-induced expectations and effects. *Neuron* 55:325–36.

Wager, T., et al. (2004). Placebo induced changes in fMRI in the anticipation and experience of pain. *Science* 303:1162–67.

Zubieta, J., et al. (2005). Placebo effects mediated by endogenous opioid activity on mu-opioid receptors. *J Neurosci* 25:7754–62.

84. Kong, J., et al. (2007). Placebo analgesia: Findings from brain imaging studies and emerging hypotheses. *Rev Neurosci* 18:173–90.

85. Lipman, J., et al. (1990). B endorphin concentration in cerebrospinal fluid: Reduced in chronic pain patients and increased during the placebo response. *Psychopharmacology* 102:112–16.

86. Colloca, L., & Benedetti, F. (2007). Nocebo hyperalgesia: How anxiety is turned into pain. *Curr Opin Anaesthesiol* 20:435–39.

87. Scott, D., et al. (2007). Individual differences in reward responding explain placebo-induced expectations and effects. *Neuron* 55:325–36.

88. Eippert, F., et al. (2009). Direct evidence for spinal cord involvement in placebo analgesia. *Science* 326:404.

89. Leuchter, A., et al. (2002). Changes in brain function of depressed subjects during treatment with placebo. *Am J Psychiatry* 159:122–29.

90. Petrovic, P., et al. (2005). Placebo in emotional processing—Induced expectations of anxiety relief activate a generalized modulatory network. *Neuron* 46:957–69.

91. Schweiger, A., et al. (1981). Nocebo: The psychologic induction of pain. *Biol Sci* 16:140–43.

92. Fielding, J., et al. (1983). An interim report of a prospective, randomized, controlled study of adjuvant chemotherapy in operable gastric cancer: British stomach cancer group. *World Journal of Surgery* 7:390–99.

93. Lynoe, N. (2005). Placebo is not always effective against nocebo bacilli. The body-mind interplay still wrapped in mystery. *Lakartidningen* 102:2627–28.

94. Rosenzweig, P., et al. (1993). The placebo effect in healthy volunteers: Influence of experimental conditions on the adverse events profile during phase 1 studies. *Clinical Pharmacology and Therapeutics* 54:578–83.

95. Wolf, S. (1962). Placebos: Problems and pitfalls. *Clinical Pharmacology and Therapeutics* 3:254–57.

96. Little, P., et al. (1999). Clinical and psychosocial predictors of illness duration from randomized controlled trial of prescribing strategies for sore throat. *BMJ* 319:736–37.

97. Di Blasi, Z., et al. (2001). Influence of context effects on health outcomes: A systematic review. *Lancet* 357:757–62.

98. Thomas, K. (1987). General practice consultations: Is there any point in being positive? *BMJ* 294:1200–1202.

99. Brown, W. (2006). Understanding and using the placebo effect. *Psychiatric Times* 23:15–17.

100. Crow, R., et al. (1999). The role of expectancies in the placebo effect and their use in the delivery of health care: A systematic review. *Health Technology Assessment* 3:1–96.

101. Baker, A., & Thorpe, J. (1957). Placebo response. *Arch Neurol Psychiatry* 78:57–60; Fisher, S., et al. (1964). Drug-set interaction: The effect of expectations on drug response in outpatients. *Neuropsychopharmacology* 3:149–56.

102. Gracely, R., et al. (1985). Clinicians' expectations influence placebo analgesia. *Lancet* 43:8419–23.

103. Cohen, P. (1996, January 27). Sugaring the pill. *New Scientist*.

104. Roberts, A., et al. (1993). The power of nonspecific effects in healing: Implications for psychosocial and biological treatments. *Clinical Psychology Review* 13:375–91.

105. Frank, J., & Frank, J. (1991). *Persuasion and healing: A comparative study of psychotherapy*. Baltimore: Johns Hopkins University Press.

106. Kaptchuk , T., et al. (2008). Components of placebo effect: Randomised controlled trial in patients with irritable bowel syndrome. *BMJ* 336:999–1003.

107. Rickels, K., et al. (1970). Pills and improvement: A study of placebo response in psychoneurotic outpatients. *Psychopharmacologia* 16:318–28.

108. Linde, K., et al. (2007). The impact of patient expectations on outcomes in four randomised controlled trials of acupuncture in patients with chronic pain. *Pain* 128:264–71.

109. Lutz, G., et al. (1999). The relation between expectations and outcomes in surgery for sciatica. *J Gen Intern Med* 12:740–44.

110. Kalauokalani, D., et al. (2001). Lessons from a trial of acupuncture and massage for low back pain: Patient expectations and treatment effects. *Spine* 26:1418–24.

111. Meade, T., et al. (1990). Low back pain of mechanical origin: Randomised comparison of chiropractic and hospital outpatient treatment. *BMJ* 300:1431–37.

112. Crum, A., & Langer, E. (2007). Mind-set matters: Exercise and the placebo effect. *Psychological Science* 18:165–71.

113. Levy, B., et al. (2006). Hearing decline predicted by elders' stereotypes. *J Gerontology: Psychological Sciences* 61:82–87; Levy, B. (2003). Mind matters: Cognitive and physical effects of aging self-stereotypes. *J Gerontology: Psychological Sciences* 58B:203–11; Levy, B., et al. (2002). Longevity increased by positive self-perceptions of aging. *J Personality and Social Psychology* 83:261–70.

114. Brody, H., & Waters, D. (1980). Diagnosis is treatment. *Journal of Family Practice* 10:445–49.

115. Sox, H., et al. (1981). Psychologically mediated effects of diagnostic tests. *Ann Intern Med* 95:680–85.

116. Petrie, K., et al. (2007). Effect of providing information about normal test results on patients' thereby making reassurance: Randomised controlled trial. *BMJ* 334:352.

117. Huibers, M., & Wessely, S. (2006). The act of diagnosis: Pros and cons of labelling chronic fatigue syndrome. *Psychological Medicine* 36:895–900.

118. Sawamoto, N., et al. (2000). Expectation of pain enhances responses to non-painful somatosensory stimulation in the anterior cingulate cortex and parietal operculum/posterior insula: An event-related functional magnetic resonance imaging study. *J Neurosci* 20:7438–45.

119. Keltner, J., et al. (2006). Isolating the modulatory effect of expectation on pain transmission: A functional magnetic resonance imaging study. *J Neurosci* 26:4437–43.

120. Amanzio, M., et al. (2001). Response variability to analgesics: A role for nonspecific activation of endogenous opioids. *Pain* 90:205–15; Benedetti, F., et al. (2003). Conscious expectation and unconscious conditioning in analgesic, motor, and hormonal placebo/nocebo responses. *J Neurosci* 23:4315–23; Colloca, L., et al. (2004). Overt versus covert treatment for pain, anxiety, and Parkinson's disease. *Lancet Neuro* 3:679–84.

121. Nitzan, U., & Lichtenberg, P. (2004). Questionnaire survey on use of placebo. *BMJ* 329:944–46.

122. Sherman, R., & Hickner, J. (2008). Academic physicians use placebos in clinical practice and believe in the mind–body connection. *J Gen Intern Med* 23:7–10.

123. Ernst, E., & Abbot, N. (1997). Placebos in clinical practice: Results of a survey of nurses. *Perfusion* 10:128–30.

124. Lichtenberg, P., et al. (2004). The ethics of the placebo in clinical practice. *J Med Ethics* 30:551–54.

125. Brown, W. (1998). The placebo effect. *Scientific American* 278:90–95.

126. Dunlop, D., et al. (1952). Survey of 17301 prescriptions on form EC10. *BMJ* 1:292–95.

127. Conboy, L., et al. (2006). Investigating placebo effects in irritable bowel syndrome: A novel research design. *Contemp Clin Trials* 27:123–34; Gruber, C. (1956). Interpreting medical data. *Arch Intern Med* 98:767–73.

128. Branthwaite, A., & Cooper, P. (1981). Analgesic effects of branding in treatment of headaches. *BMJ* 282:1576–78.

129. Buckalew, L., & Coffield, K. (1982). Drug expectations associated with perceptual characteristics: Ethnic factors. *Percept Mot Skills* 55:915–18.

130. Kaptchuk, T., et al. (2006). Sham device *v* inert pill: Randomised controlled trial of two placebo treatments. *BMJ* 332:391–97.

131. Ammirati, F., et al. (2001). Permanent cardiac pacing versus medical treatment for the prevention of recurrent vasovagal syncope: A multicenter, randomized, controlled trial. *Circulation* 104:52–57.

132. Barsky, A., et al. (2002). Nonspecific medication side effects and the nocebo phenomenon. *JAMA* 287:622–27.

133. Laska, E., & Sunshine, A. (1973). Anticipation of analgesia a placebo effect. *Headache* 13:1–11.

134. Benedetti, F., et al. (2003). Open versus hidden medical treatments: The patient's knowledge about a therapy affects the therapy outcome. *Prevention & Treatment* 6:Article 1.

135. Leuchter, A., et al. (2002). Changes in brain function of depressed subjects during treatment with placebo. *Am J Psychiatry* 159:122–29.

136. Chung, K., et al. (2007). Revelation of a personal placebo response: Its effects on mood, attitudes and future placebo responding. *Pain* 132:281–88.

137. Davison, G., et al. (1973). Attribution and the maintenance of behavior change in falling asleep. *J Abnormal Psychology* 82:124–33.

CHAPTER 9: COMPLEMENTARY AND ALTERNATIVE MEDICINE

1. Van Tulder, M., & Koes, B. (2006). Low back pain (chronic). *Clin Evid* 15:1634–53.

2. Ibid.

3. We made Dr. Jones a man for two reasons: first, most doctors are male, and second, male doctors tend to have more challenges with the interpersonal aspects of medical care than female doctors do. Mary Brown is a woman for similarly representative reasons: more women than men use CAM.

4. Chen, L., et al. (2009). Primary care visit duration and quality: Does good care take longer? *Arch Intern Med* 169:1866–72.

5. The National Center for Complementary and Alternative Medicine (NCCAM) is the federal government agency for scientific research on CAM, available online at http://nccam.nih.gov/health/whatiscam/.

6. NCCAM. (2008, December 10). According to a new government survey, 38 percent of adults and 12 percent of children use CAM, http://nccam.nih.gov/news/2008/121990.htm.

7. It is because women and people with higher education levels use CAM more that we made Mary a woman and a lawyer. The greater use by people with higher education levels may be because such people are more likely to question the authority of conventional medical practitioners and, if they are ill, to research alternative forms of treatment and/or because they have more money to spend on alternative medicine.

8. Barnes, P., et al. (2008). Complementary and alternative medicine use among adults and children: United States, 2007. National health statistics reports no. 12. Hyattsville, Md.: National Center for Health Statistics.

9. Vincent, C., & Furnham, A. (1996). Why do patients turn to complementary medicine? An empirical study. *Br J Clin Psychol* 35:37–48.

10. McGregor, K., & Peay, E. (1996). The choice of alternative therapy for healthcare: Testing some propositions. *Soc Sci Med* 43:1317–27.

11. Starfield, B. (2000). Is US health really the best in the world? *JAMA* 284:483–85.

12. Barnes et al. (2008), Complementary and alternative medicine use.

13. Furlan, A., et al. (2005). Acupuncture and dry-needling for low back pain. Cochrane Database of Systematic Reviews 2005, Issue 1. Art. No.: CD001351.

14. Cherkin, D., et al. (2009). A randomized trial comparing acupuncture, simulated acupuncture, and usual care for chronic low back pain. *Arch Intern Med* 169:858–66.

15. See, for example, Hilsden, R., et al. (2003). Complementary and alternative medicine use by Canadian patients with inflammatory bowel disease: Results from a national survey. *Am J Gastroenterol* 98:1563–68; Singh, H., et al. (2005). Understanding the motivation for conventional and complementary/alternative medicine use among men with prostate cancer. *Integr Cancer Ther* 4:187–94; Dillard, J., & Knapp, S. (2005). Complementary and alternative therapy in the emergency department. *Emerg Med Clin North Am* 23:529–49; Sirois, F. (2008). Motivations for consulting complementary and alternative medicine practitioners: A comparison of consumers from 1997–8 and 2005. *BMC Complement Altern Med* 8:16.

16. See, for example, Shih, V., et al. (2009). Complementary and alternative medicine (CAM) usage in Singaporean adult cancer patients. *Ann Oncol* 20:752–57; Langhorst, J., et al. (2007). Patterns of complementary and alternative medicine use in patients with inflammatory bowel disease: Perceived stress is a potential indicator for CAM use. *Complementary Therapies in Medicine* 15:30–37; Mak, J., & Faux, S. (2010). Complementary and alternative medicine use by osteoporotic patients in Australia: A prospective study. *J Altern Complement Med* 16:579–84; Sirois (2008), Motivations for consulting.

17. Sirois (2008), Motivations for consulting.

18. Astin, J. (1998). Why patients use alternative medicine: Results of a national survey. *JAMA* 279:1548–53. It is to represent this alignment with other values such as

environmentalism that we had our hypothetical patient work at the National Resources Defense Fund.

19. See, for example, Jean, D., & Cyr, C. (2007). Use of complementary and alternative medicine in a general pediatric clinic. *Pediatrics* 120:138–41; Wu, P., et al. (2007). Use of complementary and alternative medicine among women with depression: Results of a national survey. *Psychiatric Services* 58:349–56.

20. Astin (1998), Why patients use alternative medicine.

21. Robinson, A., & McGrail, M. (2004). Disclosure of CAM use to medical practitioners: A review of qualitative and quantitative studies. *Complementary Therapies in Medicine* 12:90–98; Richardson, M., et al. (2004). Discrepant views of oncologists and cancer patients on complementary/alternative medicine. *Support Care Cancer* 12:797–804.

22. Corbin Winslow, L., & Shapiro, H. (2002). Physicians want education about complementary and alternative medicine to enhance communication with their patients. *Arch Intern Med* 162:1176–81.

23. Milden, S., & Stokols, D. (2004). Physicians' attitudes and practices regarding complementary and alternative medicine. *Behavioral Medicine* 30:73–82.

24. Vickers, A., & Cassileth, B. (2006). Principles of complementary and alternative medicine for cancer. *Oncology*, 194–203.

25. Ruggio, M., & DeSantis, L. (2009). Complementary and alternative medicine: Longstanding legal obstacles to cutting edge treatment. *J Health & Life Sci L* 2:139–170.

26. Kaptchuk, T. (2002). The placebo effect in alternative medicine: Can the performance of healing ritual have clinical significance? *Ann Intern Med* 136:817–25.

27. Singh, S., & Ernst, E. (2008). *Trick or treatment: The undeniable facts about alternative medicine*. New York, London: Norton, at p. 245.

28. NCCAM, at http://nccam.nih.gov/health/whatiscam/#mindbody.

29. **Deep breathing**: NCCAM defines deep breathing as "slow and deep inhalation through the nose, usually to a count of ten, followed by slow and complete exhalation for a similar count." **Guided imagery**: NCCAM defines guided imagery as "any of various techniques (such as a series of verbal suggestions) used to guide another person or oneself in imagining sensations—especially in visualizing an image in the mind—to bring about a desired physical response (such as stress reduction)." **Hypnosis**: Hypnosis involves inducing a deeply relaxed state in which patients are given therapeutic suggestions. **Progressive relaxation**: Progressive relaxation involves sequentially tensing and then releasing muscle groups in order to reduce muscular tension.

Meditation: Walsh and Shapiro have defined meditation as "a family of self-regulation practices that focus on training attention and awareness in order to bring mental processes under greater voluntary control and thereby foster general mental well-being and development and/or specific capacities such as calm, clarity, and concentration." In a 2007 assessment of the research on meditation, Ospina et al. grouped meditation into five broad categories: mantra meditation, mindfulness meditation, yoga, tai chi, and qi gong.

30. Bertisch, S., et al. (2009). Alternative mind-body therapies used by adults with medical conditions. *J Psychosom Res* 66:511–19 (analyzing data from the 2002 National Health Interview Survey Alternative Medicine Supplement).

31. Ibid.

32. Izquierdo de Santiago, A., & Khan, M. (2007). Hypnosis for schizophrenia. Cochrane Database of Systematic Reviews 2007, Issue 4. Art. No.: CD004160. DOI: 10.1002/14651858.CD004160.pub3.

33. Al-Harasi, S., et al. (2010). Hypnosis for children undergoing dental treatment. Cochrane Database of Systematic Reviews 2010, Issue 8. Art. No.: CD007154. DOI: 10.1002/14651858.CD007154.pub2.

34. Webb, A., et al. (2007). Hypnotherapy for treatment of irritable bowel syndrome. Cochrane Database of Systematic Reviews 2007, Issue 4. Art. No.: CD005110. DOI: 10.1002/14651858.CD005110.pub2.

35. Barnes, J., et al. (2010). Hypnotherapy for smoking cessation. Cochrane Database of Systematic Reviews 2010, Issue 10. Art. No.: CD001008. DOI:10.1002/14651858. CD001008.pub2.

36. Ramaratnam, S., & Sridharan, K. (1999). Yoga for epilepsy. Cochrane Database of Systematic Reviews 1999, Issue 2. Art. No.: CD001524. DOI:10.1002/14651858. CD001524.

37. Krisanaprakornkit, T., et al. (2010). Meditation therapies for attention-deficit/hyperactivity disorder (ADHD). Cochrane Database of Systematic Reviews 2010, Issue 6. Art. No.: CD006507. DOI:10.1002/14651858.CD006507.pub2.

38. Krisanaprakornkit, T., et al. (2006). Meditation therapy for anxiety disorders. Cochrane Database of Systematic Reviews 2006, Issue 1. Art. No.: CD004998. DOI: 10.1002/14651858.CD004998.pub2.

39. Ospina, M., et al. (2007) Meditation practices for health: State of the research. Evidence Report/Technology Assessment No 155. AHRQ Publication No. 07-E010.

40. Ibid.

41. Ibid.

42. Ibid.

43. Ibid.

44. Ibid.

45. Smith, C., et al. (2006). Complementary and alternative therapies for pain management in labour. Cochrane Database of Systematic Reviews 2006, Issue 4. Art. No.: CD003521. DOI: 10.1002/14651858.CD003521.pub2.

46. Glazener, C., et al. (2005). Complementary and miscellaneous interventions for nocturnal enuresis in children. Cochrane Database of Systematic Reviews 2005, Issue 2. Art. No.: CD005230. DOI:10.1002/14651858.CD005230.

47. Han, A., et al. (2004). Tai chi for treating rheumatoid arthritis. Cochrane Database of Systematic Reviews 2004, Issue 3. Art. No.: CD004849. DOI:10.1002/14651858. CD004849.

48. Wang, C., et al. (2010). A randomized trial of tai chi for fibromyalgia. *N Engl J Med* 363:743–54.

49. Dickinson, H., et al. (2008). Relaxation therapies for the management of primary hypertension in adults. Cochrane Database of Systematic Reviews 2008, Issue 1. Art. No.: CD004935. DOI: 10.1002/14651858.CD004935.pub2.

50. Ospina et al. (2007), Meditation practices for health.

51. Jorm, A., et al. (2008). Relaxation for depression. Cochrane Database of Systematic Reviews 2008, Issue 4. Art. No.: CD007142. DOI: 10.1002/14651858.CD007142.pub2.

52. Ospina et al. (2007), Meditation practices for health.

53. Ibid.

54. Ibid.

CHAPTER 10: PATIENT OUTLOOK AND SOCIAL CONNECTEDNESS

1. Pressman, S., & Cohen, S. (2005). Does positive affect influence health? *Psychological Bulletin* 131:925–71.

2. Cohen, S., et al. (2003). Emotional style and susceptibility to the common cold. *Psychosom Med* 65:652–57.

3. Ostir, G., et al. (2001). The association between emotional well-being and the incidence of stroke in older adults. *Psychosom Med* 63:210–15.

4. Pressman & Cohen (2005), Does positive affect influence health?

5. Pitkalaab, K., et al. (2004). Positive life orientation as a predictor of 10-year outcome in an aged population. *J Clinical Epidemiology* 57:409–14.

6. Danner, D., et al. (2001). Positive emotions in early life and longevity: Findings from the nun study. *J Personality and Social Psychology* 80:804–13.

7. Moskowitz, J., et al. (2008). Positive affect uniquely predicts lower risk of mortality in people with diabetes. *Health Psychol* 27:S73–S82.

8. Moskowitz, J. (2003). Positive affect predicts lower risk of AIDS mortality. *Psychosom Med* 65:620–26.

9. Chida, Y., & Steptoe, A. (2008). Positive psychological well-being and mortality: A quantitative review of prospective observational studies. *Psychosom Med* 70:741–56.

10. Zautra, A., et al. (2005). Positive affect as a source of resilience for women in chronic pain. *J Consult Clin Psychol* 73:212–20.

11. Cohen et al. (2003), Emotional style and susceptibility.

12. Steptoe, A., et al. (2008). Positive affect and psychosocial processes related to health. *British Journal of Psychology* 99:211–27.

13. Chida, Y., & Steptoe, A. (2009). The association of anger and hostility with future coronary heart disease: A meta-analytic review of prospective evidence. *J Am Coll Cardiol* 53:936–46.

14. Ibid.

15. See, for example, Niaura, R., et al. (2002). Hostility, the metabolic syndrome, and incident coronary heart disease. *Health Psychol* 21:588–93; Barefoot, J., et al. (1983).

Hostility, CHD incidence, and total mortality: A 25-year follow-up study of 255 physicians. *Psychosom Med* 45:59–64.

16. Niaura et al. (2002), Hostility.

17. Kerns, R., et al. (1994). Anger expression and chronic pain. *Journal of Behavioral Medicine* 17:57–67; Carson, J., et al. (2007). Conflict about expressing emotions and chronic low back pain: Associations with pain and anger. *Journal of Pain* 8:405–11.

18. Bruehl, S., et al. (2009). Pain-related effects of trait anger expression: Neural substrates and the role of endogenous opioid mechanisms. *Neurosci Biobehav Rev* 33:475–91; Bruehl, S., et al. (2006). Anger expression and pain: An overview of findings and possible mechanisms. *Journal of Behavioral Medicine* 29:593–606.

19. Ibid.; van Middendorp, H., et al. (2010). The effects of anger and sadness on clinical pain reports and experimentally-induced pain thresholds in women with and without fibromyalgia. *Arthritis Care & Research* 62:1370–76; Fernandez, E., & Turk, D. (1995). The scope and significance of anger in the experience of chronic pain. *Pain* 61:165–75.

20. Okifuji, A., et al. (1999). Anger in chronic pain: Investigations of anger targets and intensity. *J Psychosom Res* 47:1–12.

21. Wulsin, L., et al. (2003). Do depressive symptoms increase the risk for the onset of coronary disease? A systematic quantitative review. *Psychosom Med* 65:201–10.

22. Lichtman, J., et al. (2009). Depression and coronary heart disease: Recommendations for screening, referral and treatment. *Circulation* 118:1768–75.

23. Ibid.

24. Ibid.

25. Thombs, B., et al. (2008). Depression screening and patient outcomes in cardiovascular care: A systematic review. *JAMA* 300:2161–71.

26. Irie, M., et al. (2005). Depression and possible cancer risk due to oxidative DNA damage. *J Psychiatric Research* 39:553–60.

27. Black, S., et al. (2003). Depression predicts increased incidence of adverse health outcomes in older Mexican Americans with Type 2 Diabetes. *Diabetes Care* 26:2822–28.

28. Deave, T., et al. (2008). The impact of maternal depression in pregnancy on early child development. *BJOG* 115:1043–51; Rahman, A., et al. (2004). Impact of maternal depression on infant nutritional status and illness: A cohort study. *Arch Gen Psychiatry* 61:946–52.

29. See, for example, Bair, M., et al. (2003). Depression and pain comorbidity. *Arch Intern Med* 163:2433–45; Ozalp, G., et al. (2003). Preoperative emotional states in patients with breast cancer and postoperative pain. *Acta Anaesthesiol Scand* 47:26–29.

30. Lin, E., et al. (2003). Effect of improving depression care on pain and functional outcomes among older adults with arthritis. *JAMA* 290:2428–29.

31. DiMatteo, M., et al. (2000). Depression is a risk factor for noncompliance with medical treatment: Meta-analysis of the effects of anxiety and depression on patient adherence. *Arch Intern Med* 160:2101–7.

32. Ziegelstein, R., et al. (2000). Patients with depression are less likely to follow recommendations to reduce cardiac risk during recovery from a myocardial infarction. *Arch Intern Med* 160:1818–23.

33. Rasmussen, H., et al. (2009). Optimism and physical health: A meta-analytic review. *Annals of Behavioral Medicine* 37:239–56.

34. Hudetz, J., et al. (2010). Preoperative dispositional optimism correlates with a reduced incidence of postoperative delirium and recovery of postoperative cognitive function in cardiac surgical patients. *Journal of Cardiothoracic and Vascular Anesthesia* 24:560–67.

35. Kubzansky, L., et al. (2002). Breathing easy: A prospective study of optimism and pulmonary function in the normative aging study. *Annals of Behavioral Medicine* 24:345–53.

36. Scheier, M., et al. (1999). Optimism and rehospitalization after coronary artery bypass surgery. *Arch Intern Med* 159:829–35.

37. Hudetz et al. (2010), Preoperative dispositional optimism.

38. Tindle, H., et al. (2009). Optimism, cynical hostility, and incident coronary heart disease and mortality in the Women's Health Initiative. *Circulation* 120:656–662; *Kubzansky, L., et al. (2001). Is the glass half empty or half full? A prospective study of optimism and coronary heart disease in the Normative Aging Study. Psychosom Med* 63:910–16.

39. Giltay, E., et al. (2006). Dispositional optimism and the risk of cardiovascular death: The Zutphen Elderly Study. *Arch Intern Med* 166:431–36.

40. Allison, P. (2003). Dispositional optimism predicts survival status 1 year after diagnosis in head and neck cancer patients. *J Clinical Oncology* 21:543–48.

41. Schofield, P., et al. (2004). Optimism and survival in lung carcinoma patients, *Cancer* 100:1276–82.

42. Costello, N., et al. (2002). Temporomandibular disorder and optimism: Relationships to ischemic pain sensitivity and interleukin-6. *Pain* 100:99–110; Kurtz, M., et al. (2008). Patient optimism and mastery—do they play a role in cancer patients' management of pain and fatigue? *J Pain Symptom Manage* 36:1–10.

43. Scheier, M., & Carver, C. (1985). Optimism, coping, and health: Assessment and implications of generalized outcome expectancies. *Health Psychol* 4:219–47; Wenglert, L., & Rosen, A. (1995). Optimism, self-esteem, mood and subjective health. *Personality and Individual Differences* 18:653–61; Reed, G., et al. (1999). Negative HIV specific expectancies and AIDS-related bereavement as predictors of symptom onset in asymptomatic HIV-positive gay men. *Health Psychol* 18:354–63.

44. Rasmussen et al. (2009), Optimism and physical health.

45. See, for example, Rasmussen et al. (2009), Optimism and physical health. Note that the same question arises in the literature regarding positive affect and negative affect. See, for example, Pressman & Cohen (2005), Does positive affect influence health?

46. Rasmussen et al. (2009), Optimism and physical health.

47. Peterson, C., et al. (1988). Pessimistic explanatory style is a risk factor for physical illness: A thirty-five-year longitudinal study. *J Personality and Social Psychology* 55:23–27.

48. Nabi, H., et al. (2010). Low pessimism protects against stroke: The Health and Social Support (HeSSup) prospective cohort study. *Stroke* 41:187–90.

49. Singh, J., et al. (2010). Pessimistic explanatory style. *Journal of Bone and Joint Surgery—British* 92-B:799–806.

50. Carvera, C., et al. (2010). Optimism. *Clinical Psychology Review* 30:879–89.

51. Wallston, K., et al. (1987). Perceived Control and Health. *Current Psychological Research & Reviews* 6:5–25.

52. Rodin, J., & Langer, E. (1977). Long-term effects of a control-relevant intervention with the institutionalized aged. *J Personality and Social Psychology* 35:897–902.

53. Bosma, H., et al. (1999). Socioeconomic inequalities in mortality and importance of perceived control: Cohort study. *BMJ* 319:1469–70.

54. Griffin, M., & Chen, E. (2006). Perceived control and immune and pulmonary outcomes in children with asthma. *Psychosom Med* 68:493–99; Calfree, C., et al. (2006). The influence of perceived control of asthma on health outcomes. *Chest* 130:1312–18; Katz, P., et al. (2002). Perceived control of asthma and quality of life among adults with asthma. *Ann Allergy Asthma Immuno* 89:251–58.

55. Shaw, C., & McColl, E. (2003). The relationship of perceived control to outcomes in older women undergoing surgery for fractured neck of femur. *Journal of Clinical Nursing* 12:117–23.

56. Gruber-Baldinia, A., et al. (2009). Effects of optimism/pessimism and locus of control on disability and quality of life in Parkinson's disease. *Parkinsonism and Related Disorders* 15:665–69.

57. Lachman, M., & Weaver, S. (1998). The sense of control as a moderator of social class differences in health and well-being. *J Personality and Social Psychology* 74:763–73.

58. Ibid.

59. See, for example, Schnoll, R., et al. (2011). Increased self-efficacy to quit and perceived control over withdrawal symptoms predict smoking cessation following nicotine dependence treatment. *Addictive Behaviors* 36:144–47; O'Leary, A. (1985). Self-efficacy and health: Behavioral and stress-physiological mediation. *Cognitive Theory and Research* 16:229–45.

60. Ruthig, J., et al. (2007). Comparative risk and perceived control: Implications for psychological and physical well-being among older adults. *Journal of Social Psychology* 147:345–69.

61. Berkman, L., & Syme, S. (1979). Social networks, host resistance, and mortality: A nine-year follow-up study of Alameda County residents. *Am J Epidemiol* 109:186–204.

62. Croezen, S., et al. (2010). Positive and negative experiences of social support and long-term mortality among middle-aged Dutch people. *Am J Epidemiol* 172:173–79.

63. Russek, L., & Schwartz, G. (1997). Feelings of parental caring predict health status in midlife: A 35-year follow-up of the Harvard Mastery of Stress Study. *Journal of Behavioral Medicine* 20:1–13.

64. See, for example, Rutledge, T., et al. (2004). Social networks are associated with lower mortality rates among women with suspected coronary disease: The National Heart, Lung, and Blood Institute-sponsored women's ischemia syndrome evaluation study. *Psychosom Med* 66:882–88; Orth-Gomer, K., et al. (1993). Lack of social support

and incidence of coronary heart disease in middle-aged Swedish men. *Psychosom Med* 55:37–43.

65. Brummett, B., et al. (2001). Characteristics of socially isolated patients with coronary artery disease who are at elevated risk for mortality. *Psychosom Med* 63:267–72.

66. Pinquart, M., & Duberstein, P. (2010). Associations of social networks with cancer mortality: A meta-analysis. *Critical Reviews in Oncology/Hematology* 75:122–37.

67. Lutgendorf, S., et al. (2000). Interleukin-6 and use of social support in gynecologic cancer patients. *International Journal of Behavioral Medicine* 7:127–42; see also Costanzo, E., et al. (2005). Psychosocial factors and interleukin-6 among women with advanced ovarian cancer. *Cancer* 104:305–13.

68. Leserman, J. (2000). Impact of stressful life events, depression, social support, coping, and cortisol on progression to AIDS. *Am J Psychiatry* 157:1221–28; see also Patterson, T., et al. (1996). Relationship of psychosocial factors to HIV progression. *Annals of Behavioral Medicine* 18:30–39.

69. Brummett, B., et al. (2005). Perceived social support as a predictor of mortality in coronary patients: Effects of smoking, sedentary behavior, and depressive symptoms. *Psychosom Med* 67:40–45.

70. Frasure-Smith, N., et al. (2000). Social support, depression, and mortality during the first year after myocardial infarction. *Circulation* 101:1919.

71. DiMatteo, M. (2004). Social support and patient adherence to medical treatment: A meta-analysis. *Health Psychol* 23:207–18.

72. Thomas, P. (2010). Is it better to give or to receive? Social support and the well-being of older adults. *J Gerontol B* 65B:351–57.

CHAPTER 11: HEALING ENVIRONMENTS

1. Malkin, J. (1992). *Creating healing environments for special patient populations.* Canada: Wiley.

2. Walch, J., et al. (2005). The effect of sunlight on postoperative analgesic medication use: A prospective study of patients undergoing spinal surgery. *Psychosom Med* 67:156–63.

3. Beauchemin, K., & Hays, P. (1996). Sunny hospital rooms expedite recovery from severe and refractory depressions. *J Affect Disord* 40:49–51.

4. Beauchemin, K., & Hays, P. (1998). Dying in the dark: Sunshine, gender, and outcomes in myocardial infarction. *J R Soc Med* 91:352–54.

5. Benedetti, F., et al. (2001). Morning sunlight reduces length of hospitalization in bipolar depression. *J Affect Disord* 62:221–23.

6. Federman, E., et al. (2000). Relationship between climate and psychiatric inpatient length of stay in Veterans Health Administration hospitals. *Am J Psychiatry* 157:1669.

7. Keep, P., et al. (1980). Windows in the intensive therapy unit. *Anaesthesia* 35:257–62.

8. Golden, R., et al. (2005). The efficacy of light therapy in the treatment of mood disorders: A review and meta-analysis of the evidence. *Am J Psychiatry* 162:656–62.

9. Partonen, T., & Lonnqvist, J. (2000). Bright light improves vitality and alleviates distress in healthy people. *J Affect Disord* 57:55–61.

10. Leppämäki, S., et al. (2002). Bright-light exposure combined with physical exercise elevates mood. *J Affect Disord* 72:139–44.

11. Beauchemin & Hays (1998), Dying in the dark.

12. Mroczek, J., et al. (2005). Hospital design and staff perceptions: An exploratory analysis. *Health Care Manag* 24:233–44.

13. Alimoglu, M., & Donmez, L. (2005). Daylight exposure and the other predictors of burnout among nurses in a university hospital. *Int J Nurs Stud* 42:549–55.

14. Mroczek et al. (2005), Hospital design.

15. Buchanan, T., et al. (1991). Illumination and errors in dispensing. *American Journal of Hospital Pharmacy* 48:2137–45.

16. Booker, J., & Roseman, C. (1995). A seasonal pattern of hospital medication errors in Alaska. *Psychiatry Research* 57:251–57.

17. Verderber, S., & Reuman, D. (1987). Windows, views, and health status in hospital therapeutic environments. *Journal of Architectural and Planning Research* 4:120–33.

18. Moore, E. (1981). A prison environment's effect on health care service demands. *Journal of Environmental Systems* 11:17–34.

19. Ulrich, R. (1984). View through a window may influence recovery from surgery. *Science* 224:420–21.

20. Ulrich, R., et al. (2008). A review of the research literature on evidence-based healthcare design, *HERD* 1 (3).

21. Heerwagen, J., & Orians, G. (1986). Adaptations to windowlessness: A study of the use of visual decor in windowed and windowless offices. *Environment and Behavior* 18:623–39.

22. Ulrich, R., et al. (1993). Effects of exposure to nature and abstract pictures on patients recovery from heart surgery. *Psychophysiology* S1–7.

23. Tse, M., et al. (2002). The effect of visual stimuli on pain threshold and tolerance. *Journal of Clinical Nursing* 11:264–69.

24. Diette, G., et al. (2003). Distraction therapy with nature sights and sounds reduces pain during flexible bronchoscopy: A complementary approach to routine analgesia. *Chest* 123:941–48.

25. Ulrich, R. S. (1999). Effects of gardens on health outcomes: Theory and research. In C. Cooper-Marcus & M. Barnes (eds.), *Healing gardens: Therapeutic benefits and design recommendations* (pp. 27–86). New York: Wiley.

26. Ulrich et al. (2008), A review of the research literature.

27. Berglund, B., Lindvall, T., & Schwela, D. (eds.). (1999). *Guidelines for Community Noise*. World Health Organization. A-weighted decibels ("dB(A)") are typically used for environmental noise measurement.

28. Allaouchiche, B., et al. (2002). Noise in the postanaesthesia care unit. *British Journal of Anaesthesia* 88:369–73; McLaughlin, A., et al. (1996). Noise levels in a cardiac

surgical intensive care unit: A preliminary study conducted in secret. *Intensive &
Critical Care Nursing* 12:226–30; Busch-Vishniac, I., et al. (2005). Noise levels in Johns
Hopkins Hospital. *Journal of the Acoustical Society of America* 118:3629–45; Robertson,
A., et al. (1998). Peak noise distribution in the neonatal intensive care nursery. *Journal
of Perinatology* 18:361–64.

29. McLaren, E., & Maxwell-Armstrong, C. (2008). Noise pollution on an acute
surgical ward. *Ann R Coll Surg Engl* 90:136–39.

30. Chaudhury, H., et al. (2006). Nurses' perception of single-occupancy versus multioccupancy rooms in acute care environments: An exploratory comparative assessment.
Applied Nursing Research 19:118–25.

31. Topf, M. (1992). Effects of personal control over hospital noise on sleep. *Research in Nursing & Health* 15:19–28.

32. Hweidi, I. (2007). Jordanian patients' perception of stressors in critical care units:
A questionnaire survey. *Int J Nurs Stud* 44:227–35.

33. Ulrich et al. (2008), A review of the research literature.

34. Freedman, N., et al. (1999). Patient perception of sleep quality and etiology of
sleep disruption in the intensive care unit. *American Journal of Respiratory and Critical
Care Medicine* 159:1155–62.

35. Topf, M., et al. (1996). Effects of critical care unit noise on the subjective quality
of sleep. *Journal of Advanced Nursing* 24:545–51.

36. Hurtley, C. (ed.). (2009). *Night noise guidelines for Europe*. WHO Regional Office for Europe.

37. Hagerman, I., et al. (2005). Influence of intensive coronary care acoustics on the
quality of care and physiological state of patients. *International Journal of Cardiology*
98:267–70.

38. Zahr, L., & de Traversay, J. (1995). Premature infant responses to noise reduction by earmuffs: Effects on behavioral and physiologic measures. *Journal of Perinatology* 15:448–55.

39. Morrison, W., et al. (2003). Noise, stress, and annoyance in a pediatric intensive
care unit. *Critical Care Medicine* 31:113–19.

40. Blomkvist, V., et al. (2005). Acoustics and psychosocial environment in intensive
coronary care. *Occup Environ Med* 62 (3): e1.

41. Topf, M., & Dillon, E. (1988). Noise-induced stress as a predictor of burnout in
critical care nurses. *Heart Lung* 17:567–74.

42. Nagar, D., & Pandey, J. (1987). Affect and performance on cognitive task as a
function of crowding and noise. *J Applied Psychology* 17:147–57; Fisher, S. (1972). A
"distraction effect" of noise bursts. *Perception* 1:223–36.

43. Bayo, M., et al. (1995). Noise levels in an urban hospital and workers' subjective
responses. *Archives of Environmental Health* 50:247–51.

44. Flynn, E., et al. (1999). Impact of interruptions and distractions on dispensing errors in an ambulatory care pharmacy. *Pharmacy* 56:1319–25; Pape, T. (2003). Applying
airline safety practices to medication administration. *Medsurg Nurs* 12:77–93.

45. Cropp, A., et al. (1994). Name that tone: The proliferation of alarms in the intensive care unit. *Chest* 105:1217–20.

46. Ulrich et al. (2008), A review of the research literature.

47. Bradt, J., & Dileo, C. (2009). Music for stress and anxiety reduction in coronary heart disease patients. Cochrane Database Syst Rev:CD006577.

48. Kanpp, C., et al. (2009). Music therapy in an integrated pediatric palliative care program. *Am J Hosp Palliat Care* 26:449–55.

49. Williams, J. (1992). The effects of ocean sounds on sleep after coronary artery bypass surgery. *Am J Crit Care* 1:91–97.

50. Ulrich et al. (2008), A review of the research literature.

51. Ibid.

52. Chaudhury, H., et al. (2006). Nurses' perception of single-occupancy versus multioccupancy rooms in acute care environments: An exploratory comparative assessment. *Applied Nursing Research* 19:118–25.

53. Ulrich et al. (2008), A review of the research literature.

54. Koivula, M., et al. (2002). Social support and its relation to fear and anxiety in patients awaiting coronary artery bypass grafting. *Journal of Clinical Nursing* 11:622–33; Ulrich et al. (2008), A review of the research literature; DiMatteo, M. (2004). Social support and patient adherence to medical treatment: A meta-analysis. *Health Psychol* 23:207–18; Uchino, B., et al. (1996). The relationship between social support and physiological processes: A review with emphasis on underlying mechanisms and implications for health. *Psychological Bulletin* 119:488–531.

55. Ulrich et al. (2008), A review of the research literature.

56. Holahan, C. (1972). Seating patterns and patient behavior in an experimental dayroom. *J Abnormal Psychology* 80:115–24; Baldwin, S. (1985). Effects of furniture re-arrangement on the atmosphere of wards in a maximum-security hospital. *Hospital and Community Psychiatry* 36:525–28.

57. Leather, P., et al. (2003). Outcomes of environmental appraisal of different hospital waiting areas. *Environment and Behavior* 35:842–69.

58. Swan, J., et al. (2003). Do appealing hospital rooms increase patient evaluations of physicians, nurses, and hospital services? *Health Care Manage Rev* 28:254–64.

59. Douglas, C., & Douglas, M. (2004). Patient-friendly hospital environments: Exploring the patients' perspective. *Health Expectations* 7:61–73.

60. Carpman, J. (2000). Wayfinding in health facilities. Carpman Grant Associates LLC.

61. Carpman, J., & Grant, M. (2001). *Design that cares*. San Francisco: Jossey-Bass.

62. Zimring, C. (1990). The cost of confusion: Non-monetary and monetary cost of the Emory University hospital wayfinding system. Atlanta: Georgia Institute of Technology.

APPENDIX 1: PSYCHIATRIC DIAGNOSIS

1. Rosenhan, D. (1973). On being sane in insane places. *Science* 179:250–58.

2. Spitzer, R., & Fleiss, J. (1974). A re-analysis of the reliability of psychiatric diagnosis. *British J Psychiatry* 125:341–47.

3. Riskind, J., et al. (1987). Reliability of DSM-III diagnoses for major depression and general anxiety disorder using the structured clinical interview for DSM-III. *Arch Gen Psychiatry* 44:817–20.

4. Cosgrove, L., et al. (2006). Financial ties between DSM-IV panel members and the pharmaceutical industry. *Psychotherapy and Psychosomatics* 75:154–60.

5. Westly, E. (2010, May/June). Different shades of blue. *Scientific American Mind* (pp. 30–37).

APPENDIX 2: DARWINIAN MEDICINE

1. Williams, G., & Nesse, R. (1991). The dawn of Darwinian medicine. *Quarterly Review of Biology* 66:1–22. Nesse, R. & Williams, G. (1995). *Why we get sick: The new science of Darwinian medicine*. New York: Vintage Books.

2. Nesse, R., & Stearns, S. (2007). The great opportunity: Evolutionary applications to medicine and public health. DOI:10.1111/j.1752–4571.2007.00006.x.

3. Nesse, R. (2008). Evolution: Medicine's most basic science. *Lancet* 372:S21–27.

4. Eaton, S., et al. (1966). An evolutionary perspective enhances understanding of human nutritional requirements. *J Nutr* 126:1732–40.

5. Kluger, M., et al. (1996). The adaptive value of fever. *Infect Dis Clin North Am* 10:1–20.

6. Styrt, B., & Sugarman, B. (1990). Antipyresis and fever. *Arch Intern Med* 150:1589–97.

7. Doran, T., et al. (1989). Acetaminophen: More harm than good for chickenpox? *J Pediatr* 114:1045–48.

8. Graham, N., et al. (1990). Adverse effects of aspirin, acetaminophen and ibuprophen on immune function, viral shedding and clinical status in rhinovirus-infected volunteers. *J Infect Dis* 162:1277–82.

9. Barlow, G., et al. (2010). Letter: Fever as nature's engine: Some clinical data. *BMJ* 340, DOI:10.1136/bmj.c905.

10. DuPont, H., & Hornick, R. (1973). Adverse effect of Lomotil therapy in shigellosis. *JAMA* 226:1525–28.

11. Murray, M., et al. (1978). The adverse effect of iron repletion on the course of certain infections. *BMJ* 2:1113–15.

12. Pepper, G., et al. (2006). Rates of nausea and vomiting in pregnancy and dietary characteristics across populations. *Proceedings of the Royal Society B* 273(1601): 2675–79; Chan, R., et al. (2010). Severity and duration of nausea and vomiting symptoms in pregnancy and spontaneous abortion. *Hum Reprod* 25:2907–12.

13. Jones, D. (2010, August 14). Heal thyself. *New Scientist*.

14. http://www-personal.umich.edu/~nesse.

15. Kliukiene, J. et al. (2001) Risk of breast cancer among Norwegian women with visual impairment. *Brit J of Cancer* 84:397–99.

16. Stevens, R. (2005) Circadian disruption and breast cancer: from melatonin to clock genes. *Epidemiology* 16:254-8.

17. Medeiros, M., et al. (2003). *Schistosoma mansoni* infection is associated with a reduced course of asthma. *J Allergy Clinical Immunology* 111:947-51.

18. Hunter, M., & McKay, D. (2004). Review article: Helminths as therapeutic agents for inflammatory bowel disease. *Aliment Pharmacol Ther* 19:167-77; Summers, R., et al. (2005). Trichuris suis therapy in Crohn's disease. *Gut* 54:87-90.

19. Feary, J. (2010). Experimental hookworm infection: A randomized placebo-controlled trial in asthma. *Clin Exp Allergy* 40:299-306.

20. Ewald, P. (1993). *Evolution of infectious disease*. New York: Oxford University Press; Ewald, P. (1995). Emerging pathogens: Insights from evolutionary biology. *Emerging Infectious Diseases* 2:245-57; Ewald, P. (2002). *Plague time: The new germ theory of disease*. New York: Anchor.

APPENDIX 3: WELLNESS STRATEGIES

1. Glassner, B. (2007). *The gospel of food: Why we should stop worrying and enjoy what we eat*. New York: HarperPerennial.

2. Hallberg, L., et al. (1977). Iron absorption from Southeast Asian diets II. Role of various factors that might explain low absorption. *Am J Clin Nutr* 30: 539-48; Bjorn-Rasmussen, E., et al. (1976). Measurement of iron absorption from composite meals. *Am J Clin Nutr* 29:772-78.

3. Comparing life spans of different countries is not an accurate measure of the effectiveness of the countries' health-care systems. Many deaths, such as from motor vehicle accidents and homicides, occur independently of the health-care systems. Also, countries differ in the age at which infants are considered live-born—which results in differences in infant mortality rates. Doctors in different countries differ in their willingness to perform heroic measures to prolong life that result in greatly reduced quality of life.

4. Rozin, P., et al. (1999). Attitudes to food and the role of food in life: Comparisons of Flemish Belgium, France, Japan and the United States. *Appetite* 33:163-180; Rozin, P., et al. (2003). The ecology of eating: Part of the French paradox results from lower food intake in French than Americans, because of smaller portion sizes. *Psychological Science* 14:450-54; Girard Eberle, S. (2009). The pleasure principle—Can you really have your cake and eat it, too? *Environmental Nutrition* 32:1, 6.

5. Lee, I., & Paffenbarger, R. (1998). Life is sweet: Candy consumption and longevity. *BMJ* 317:1683-84.

6. Adamson, G., et al. (1999). HPLC method for the quantification of procyanidins in cocoa and chocolate samples and correlation to total antioxidant capacity. *J Agric Food Chem* 47:4184-88.

7. Rein, D., et al. (2000). Cocoa inhibits platelet activation and function. *Am J Clin Nutr* 72:30-35.

8. Flammer, A., et al. (2007). Dark chocolate improves coronary vasomotion and reduces platelet reactivity. *Circulation* 116:2376–82.

9. Knekt, P., et al. (1996). Flavonoid intake and coronary mortality in Finland: A cohort study. *Brit Med J* 312:478–81; Hertog, M., et al. (1993). Dietary antioxidant flavonoids and risk of coronary heart disease: The Zutphen Elderly Study. *Lancet* 342:1007–11; Hollman, P., et al. (1996). Role of dietary flavonoids in protection against cancer and coronary heart disease. *Biochem Soc Transact* 24:785–89.

10. Vinson, J., et al. (1999). Phenol antioxidant quantity and quality in foods: Cocoa, dark chocolate, and milk chocolate. *J Agric Food Chem* 47:4821–24.

11. Martin, F., et al. (2009). Metabolic effects of dark chocolate consumption on energy, gut microbiota and stress-related metabolism in free-living subjects. *J Proteome Research* 8:5568–79.

12. Akbaraly, T., et al. (2009). Dietary pattern and depressive symptoms in middle age. *British J Psychiatry* 195:408–13.

13. http://www.mayoclinic.com/health/water/NU00283 (accessed January 10, 2010).

14. Holahan, C., et al. (2010). Late-life alcohol consumption and 20-year mortality. *Alcoholism Clinical and Experimental Research* 34:1961–71, DOI:10.1111/j.1530-0277.2010.01286.x.

15. Marques-Vidal, P., et al. (2001). Different alcohol drinking and blood pressure relationships in France and Northern Ireland. *Hypertension* 38:1361–66.

16. Arriola, L., et al. (2009). Alcohol intake and the risk of coronary heart disease in the Spanish EPIC cohort study. *Heart*. DOI:10.1136/hrt.173419.

17. Spaak, J., et al. (2008). Dose-related effects of red wine and alcohol on hemodynamics, sympathetic nerve activity, and arterial diameter. *Amer J Physiology, Heart and Circulatory Physiology* 294:H582–83.

18. Streppel, M., et al. (2009). Long-term wine consumption is related to cardiovascular mortality and life expectancy independently of moderate alcohol intake: The Zutphen Study. *J Epidemiol Community Health* 63:534–40.

19. Brown, L., et al. (2009). The biological responses to resveratrol and other polyphenols from alcoholic beverages. *Alcoholism Clinical and Experimental Research* 33:1513–23.

20. Allen, N., et al. (2009). Moderate alcohol intake and cancer incidence in women. *J National Cancer Institute* 101:296–305.

21. Janecka, L. (2010). The roast with the most. *Psychology Today* 43:44–45.

22. Rasmussen, J., & Gallino, M. (1997). Effects of caffeine on subjective reports of fatigue and arousal during mentally demanding activities. *European J Clinical Pharmacology* 37:61–90.

23. Graham, T., & Spriet, L. (1991). Performance and metabolic responses to a high caffeine dose during prolonged exercise. *J Appl Physiol* 71:2292–98.

24. Wyatt, J., et al. (2004). Low-dose repeated caffeine administration for circadian-phase–dependent performance degradation during extended wakefulness. *Sleep* 27:374–81.

25. Rogers, P., et al. (2010). Association of the anxiogenic and alerting effects of caffeine with adora2a and adora1 polymorphisms and habitual level of caffeine consumption. DOI:10.1038/npp.2010.71.

26. Inoue, M., et al. (2005). Influence of coffee drinking on subsequent risk of hepatocellular carcinoma: A prospective study in Japan. *J National Cancer Institute* 97:293–300.

27. Williams, Sarah. (2005, September 16). Coffee contains many antioxidants. *Johns Hopkins News-Letter*, at http://media.www.jhunewsletter.com/media/storage/paper932/news/2005/09/16/Science/Coffee.Contains.Many.Antioxidants-2243286.shtml (accessed January 21, 2010).

28. Frost Andersen, L., et al. (2006). Consumption of coffee is associated with reduced risk of death attributed to inflammatory and cardiovascular diseases in the Iowa Women's Health Study. *Am J Clin Nutr* 83:1039–46.

29. Ritchie, K., et al. (2007). A prospective population study (the Three City Study). *Neurology* 69:536–45.

30. Eskelinen, M., et al. (2009). Midlife coffee and tea drinking and the risk of late-life dementia: A population-based CAIDE study. *J Alzheimers Dis* 16:85–91.

31. Science Daily. (2007, June 15). How coffee raises cholesterol. *Science Daily*, at http://www.sciencedaily.com/releases/2007/06/070614162223.htm (accessed January 21, 2010).

32. Wallop, H. (2008, April 10). Peter Jones' cat dung coffee, £50 a cup. *Telegraph*, at http://www.telegraph.co.uk/news/uknews/1584553/Peter-Jones-cat-dung-coffee-50-a-cup.html (accessed January 26, 2010).

33. Rosengren, A., & Wilhelmsen, L. (1997). Physical activity protects against coronary death and deaths from all causes in middle-aged men. Evidence from a 20-year follow-up of the primary prevention study in Göteborg. *Ann Epidemiol* 7:69–75.

34. Hoffman, M., & Hoffman, D. (2007). Does aerobic exercise improve pain perception and mood? A review of the evidence related to healthy and chronic pain subjects. *Current Pain and Headache Reports* 11:93–97.

35. Boecker, H., et al. (2008). The runner's high: Opioidergic mechanisms in the human brain. *Cerebral Cortex*, DOI:10.1093/cercor/bhn013.

36. Wu, C., et al. (2007). Treadmill exercise counteracts the suppressive effects of peripheral lipopolysaccharide on hippocampal neurogenesis and learning and memory. *J Neurochem* 103:2471–81.

37. Murphy, E., et al. (2008). Exercise stress increases susceptibility to influenza infection. *Brain Behav Immun* 22:1152–55.

38. Helliker, K. (2010, January 4). Why you should step up your workout. *Wall Street Journal*, at http://online.wsj.com/article/SB100014240527487043503045746385500590 84962.html (accessed February 2, 2010).

39. McGonigal, K. (2009, October 5). Change your posture. *Psychology Today*, at http://www.psychologytoday.com (accessed September 14, 2010).

40. Briñol, P., et al. (2009). Body posture effects on self-evaluation: A self-validation approach. *European J Social Psychology* 39:1053–64.

41. Rechtschaffen, A. (1998). Current perspectives on the function of sleep. *Perspectives in Biology and Medicine* 41:359–90.

42. Patlak, M. (2005). Your guide to healthy sleep. NIH Publication No. 06-5271.

43. http://harvardmagazine.com/2005/07/deep-into-sleep.html; http://www.utne.com/Spirituality/The-No-Wake-Zone-Insomnia-Sleep.aspx (both accessed January 26, 2010).

44. Milner, C., & Cote, K. (2009). Benefits of napping in healthy adults: Impact of nap length, time of day, age, and experience with napping. *J Sleep Res* 18:272–81.

45. Horne, J., et al. (2008). Sleep extension versus nap or coffee, within the context of sleep debt. *J Sleep Res* 17:432–36.

46. Naska, A., et al. (2007). Siesta in healthy adults and coronary mortality in the general population. *Arch Intern Med* 167:296–301.

47. Dhand, R., & Sohal, H. (2006). Good sleep, bad sleep! The role of daytime naps in healthy adults. *Curr Opin Pulm Med* 12:379–82.

48. Science Daily. Midday nap markedly boosts the brain's learning capacity. *Science Daily*, at http://www.sciencedaily.com/releases/2010/02/100221110338.htm (accessed January 2010).

49. Reyner, L., & Horne, J. (1997). Caffeine combined with a short nap effectively counteracts driver sleepiness. *Sleep Research* 34:721–25.

50. Nilsson, U. (2008). The anxiety- and pain-reducing effects of music interventions: A systematic review. *AORN J* 87:780–807; Conrad, C., et al. (2007). Overture for growth hormone: Requiem for interleukin–6? *Critical Care Medicine* 35:2709–13; Teng, X., et al. (2007). The effect of music on hypertensive patients. *Conf Proc IEEE Eng Med Biol Soc* 4649–51; Siedliecki, S., & Good, M. (2006). Effect of music on power, pain, depression and disability. *Journal of Advanced Nursing* 54:553–62.

51. Cepeda, M., et al. (2006). Music for pain relief. The Cochrane Database of Systematic Reviews, Issue 2.

52. Grant, W. (2002). An estimate of premature cancer mortality in the United States due to inadequate doses of solar ultraviolet-B radiation. *Cancer* 94:1867–75.

53. World Health Organization. (2005). WHO guidelines on hand hygiene in health care, at http://www.who.int/patientsafety/events/05/HH_en.pdf (accessed January 12, 2010).

54. Lipsky, B., et al. (2006). Epidemiology of community and healthcare associated musculoskeletal infections (MSI) in hospitalized patients: Results from a US database of culture-proven cases (Abstract K-1178). 46th Interscience Conference on Antimicrobial Agents and Chemotherapy. September 27–30, San Francisco.

55. Meengs, M., et al. (1994). Hand washing frequency in an emergency department. *J Emergency Nursing* 20:183–88.

56. Widmer, A., et al. (2007). Introducing alcohol-based hand rub for hand hygiene: The critical need for training. *Infect Control Hosp Epidemiol* 28:50–54.

57. Jones, J., et al. (1995). Stethoscopes: A potential vector of infection? *Annals of Emergency Medicine* 26:296–99.

58. Embil, J., et al. (2002). Scissors: A potential source of nosocomial infection. *Infect Control Hosp Epidemiol* 23:147–51.

59. Phillips, D., & Barker, G. (2010). A July spike in fatal medication errors: A possible effect of new medical residents. *J Gen Intern Med* 25:774–79.

60. Banks, L. W. (2008, October 9). They call him Dr. Germ. *Tucson Weekly*, at http://www.tucsonweekly.com/tucson/they-call-him-dr-germ/Content?oid=1092882 (accessed January 15, 2010).

61. Centers for Disease Control and Prevention. (2010, May 21). Violations identified from routine swimming pool inspections—selected states and counties, United States, 2008. *Morbidity and Mortality Weekly Report*, at http://www.cdc.gov/mmwr/preview/mmwrhtml/mm5919a2.htm (accessed September 23, 2010).

62. Winther, B., et al. (2007). Environmental contamination with rhinovirus and transfer to fingers of healthy individuals by daily life activity. *J Med Virol* 79:1606–10.

63. Pappas, D., et al. (2010). Respiratory viral RNA on toys in pediatric office waiting rooms. *Pediatr Infect Dis J* 29:102–4; Winther, B., et al. (2011). Rhinovirus contamination of surfaces in homes of adults with natural colds: Transfer of virus to fingertips during normal daily activities. *J Medical Virology* 83:906–9.

64. Martin, R. (2001). Humor, laughter, and physical health: Methodological issues and research findings. *Psychological Bulletin* 127:504–19.

65. According to the laws of probability, a fair coin should turn up heads five times in a row about 3 percent of the time. The likelihood is small enough that an observer could reasonably conclude that such a coin is biased toward heads. But if fifty coins are each flipped five times, even if all are fair, the likelihood that at least one will turn up heads on each flip is almost 80 percent. Under those conditions, it would be premature to conclude that a five-heads-in-a-row coin is biased. Similarly, with a single outcome measure and standard statistical analysis, the likelihood that an ineffective treatment will appear effective is quite small. But if several outcomes are measured, a statistical correction is necessary so that a treatment does not appear effective by chance alone.

66. Secretory IgA (SIgA) is found in saliva, throughout the gastrointestinal tract, and in mucous secretions throughout the body. SIgA is part of the immune system and helps provide the first line of defense against bacteria, food toxins, fungus, parasites, and viruses.

67. Berkman, L., & Syme, S. (1979). Social networks, host resistance, and mortality: A nine-year follow-up study of Alameda County residents. *Am J Epidemiol* 109:186–204.

68. Emmons, R., & McCullough, M. (2003). Counting blessings versus burdens: An experimental investigation of gratitude and subjective well-being in daily life. *J Personality and Social Psychology* 84:377–89.

69. Alspach, G. (2009). Extending the tradition of giving thanks: Recognizing the health benefits of gratitude. *Critical Care Nurse* 29:12–18; Medical News Today. (2007, August 19). Expressing gratitude improves well-being and quality of life of organ recipients. *Medical News Today*, at http://www.medicalnewstoday.com/articles/79849.php.

70. Kurtz, J., & Lyubomirsky, S. (2008). Towards a durable happiness. In S. Lopez & J. Rettew (eds.), *The positive psychology perspective series*. Vol. 4. Westport, Conn.: Greenwood.

71. Brydon, L., et al. (2009). Dispositional optimism and stress-induced changes in immunity and negative mood. *Brain Behav Immun* 23:810–16; Sheldon, K., & Lyubomirsky, S. (2006). How to increase and sustain positive emotion: The effects of expressing gratitude and visualizing best possible selves. *J Positive Psychol* 1:73–82.

72. Ten Eyck, L., et al. (2008). Effects of directed thinking on exercise and cardiovascular fitness. *J Applied Biobehavioral Research* 12:237–58.

INDEX

absolute vs. relative risks, 38
academic detailing, 133
acupuncture, 145, 158, 165
adherence to treatment, 4–8, 11,
    14–15, 18, 20, 193, 196, 198,
    211
advertisements, 25, 125–26, 135–36
affect, positive and negative, 8,
    189–191
against diagnosis, 96–97
agenda setting, 14–15
alcohol, 24, 33, 148, 233–36
audit and feedback, 132–33

bad news, delivering, 19–20
bedside manner, 162
bias: against adopting beneficial
    therapies, 69–70; against losses,
    74; hindsight bias, 72–73;
    optimism bias, 69; projection
    bias, 70–72; selection bias, 65–67;
    toward certainty, 64–65; toward

normalization, 73. *See also*
    heuristics

caffeine, 236–39
chocolate, 231–32
classical conditioning, 153–54
clinical vs. statistical significance,
    35–36, 261
Cochrane collaboration, 16, 116, 137,
    260
cognitive errors, 102–5
comparative effectiveness studies,
    133–34
computer-based decision support
    systems, 108–9
conflicts of interest, 122, 130
contextual decision-making errors,
    53–54
continuing medical education
    courses, 124–25
correlational studies, 31–33, 229,
    231–34, 237, 241, 243

cultural competence, 10–11
cultural differences, outcomes, 10, 158

Darwinian medicine, 219–28; infectious disease control, 227–28; intensive care management, 224–25; novel factors in the modern environment, 226–27; symptoms as positive bodily defenses, 221–26
decision aids: doctors, 76, 108–9; patients, 16–17
decision experts, 110–12
decision making: emotions, 47–48; framing, 62–64; immediate needed, 45–47; intuition, 44–45; number of alternatives, 50–52. *See also* bias; heuristics
decision support systems, 108–9
deliberate practice, 111–12
diagnosis: cultural factors, 83–84; diagnostic aids, 108–10; diagnostic error rate, 88–89; diagnostic tests as treatment, 167–68; diagnostic tests that should be used judiciously, 91–93; feedback, importance of, 101–2, 104, 107, 110–12, 132; frequently overdiagnosed diseases, 90–91; frequently underdiagnosed diseases, 93–96; sensitivity, 75, 116; specificity, 75, 116
Diagnostic and Statistical Manual, 215–17
direct-to-consumer advertising, 130, 135–36
doctor communication styles, 3–4, 13
doctor job satisfaction, 8–9, 204

doctor-patient relationship, 8, 135, 180, 185
double-blind studies, 33–34
drug companies, x, 26–28, 30–31, 39–41, 52, 122–35, 217
drug company representatives (detailmen), 128–30
drugs, comparing new with old, 28

educational outreach visits (academic detailing), 133
effect size, 36–38, 194, 204
endorphin system, 159
epidemiologists, 33
evolutionary principles applied to psychiatric disorders, 225–26
evolutionary trade-offs, 220–21
expectancy-value theory, 155–56
expectation effects, 139–73
experimental vs. correlational studies, 31–33
expert panels, 131
expert performance, 111–12

FDA committees, 130–31
FDA scientists, 30
financial ties with industry, 29, 122, 131, 217
formularies, 132
free samples, 53
funding, source of, 28, 30–31

ghostwriters, 25–26

healing environments, 201–13; layout and décor, 210–12; lighting, 202–5; nature, 205–7; sound, 207–10; wayfinding, 212–13
health literacy, 5–6, 255
health practices, overturned, 23–24

heuristics, 57–62; anchoring and adjustment heuristic, 60–62; availability heuristic, 57–59; representative heuristic, 59–60; smart heuristics, 74–75
history taking, 105–7

lifespans, calculating average, 83, 221, 297
likelihood ratios, 116–18

malpractice complaints, 2, 9, 72, 83, 89–90, 106, 114–15
marketing, x, 29, 53, 123–130, 133
meaning of treatments, 157–59
medical literature, 24–25, 41, 46, 108
medical schools, 24, 122–23, 219
menopause, 144
mind-body therapies, 185–88

nocebo, 158, 161–62
no-fault errors, 100
noise, in hospitals, 207–10
nonspecific factors affecting response, ix
nucleus accumbens, 149, 160
number needed to treat, 36–38

odds ratios, 38
off-label prescribing, 129, 137, 259
optimism vs. pessimism, 69, 77, 191, 193–95
order effects, 104
overconfidence, 102–4

pain, discussing, 18–19
parasitic worms, 226–27
Parkinson's disease, 150, 195, 238
patents on drugs, 28, 41, 122–24, 129

patient-centered care, 5, 9–12, 17, 256
patient characteristics affecting treatment decisions, 12–13, 50, 81, 84–86, 97
patient decision aids, 16–17
patient satisfaction, 2–3, 16–17, 202, 211
peak-end rule, 68–69
perceived control, 195–96
physical examination, 80, 105–7
Physicians' Desk Reference, 52, 123
placebos, 27, 34–35, 37, 127, 146–73, 185; active placebos, 150; mechanisms, 152–61; placebo responders, 147, 158–61
positive emotions, 99
premature closure, 104–5
probabilities of disease, calculating, 113–18
pseudopatients, 215–16
psychiatric diagnosis, 215–17
publication bias, 36

race, 12, 50, 81, 84–86

second opinions, 105, 110, 118
shared decision making, 7, 17–18, 199
simulation training, 76, 112
statistical vs. clinical significance, 24, 35–36, 261
stereotypes, 142–43, 167
stress, 1–2, 8–9, 23, 48–49, 152, 187–88, 193, 202–4, 206–9, 211–12, 232, 234, 240, 243
surgery, 18, 23–24, 51, 62, 76, 83, 85, 92, 118, 136, 143–46, 150, 152, 165, 170, 193, 195, 202, 205–6, 244–45
survival vs. mortality rates, 40
system errors, 100–102

telemedicine, 109–10
terminating treatment, 172
treatment plans, 4–5, 7, 11, 17–18,
    21, 87, 109, 193, 211

unfair comparisons of drugs, 27–28,
    276
Union of Concerned Scientists,
    30

variability, 88, 113
voodoo death, 146

waiting areas, 206, 211
wellness strategies, 229–52; eating,
    230–32; exercise, 239–41; friends,
    250; gratitude, 250–52; laughter,
    249–50; music, 244; naps, 242–44;
    sleep, 241–42; water, 232–33

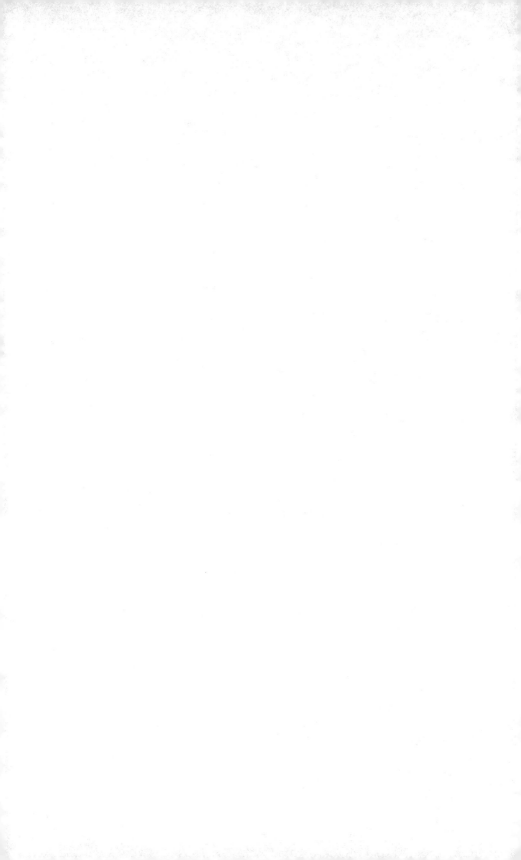